AN ILLUSTRATED COLOUR TEXT

Clinical Biochemistry

AN ILLUSTRATED COLOUR TEXT

Clinical Biochemistry

SECOND EDITION

Allan Gaw MD PhD
Deputy Study Director

Robert A. Cowan BSc PhD
Lecturer in Pathological Biochemistry

Denis St. J. O'Reilly MSc MD FRCPath
Consultant Clinical Biochemist

Michael J. Stewart PhD FRCPath
Consultant Scientist

James Shepherd PhD FRCP FRCPath FRSE
Professor of Pathological Biochemistry

Department of Pathological Biochemistry
University of Glasgow and
Glasgow Royal Infirmary University NHS Trust
Glasgow, UK

Illustrated by Robert Britton

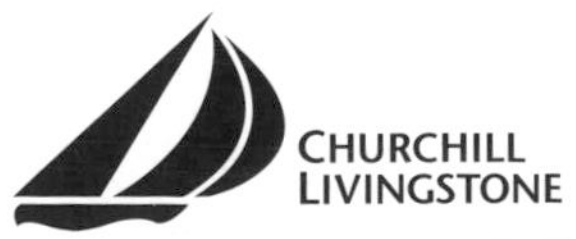

CHURCHILL
LIVINGSTONE

EDINBURGH LONDON NEW YORK PHILADELPHIA SYDNEY TOKYO 1999

CHURCHILL LIVINGSTONE
An imprint of Elsevier Science Limited

First published 1995
Second Edition 1999
Reprinted 2001, 2002

ISBN 0443 06183 1

British Library of Cataloguing in Publication Data
A catalogue record for this book is available from the British Library.

Library of Congress Cataloging in Publication Data
A catalog record for this book is available from the Library of Congress.

Note to the reader

The reference ranges quoted in this book are for use with the case histories only and should not be used for any other purpose. Each laboratory issues its own reference ranges appropriate to its assay methods and these should always be used in the interpretation of biochemical tests performed in that laboratory.

While every effort has been made to ensure that the drug doses quoted in this book are correct, indications and regimens change with time. Therefore, it remains the responsibility of the reader to check dosage details for each drug on the current data sheet.

For Churchill Livingstone

Publisher: Timothy Horne
Project Editor: Jim Killgore
Design: Sarah Cape
Electronic page make-up: Sarah Cape, Pat Miller, Charles Simpson
Production: Nancy Arnott

Printed in China by RDC Group Limited
C/03

The publisher's policy is to use **paper manufactured from sustainable forests**

PREFACE TO THE FIRST EDITION

Medical education is changing, so the educational tools we use must change too. This book was designed and written for those studying Clinical Biochemistry for the first time. We have placed the greatest emphasis on the foundations of the subject, while covering all those topics found in a medical undergraduate course on Clinical Biochemistry. The format is not that of a traditional textbook. By arranging the subject in double-page learning units we offer the student a practical and efficient way to assimilate the necessary facts, while presenting opportunities for problem solving and self-testing with case histories. Clinical notes present channels for lateral thinking about each learning unit, and boxes summarizing the key points may be used by the student to facilitate rapid revision of the text.

The book is divided into four main sections. *Introducing clinical biochemistry* outlines the background to our subject. In *Core biochemistry* we cover the routine analyses that would form the basic repertoire of most hospital laboratories. The *Endocrinology* section covers thyroid, adrenal, pituitary and gonadal function testing, and in *Specialized investigations* we discuss less commonly requested, but important, analyses.

This book relies on illustrations and diagrams to make many of its points and these should be viewed as integral to the text. The reader is assumed to have a basic knowledge of anatomy, physiology and biochemistry and to be primarily interested in the subject of Clinical Biochemistry from a user's point of view rather than that of a provider. To this end we have not covered analytical aspects except in a few instances where these have direct relevance to the interpretation of biochemical tests. What we have tried to do is present Clinical Biochemistry as a subject intimately connected to Clinical Medicine, placing emphasis on the appropriate use of biochemical tests and their correct interpretation in a clinical setting.

Glasgow
1995

Allan Gaw, Robert A. Cowan,
Denis St. J. O'Reilly,
Michael J. Stewart and James Shepherd

PREFACE TO THE SECOND EDITION

There is a great temptation when writing the second edition of a textbook to start again and write a new first edition. To the authors, perhaps because of their proximity, the original textbook has become a little jaded. However, if we were to believe that we would be ignoring the many letters and communications we have received from teachers and students around the world, all of whom have congratulated us on producing a textbook of Clinical Biochemistry that is interesting, relevant and, above all, easy to access.

In this context the preparation of a new edition takes on a different meaning. To redraft and redesign a successful and useful text book would be nothing short of vandalism. Instead we were charged with updating the outmoded, clarifying the equivocal and correcting the errors which were thankfully very few in the original, but without destroying the spirit of a successful book. If it wasn't broken we didn't fix it. What we have done is make changes to every single double-page spread of the text: some small, some large.

Clinical Biochemistry is a truly international subject, attested to by our global readership and now by the geographical distribution of our authors. Since the first editon was published two of our team have moved away to work in South Africa and Thailand, respectively. Living and working on three different continents has not made the writing of this new edition any easier but it has made it more fun.

In the preface to our first edition we wrote that medical education is changing, so the educational tools we use must change too. Nothing could have been more true. Many medical schools, including our own, have in the last few years switched to a problem based learning approach in the education of their medical students. With this concept comes much that is good. But it also brings a need for a new kind of textbook: one that can integrate the traditional material into a clear clinical context and also place it side by side with information from other specialties. Our first edition of Clinical Biochemistry already had this objective and our new edition continues very much in this vein. We believe this new edition is a significant improvement over the first, but we have not sacrificed what was good about the original for the sake of change.

1998

Allan Gaw, Robert A. Cowan,
Denis St. J. O'Reilly,
Michael J. Stewart and James Shepherd

ACKNOWLEDGEMENTS

The following have helped in many different ways in the preparation of the first and second editions of this book: in providing illustrations, in discussions, and in suggesting improvements to the manuscript.

Bryan Adamson
Sally Beard
Graham Beastall
Iain Boyle
Brian Cook
Frances Dryburgh
Andy Duncan
Gordon Fell
Alan Foulis
Moira Gaw
Dairena Gaffney
Christina Gray
David Halls
John Hinnie
Jennie Johnston
Witsanu Kumthornthip
Kim Lim
Grace Lindsay
Greig Louden
Jean McAllister
Derek McLean
Hazel Miller
Michael Murphy
Heather Murray
Brian Neilly
Nigel Rabie
Margaret Rudge
Naveed Sattar
Ian Stewart
Mike Wallace
Janet Warren
Philip Welsby
Peter H. Wise
Helen Wright

Special mention must be made of our editorial and design team at Harcourt Brace without whose encouragement and wise counsel this book would not have been written.

CONTENTS

INTRODUCING CLINICAL BIOCHEMISTRY 1

CORE BIOCHEMISTRY 11

ENDOCRINOLOGY 73

SPECIALIZED INVESTIGATIONS 95

INTRODUCING CLINICAL BIOCHEMISTRY

THE CLINICAL BIOCHEMISTRY LABORATORY

Clinical biochemistry, chemical pathology and clinical chemistry are all names for the subject of this book, that branch of laboratory medicine in which chemical and biochemical methods are applied to the study of disease (Fig. 1). While in theory this embraces all non-morphological studies, in practice it is usually, though not exclusively, confined to studies on blood and urine because of the relative ease in obtaining such specimens although analyses are made on other body fluids such as gastric aspirate and cerebrospinal fluid. Clinical biochemical tests comprise over one-third of all hospital laboratory investigations.

THE USE OF BIOCHEMICAL TESTS

Biochemical investigations are involved, to varying degrees, in every branch of clinical medicine. The results of biochemical tests may be of use in diagnosis and in the monitoring of treatment. Biochemical tests may also be of value in screening for disease or in assessing the prognosis once a diagnosis has been made (Fig. 2). The biochemistry laboratory is often involved in research into the biochemical basis of disease and in clinical trials of new drugs.

History

Clinical examination

Diagnostic services

Imaging

Physiological tests: ECG, EEG, lung function

Laboratory services

Haematology

Histopathology

Immunology

Microbiology

Clinical biochemistry

Emergency services

Core biochemistry

Specialized tests

Fig. 1 **The place of clinical biochemistry in medicine.**

CORE BIOCHEMISTRY

Biochemical facilities are provided in every hospital, although not necessarily to the same extent. Most biochemistry laboratories provide the 'core analyses', commonly requested tests which are of value in many patients, on a frequent basis (Table 1). The clinician will often request specific groupings of tests, and clinical biochemistry assumes a cryptic language of its own as request forms arrive at laboratory reception for 'U and Es' (urea and electrolytes), 'LFTs' (liver function tests) or 'blood gases'.

SPECIALIZED TESTS

There are a variety of specialties within clinical biochemistry (Table 1). Not every laboratory is equipped to carry out all possible biochemistry requests. Large departments may act as reference centres where less commonly asked for tests are performed. For some tests which are needed in the diagnosis of rare diseases, there may be just one or two laboratories in the country offering the service.

Table 1 **The clinical biochemistry repertoire**

Core biochemical tests
Sodium, potassium, chloride and bicarbonate
Urea and creatinine
Calcium and phosphate
Total protein and albumin
Bilirubin and alkaline phosphatase
Alanine aminotransferase (ALT) and aspartate aminotransferase (AST)
Thyroxine (T_4) and Thyroid Stimulating Hormone (TSH)
γ-glutamyl transpeptidase (γGT)
Creatine kinase (CK)
H^+, PCO_2 and PO_2 (blood gases)
Glucose
Amylase

Specialized tests	Emergency tests
Hormones	Urea and electrolytes
Specific proteins	Blood gases
Trace elements	Amylase
Vitamins	Glucose
Drugs	Salicylate
Lipids and lipoproteins	Paracetamol
DNA analyses	Calcium

THE EMERGENCY LAB

All clinical biochemistry laboratories provide facilities for urgent tests. Only a small number of test types are available from the 'emergency laboratory'. These are processed rapidly and reports phoned

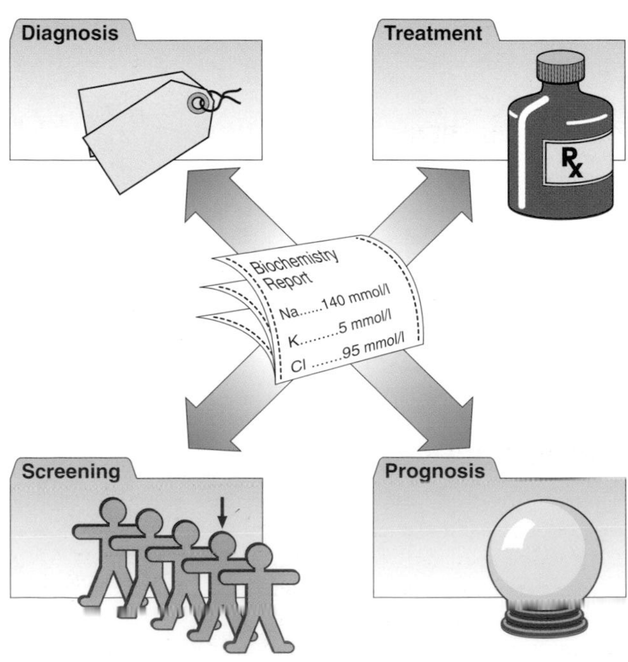

Fig. 2 **How biochemical tests are used.**

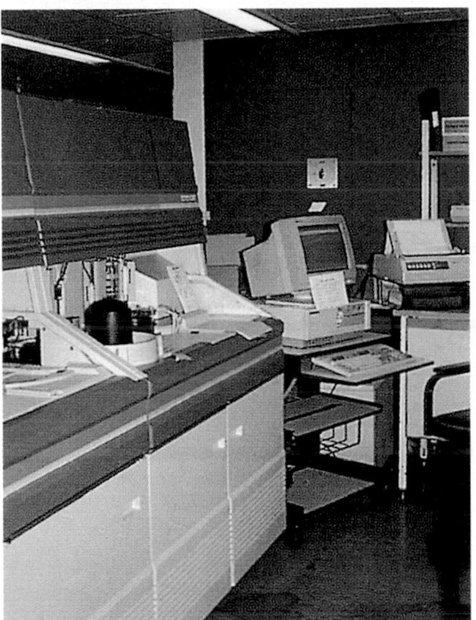
(a)

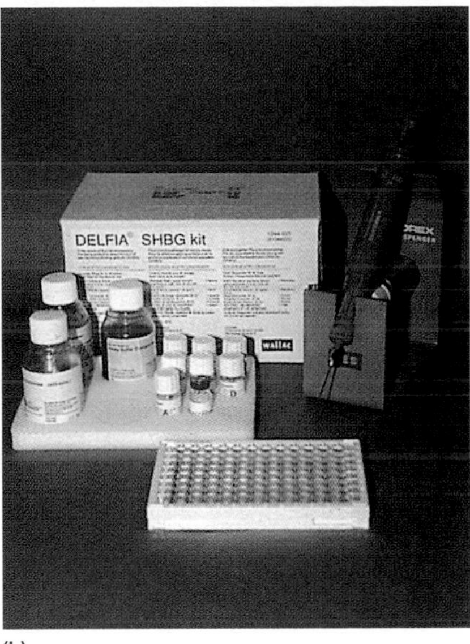

(b)

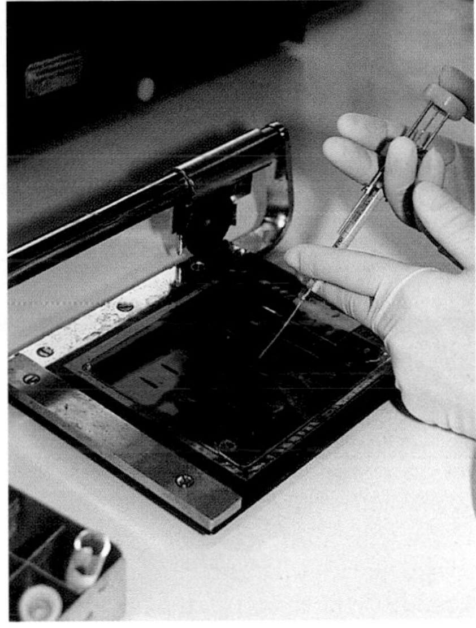
(c)

Fig. 3 **Analysing the samples: (a)** the automated analyser, **(b)** 'kit' analyses and **(c)** manual methods.

to the requesting clinician or ward. An urgent test is designated as one on which the clinician is likely to take immediate action. An 'on call' service may be provided to ensure that such requests can be done outside the normal working hours of the laboratory. Table 1 shows some of the tests available on an emergency basis.

IN THE OPERATING SUITE OR CLINIC

In some large hospitals, the facilities to perform biochemistry analyses are sited close to where they are needed, for example monitoring of patients undergoing major surgery, such as transplantation, or providing blood glucose results at the diabetic clinic. Many biochemical tests are now being performed away from the laboratory (see pp. 8–9).

AUTOMATION AND COMPUTERIZATION

Most laboratories are now computerized, and the use of bar-coding of specimens and automated methods of analysis allows a high degree of productivity and improves the quality of service. Links to computer terminals on wards and GP surgeries allow direct access to results by the requesting clinician.

TEST REPERTOIRE

There are over 400 different tests which may be carried out in clinical biochemistry laboratories. They vary from the very simple, such as the measurement of sodium, to the highly complex, such as DNA analysis, screening for drugs, or differentiation of lipoprotein variants. Many high volume tests are done on large automated machines. Less frequently performed tests may be conveniently carried out by using commercially prepared reagents packaged in 'kit' form. Some analyses are carried out manually (Fig. 3). Increasing workload, and budgetary constraints, mean that all laboratories continually reassess what is the most cost-effective way of providing the best service.

Dynamic tests require several specimens, timed in relation to a biochemical stimulus, such as a glucose load in the glucose tolerance test for the diagnosis of diabetes mellitus. Some tests provide a clearcut answer to a question; others are only a part of the diagnostic jigsaw.

This book describes how the results of biochemistry analyses are interpreted, rather than how the analyses are performed in the laboratory. An important function of many departments is research and development. Advances in analytical methodology and in our understanding of disease continues to change the test repertoire of the biochemistry department as the value of new tests is appreciated.

LABORATORY PERSONNEL

As well as performing the analyses, the clinical biochemistry laboratory also provides a consultative service. The laboratory has on its staff both medical and scientific personnel who are familiar with the clinical significance and the analytical performance of the test procedures, and they will readily give advice on the interpretation of the results. Do not be hesitant to take advantage of this advice, especially where a case is not straightforward.

Clinical note

The clinical biochemistry laboratory plays only a part in the overall assessment and management of the patient. For some patients, biochemical analyses may have little or no part in their diagnosis or the management of their illness. For others, many tests may be needed before a diagnosis is made, and repeated analyses required to monitor treatment over a long period.

The clinical biochemistry laboratory

- Biochemical tests are used in diagnosis, monitoring treatment, screening and for prognosis.
- Core biochemical tests are carried out in every biochemistry laboratory. Specialized tests may be referred to larger departments. All hospitals provide for urgent tests in the 'emergency laboratory'.
- Laboratory personnel will readily give advice, based on their knowledge and experience, on the use of the biochemistry laboratory, on the appropriate selection of tests, and about the interpretation of results.

THE USE OF THE LABORATORY

Every biochemistry analysis should attempt to answer a question which the clinician has posed about the patient. Obtaining the correct answers can often seem to be fraught with difficulty.

SPECIMEN COLLECTION

In order to carry out biochemical analyses, it is necessary that the laboratory be provided with both the correct specimen for the requested test, and also information which will ensure that the right test is carried out and the result returned to the requesting clinician with the minimum of delay. As much detail as possible should be included on the request form to help both laboratory staff and the clinician in the interpretation of results. This information can be very valuable when assessing a patient's progress over a period, or reassessing a diagnosis. Patient identification must be correct, and the request form should include some indication of the suspected pathology. The requested analyses should be clearly indicated. Request forms differ in design. Clinical biochemistry forms in Europe are conventionally coloured green.

A variety of specimens are used in biochemical analysis and these are shown in Table 1. However, the majority of biochemical tests are performed on serum from venous blood or urine.

Blood specimens

If blood is collected into a plain tube and allowed to clot, after centrifugation a *serum* specimen is obtained (Fig. 1). For many biochemical analyses this will be the specimen recommended. In other cases, especially when the analyte in question is unstable and speed is necessary to obtain a specimen which can be frozen quickly, the blood is collected into a tube containing an anticoagulant such as heparin. When centrifuged, the supernatant is called *plasma* which is almost identical to the cell-free fraction of blood but contains the anticoagulant as well.

Urine specimens

Urine specimen containers may include a preservative to inhibit bacterial growth, or acid to stabilize certain metabolites. They need to be large enough to hold a full 24 h collection. Random urine samples are collected into small 'universal' containers.

Other specimen types

For some tests, specific body fluids or tissue may be required. There will be specific protocols for the handling and transport of these samples to the laboratory. Consult the local lab for advice.

Table 1 **Specimens used for biochemical analyses**

Specimens
Venous blood, serum or plasma
Arterial blood
Capillary blood
Urine
Faeces
Cerebrospinal fluid (CSF)
Sputum and saliva
Tissue and cells
Aspirates, e.g. pleural fluid ascites joint (synovial) fluid intestinal (duodenal) pancreatic pseudocysts
Calculi (stones)

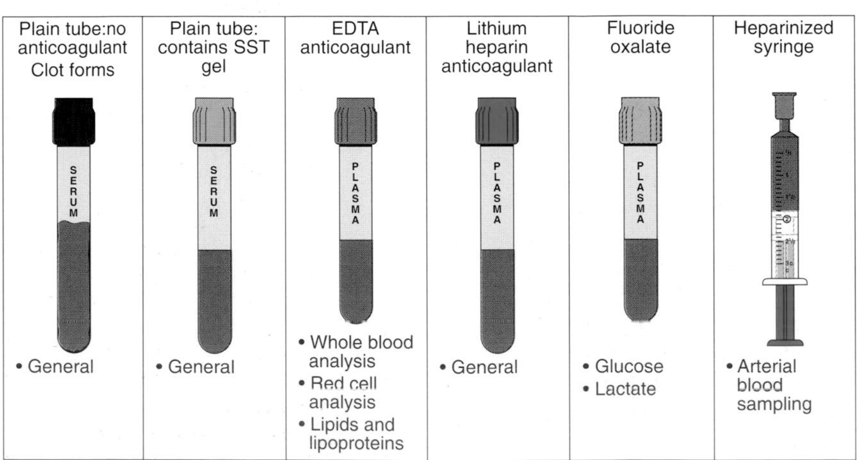

Fig. 1 **Blood specimen tubes for specific biochemical tests.** The colour-coded tubes are the vacutainers in use in the authors' hospital and laboratory.

Dangerous specimens

All specimens from patients with dangerous infections should be labelled with a yellow 'dangerous specimen' sticker. A similar label should be attached to the request form. Of most concern to the laboratory staff are hepatitis B and HIV, but *all* specimens should always be treated both by clinicians and biochemistry staff as potentially hazardous.

SAMPLING ERRORS

There are a number of potential errors which may contribute to the success or failure of the laboratory to provide the correct answers to the clinician's questions. Some of these problems arise when a clinician first obtains specimens from the patient.

- *Blood sampling technique.* Difficulty in obtaining a blood specimen may lead to haemolysis with consequent release of potassium and other red cell constituents. Results for these will be falsely elevated.
- *Prolonged stasis during venepuncture.* Plasma water diffuses into the interstitial space and the serum or plasma sample obtained will be concentrated. Proteins and protein-bound components of plasma such as calcium or thyroxine will be falsely elevated.
- *Insufficient specimen.* Each biochemical analysis requires a certain volume of specimen to enable the test to be carried out. It may prove to be impossible for the laboratory to measure everything requested on a small volume specimen.
- *Errors in timing.* The biggest source of error in the measurement of any analyte in a 24-hour urine specimen is in the collection of an accurately timed volume of urine.
- *Incorrect specimen container.* For many analyses the blood must be collected into a container with anticoagulant and preservative. For example, samples for glucose should be collected into a special container containing fluoride which inhibits glycolysis; otherwise the time taken to deliver the sample to the laboratory can affect the result. If a sample is collected into the wrong container, it should never be decanted into another type of tube. For example, blood which has been exposed even briefly to EDTA (an anticoagulant used in sample containers for lipids) will have a markedly reduced calcium concentration, approaching zero.

- *Inappropriate sampling site.* Blood samples should not be taken 'downstream' from an intravenous drip. It is not unheard of for the laboratory to receive a blood glucose request on a specimen taken from the same arm into which 5% glucose is being infused. Usually the results are biochemically incredible but it is just possible that they may be acted upon, with disastrous consequences for the patient.
- *Incorrect specimen storage.* A blood sample stored overnight before being sent to the laboratory will show falsely high potassium, phosphate and red cell enzymes such as lactate dehydrogenase, because of leakage into the extracellular fluid from the cells.

HOW OFTEN TO INVESTIGATE

Many biochemical tests are repeated at intervals. How often depends on how quickly significant changes are liable to occur, and there is little point in requesting tests if a numerical change will *not* have an influence on treatment.

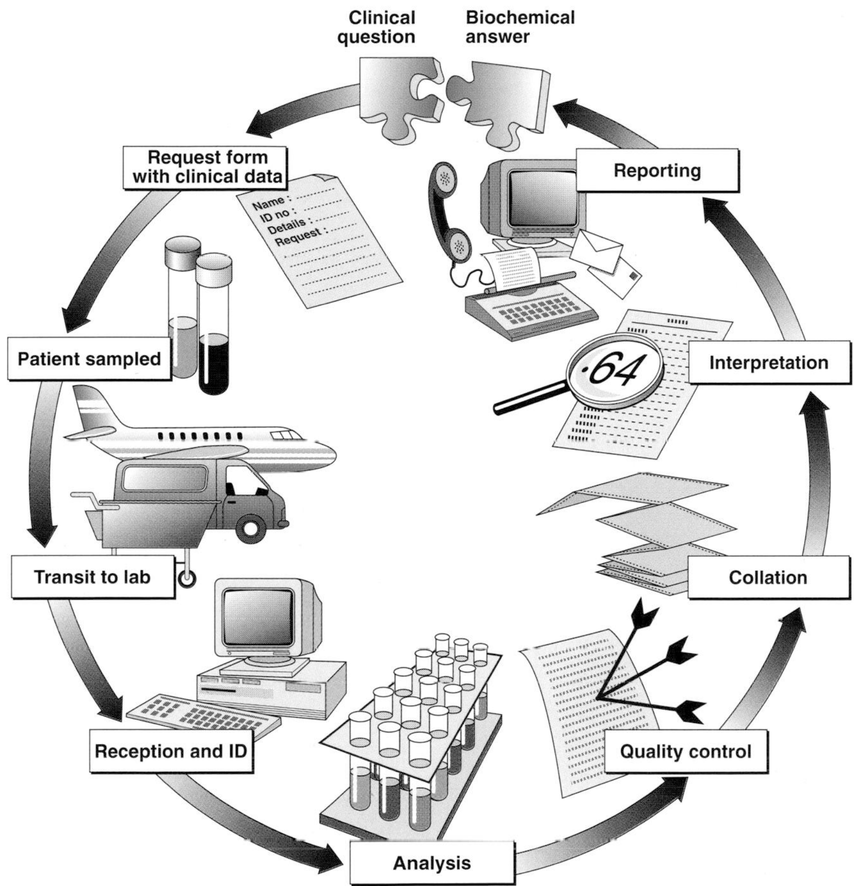

Fig. 2 **Circuit diagram of the clinical biochemistry process.**

URGENT REQUESTS

The main reason for asking for an analysis to be performed on an urgent basis is that immediate treatment depends on the result.

ANALYSING THE SPECIMEN

Once the form and specimen arrive at the laboratory reception, they are matched with a unique identifying number or bar code. The average lab receives many thousands of requests and samples each day and it is important that all are clearly identified and never mixed up. Samples proceed through the laboratory as shown in Figure 2. All analytical procedures are quality controlled and the laboratory strives for reliability.

Once the results are available they are collated and a report is issued. Cumulative reports allow the clinician to see at a glance how the most recent result(s) compare with those tests performed previously, providing an aid to the monitoring of treatment.

UNNECESSARY TESTING

There can be no definite rules about the appropriateness, or otherwise, of laboratory testing because of the huge variety of clinical circumstances which may arise. Clinicians should always bear in mind that in requesting a biochemical test they should be asking a question of the laboratory. If not, both the clinician and the laboratory may be performing unnecessary work, with little benefit to the patient.

Case history 1

A blood specimen was taken from a 65-year-old woman to check her serum potassium concentration as she had been on thiazide diuretics for some time. The GP left the specimen in his car and dropped it off at the laboratory on the way to the surgery the next morning.

Immediately on analysing the sample, the biochemist was on the phone to the GP. Why?

Comment on page 152.

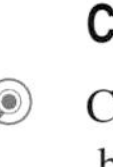

Clinical note

Clinical biochemistry is but one branch of laboratory medicine. Specimens may be required for haematology, microbiology, virology, immunology and histopathology, and all require similar attention to detail in filling out request forms and obtaining the appropriate samples for analysis.

The use of the laboratory

- Each biochemistry test request should be thought of as a question about the patient; each biochemical result as an answer.
- Request forms and specimens must be correctly labelled to ensure that results can be communicated quickly to the clinician.
- Many biochemical tests are performed on serum, the supernatant obtained from centrifugation of clotted blood collected into a plain container. Others require 'plasma', the supernatant obtained when blood is prevented from clotting by an anticoagulant.
- A variety of sampling errors may invalidate results.

THE INTERPRETATION OF RESULTS

THE LABORATORY REPORT

It can take considerable effort, and expense, to produce what may seem to be just numbers on pieces of paper. Understanding what these numbers mean is of crucial importance if the correct diagnosis is to be made, or if the patient's treatment is to be changed.

HOW BIOCHEMICAL RESULTS ARE EXPRESSED

Most biochemical analyses are quantitative, although simple qualitative or semi-quantitative tests such as those for the presence of glucose in urine are commonly encountered in methods used for biochemistry testing away from the laboratory. Many tests measure the amount of the analyte in a small volume of the sample, whether that is blood, plasma, serum, urine or some other fluid or tissue. The test results are commonly expressed in molar units. A mole of any compound always contains 6×10^{23} molecules. Describing how much of an analyte is present in 'moles' indicates how many molecules of the substance are present. Molar units can be converted to mass units; one mole is the molecular weight of the substance in grams.

Results are reported as concentrations, usually in terms of the number of moles in one litre (mol/l) (Table 1).

The concept of concentration is illustrated in Figure 1. The concentration of any analyte in a body compartment is a ratio: the amount of the substance dissolved in a known volume. Changes in concentration can occur for two reasons:

- The amount of the analyte can increase or decrease.
- The volume of fluid in which the analyte is dissolved can similarly change.

Enzymes are not usually expressed in moles but as enzyme activity in 'units'. Enzyme assays are carried out in such a way that the activity measured is directly proportional to the amount of enzyme present. Some hormone measurements are expressed as 'units' by comparison to standard reference preparations of known biological potency. Large molecules such as proteins are reported as grams or milligrams. Blood gas results (PCO_2 or PO_2) are expressed in kilopascals (kPa), the units in which partial pressures are measured.

Table 1 **Molar units**

Mole	Abbreviation	Definition
Millimole	mmol	$\times 10^{-3}$ of a mole
Micromole	µmol	$\times 10^{-6}$
Nanomole	nmol	$\times 10^{-9}$
Picomole	pmol	$\times 10^{-12}$
Femtomole	fmol	$\times 10^{-15}$

VARIATION IN RESULTS

Biochemical measurements vary for two reasons. There is analytical variation, and also biological variation.

Laboratory analytical performance

A number of terms describe biochemical results. These include:

- precision and accuracy
- sensitivity and specificity
- quality assurance
- reference ranges.

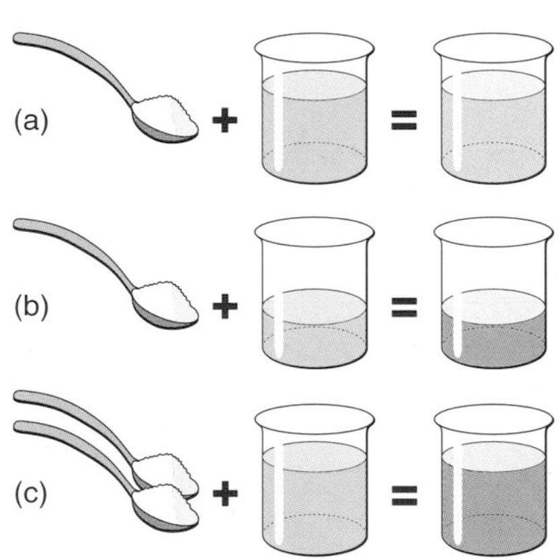

Fig. 1 **Understanding concentrations.** Concentration is always dependent on two factors: the amount of solute and the amount of solvent. The concentration of the sugar solution in the beaker can be increased from 1 spoon/beaker **(a)** to 2 spoons/beaker by either decreasing the volume of solvent **(b)** or increasing the amount of solute **(c)**.

Precision and accuracy

Precision is the reproducibility of an analytical method. Accuracy defines how close the measured value is to the actual value. A good analogy is that of the shooting target. Figure 2 shows the scatter of results which might be obtained by someone with little skill, compared with that of someone with good precision where the results are closely grouped together. Even when the results are all close, they may not hit the centre of the target. Accuracy is therefore poor, as if the 'sights' are off. It is the objective in every biochemical method to have good precision and accuracy.

Sensitivity and specificity

Sensitivity of an assay is a measure of how little of the analyte the method can detect. As new methods are developed they may offer improved detection limits which may help in the discrimination between normal results and those in patients with the suspected disease. Specificity of an assay relates to how good the assay is at discriminating between the requested analyte and potentially interfering substances.

Quality assurance

Every laboratory takes great pains to ensure that the methods in use continue to produce reliable results. Laboratory staff monitor performance of assays using quality control samples to give reassurance that the method is performing satisfactorily with the patients' specimens. These are internal quality controls which are analysed every day or every time an assay is run. The expected values are known and the actual results obtained are compared with previous values to monitor performance. In external quality assurance schemes, identical samples are distributed to laboratories; results are then compared.

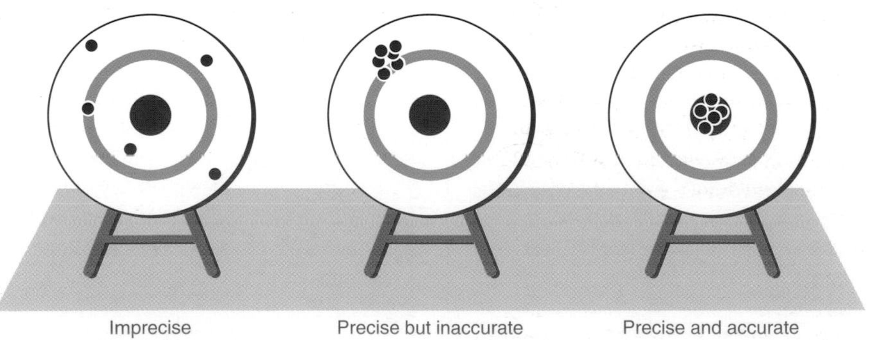

Fig. 2 **Precision and accuracy.**

In this way, the laboratory's own internal standards are themselves assessed.

Reference ranges

Analytical variation is generally less than that from biological variables. Biochemical test results are usually compared to a reference range considered to represent the normal healthy state (Fig. 3). Most reference ranges are chosen arbitrarily to include 95% of the values found in healthy volunteers, and hence, by definition, 5% of the population will have a result outwith the reference range. In practice there are no rigid limits demarcating the diseased population from the healthy; however, the further a result is from the limits of the range, the more likely it is to represent pathology. In some situations it is useful to define 'action limits', where appropriate intervention should be made in response to a biochemical result.

There is often a degree of overlap between the disease state and the 'normal value' (Fig. 4). A patient with an abnormal result who is found not to have the disease is a *false positive*. A patient who has the disease but has a 'normal' result is a *false negative*.

Biological factors affecting the interpretation of results

The discrimination between normal and abnormal results is affected by various physiological factors which must be considered when interpreting any given result. These include:

- *Sex of the patient.* Reference ranges for some analytes such as serum creatinine are different for men and women.
- *Age of the patient.* There may be different reference ranges for neonates, children, adults and the elderly.
- *Effect of diet.* The sample may be inappropriate if taken when the patient is fasting or after a meal.
- *Time when sample was taken.* There may be variations during the day and night.
- *Stress and anxiety.* These may affect the analyte of interest.
- *Posture of the patient.* Redistribution of fluid may affect the result.
- *Effects of exercise.* Strenuous exercise can release enzymes from tissues.
- *Medical history.* Infection and/or tissue injury can affect biochemical values independently of the disease process being investigated.
- *Pregnancy.* This alters some reference ranges.
- *Menstrual cycle.* Hormone measurements will vary through the menstrual cycle.

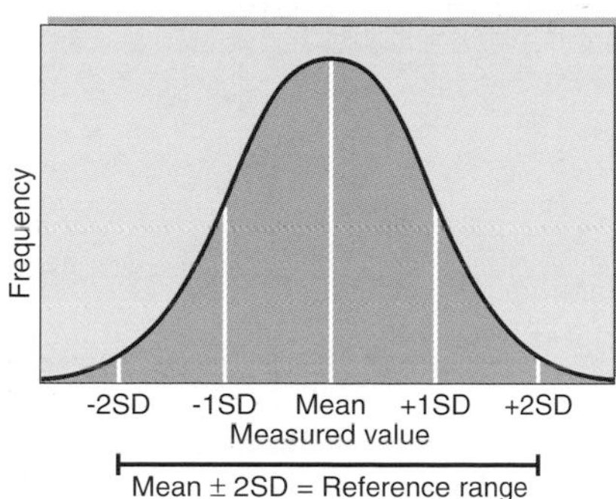

Fig. 3 **Reference range in a normal healthy population.**

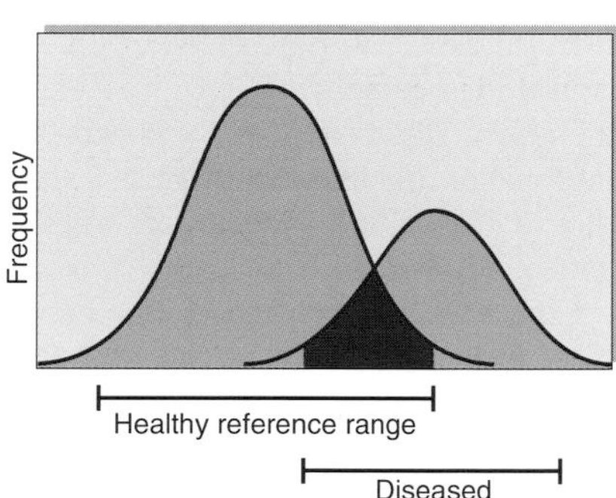

Fig. 4 **Overlap of biochemical results in health and disease.**

- *Drug history.* Drugs may have specific effects on the plasma concentration of some analytes.

Other factors

When the numbers have been printed on the report form, they still have to be interpreted in the light of a host of variables. Analytical and biological variations have already been considered. Other factors relate to the patient. The clinician can refer to the patient or to the clinical notes, whereas the biochemist has only the information on the request form to consult. The cumulation of biochemistry results is often helpful in patient management.

Case history 2

A serum potassium concentration of 45 mmol/l was recorded in the notes of a 35-year-old man being prepared for appendicectomy. The set of electrolyte results had been phoned from the laboratory. The consultant surgeon was unperturbed, although he did check the results on the ward terminal himself. Why?

Comment on page 152.

The clinician may well ask the following questions on receiving a biochemistry report:

- 'Does the result fit in with what I expected on the basis of the clinical examination and history of the patient?'
- 'If the result is not what I expected, can I explain the discrepancy?'
- 'How can the result change my diagnosis or the way I am managing the patient?'
- 'What should I do next?'

What is done in response to a biochemistry report rests with the clinical judgement of the doctor. There is a maxim that doctors should always 'treat the patient, rather than the laboratory report'. The rest of this book deals with the biochemical investigation of patients and the interpretation of the results obtained.

Clinical note

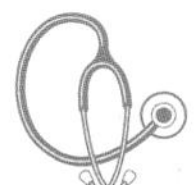

It is important to realize that an abnormal result does not always indicate that a disease is present, nor a normal result that it is not. Beware of over-reacting to the slightly abnormal result in the otherwise healthy individual.

The interpretation of results

- Biochemistry results are often reported as concentrations. Concentrations change if the amount of the analyte changes, or if the volume of solution changes.
- Variability of results is caused by both analytical factors and biological factors.
- The reference range supplied with the test result is only a guide to the probability of the results being statistically 'normal' or 'abnormal'.
- Different reference ranges may apply depending on the age or sex of the patient.
- Sequential changes observed in cumulative reports when placed in clinical context are as important as the absolute value of the result.
- If a result does not accord with that expected for the patient the finding should be discussed with the laboratory reporting office and a repeat test arranged.

BIOCHEMICAL TESTING OUTSIDE THE LABORATORY

INTRODUCTION

The methods for measuring some biological compounds in blood and urine have become so robust and simple to use that measurements can be made away from the laboratory—by the patient's bedside, in the ward sideroom, at the GP's surgery, in the home or even in the shopping centre! Convenience and the desire to know results quickly, as well as expectation of commercial profit by the manufacturers of the tests, have been the major stimuli for these developments. Experience has shown that motivated individuals, e.g. diabetics, frequently perform the tests as well as highly qualified professionals.

The immediate availability of results can enable the appropriate treatment to be instituted quickly. Patients' fears can be allayed. However, it is important to ensure that the limitations of any test and the significance of the results are appreciated by the tester to avoid inappropriate intervention or unnecessary anxiety.

TESTS PERFORMED AWAY FROM THE LABORATORY

Table 1 shows what can be measured in a blood sample outwith the normal laboratory setting. The most common blood test outside the laboratory is the determination of glucose concentration, in a finger stab sample, at home or in the clinic. Diabetic patients who need to monitor their blood glucose on a regular basis can do so at home or at work using one of many commercially available pocket-sized instruments.

Figure 1 shows a portable bench analyser. This instrument may be used to monitor patients' glucose and cholesterol, and is frequently used in many outpatient clinics and in screening centres.

Table 2 lists urine constituents that can be measured away from the laboratory. Many are conveniently measured, semi-quantitatively, using test strips which are dipped briefly into a fresh urine sample. Any excess urine is removed, and the result assessed after a specified time by comparing a colour change with a code on the side of the test strip container. The information obtained from such tests is of variable value to the tester, whether patient or clinician.

The tests commonly performed away from the laboratory can be categorized as follows:

A. *Tests performed in medical or nursing settings.* They clearly give valuable information and allow the practitioner to reassure the patient or family, or initiate further investigations or treatment.
B. *Tests performed in the home, shopping centre or clinical setting.* They can give valuable information when properly and appropriately used.
C. *Alcohol tests.* These are sometimes used to assess fitness to drive. In clinical practice alcohol measurements need to be carefully interpreted. In the Accident and Emergency setting, extreme caution must be taken before one can fully ascribe confusion in a patient with head injury to the effects of alcohol, a common complicating feature in such patients.

Table 1 **Common tests on blood performed away from the laboratory**

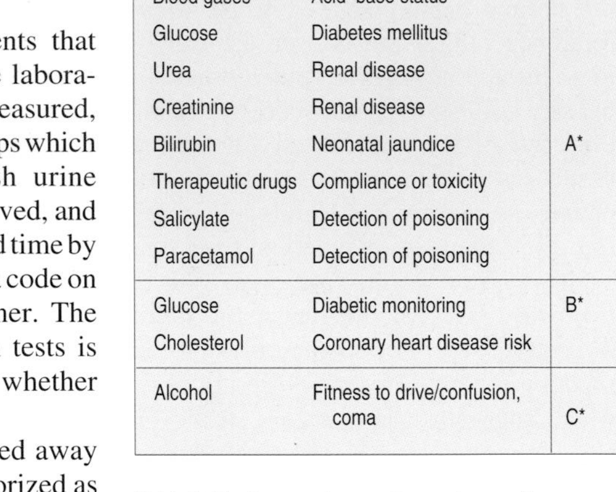

Analyte	Used when investigating	
Blood gases	Acid–base status	
Glucose	Diabetes mellitus	
Urea	Renal disease	
Creatinine	Renal disease	
Bilirubin	Neonatal jaundice	A*
Therapeutic drugs	Compliance or toxicity	
Salicylate	Detection of poisoning	
Paracetamol	Detection of poisoning	
Glucose	Diabetic monitoring	B*
Cholesterol	Coronary heart disease risk	
Alcohol	Fitness to drive/confusion, coma	C*

Table 2 **Tests on urine performed away from the laboratory**

Analyte	Used when investigating	
Ketones	Diabetic ketoacidosis	
Protein	Renal disease	
Red cells/ haemoglobin	Renal disease	
Bilirubin	Liver disease and jaundice	A*
Urobilinogen	Jaundice/haemolysis	
pH	Renal tubular acidosis	
Glucose	Diabetes mellitus	B*
hCG	Pregnancy test	

**See main text*

METHODOLOGY OF SIDEROOM TESTS

It is a feature of many sideroom tests that their simplicity disguises the use of sophisticated methodology. A home pregnancy test method involves an elegant application of monoclonal antibody technology to detect the human chorionic gonadotrophin (hCG) which is produced by the developing embryo (Fig. 2). The test is simple to carry out; a few drops of urine are placed in the sample window, and the result is shown within five minutes. The addition of the urine solubilizes a mono-clonal antibody for hCG which is covalently bound to tiny blue beads. A second monoclonal, specific for another region of the hCG molecule, is firmly attached in a line at the result window. If hCG is present in the sample it is bound by the first antibody, forming a blue bead–antibody–hCG complex. As the urine diffuses through the strip, any hCG present becomes bound at the second antibody site and this concentrates the

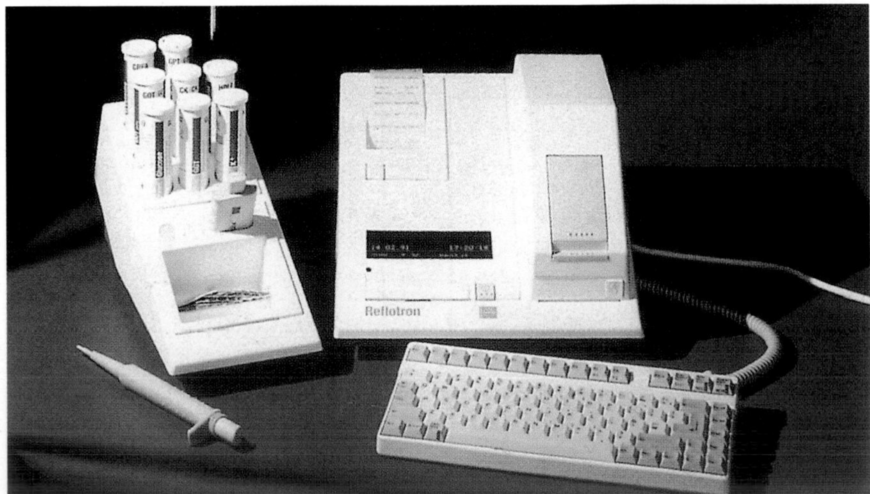

Fig. 1 **A portable bench analyser (Courtesy of Boehringer Mannheim GmbH.).**

blue bead complex in a line—a positive result. A third antibody recognizes the constant region of the first antibody and binds the excess, thus providing a control to show that sufficient urine had been added to the test strip, the most likely form of error.

GENERAL PROBLEMS

The obvious advantages in terms of time saving and convenience to both patient and clinician must be balanced by a number of possible problems in the use of these tests. They include:

- *Cost.* Many of these tests are expensive alternatives to the traditional methods used in the laboratory. This additional expense must be justified, for example, on the basis of convenience or speed of obtaining the result.
- *Responsibility.* The person performing the assay outwith the laboratory (the operator) must assume a number of responsibilities which would normally be those of the laboratory staff. There is the responsibility to perform the assay appropriately and to provide an answer that is accurate, precise and meaningful. The operator must also record the result, so that others may be able to find it (e.g. in the patient's notes), and interpret the result in its clinical context.

ANALYTICAL PROBLEMS

Many problems under this heading will have little to do with the assay technology but will be due to operator errors. Tests designed for use outwith the laboratory are robust but are by no means foolproof. Most operators will not be trained laboratory technicians but patients, nurses or clinicians. If an assay is to be performed well these individuals must be trained in its use. This may require the reading of a simple set of instructions (e.g. a home pregnancy test) or attending short training sessions (e.g. the ward-based blood gas analyser). The most commonly encountered analytical errors arise because of failure to:

- calibrate an instrument
- clean an instrument
- use quality control materials
- store reagents or strips in appropriate conditions.

All of these problems can be readily overcome by following instructions carefully. Regular maintenance of the equipment may be necessary, and simple quality control checks should be performed. It should always be possible to arrange simple quality control cross checks with the main biochemistry laboratory.

INTERPRETIVE PROBLEMS

Even when analytically correct results are obtained, there are other problems which must be overcome before the exercise can be considered a success. The general appropriateness of the test must be considered. If an assay is performed in an individual of inappropriate age, sex, or at the wrong time of day, or month, then the result may be clinically meaningless.

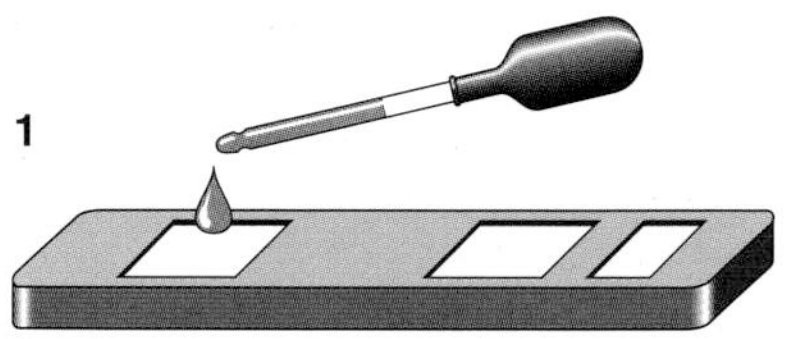

A urine sample is applied to the test strip.

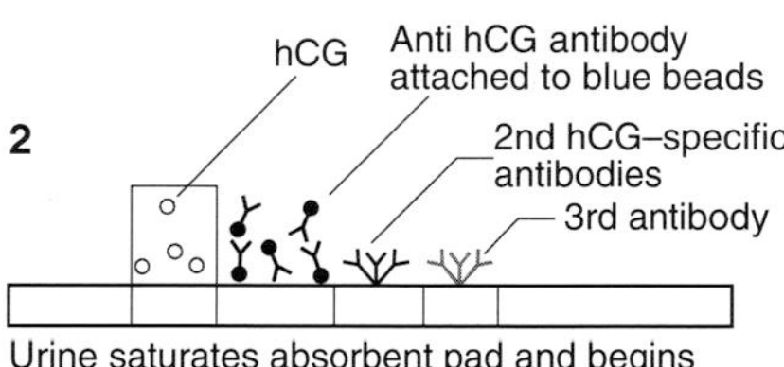

Urine saturates absorbent pad and begins to move along test strip.

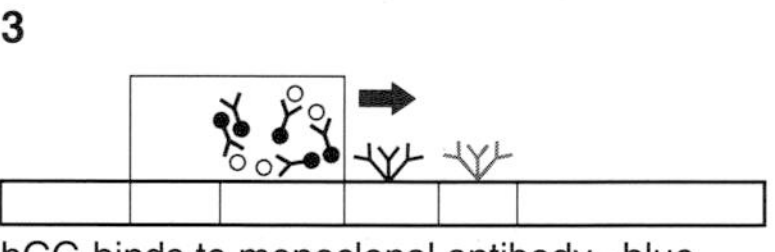

hCG binds to monoclonal antibody–blue bead complex, which then moves along the plate as the urine diffuses.

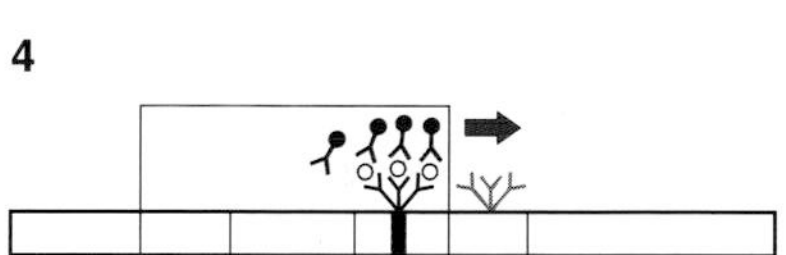

The hCG–antibody–blue bead complex binds to a 2nd hCG specific antibody fixed to the plate along a straight line. This produces a blue line on the plate.

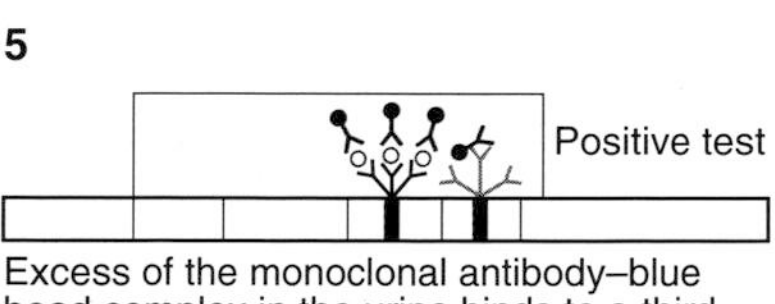

Excess of the monoclonal antibody–blue bead complex in the urine binds to a third antibody forming another blue line. This signals the test is complete.

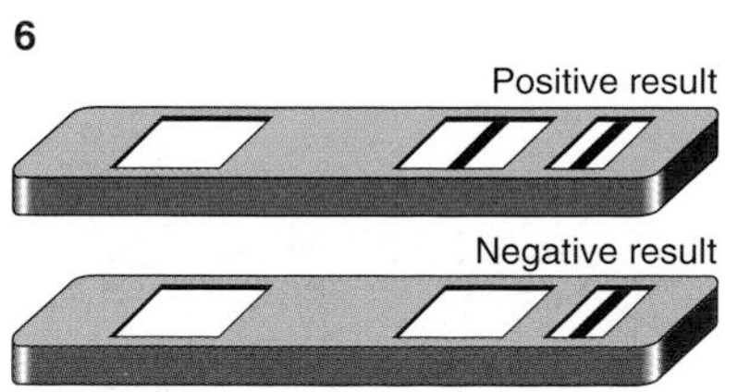

A positive result is shown by 2 blue lines; a negative result is shown by 1 blue line.

Fig. 2 **How a pregnancy test kit works.**

Similarly, the nature of the sample collected for analysis should be considered when interpreting the result. Where the results seem at odds with the clinical situation, interference from contaminants (e.g. detergents in urine containers) should be considered as should cross reactivity of the assay with more than one analyte (e.g. haemoglobin and myoglobin).

Any biochemical assay takes all these potential problems into account. However, with extra-laboratory testing, correct interpretation of the result is no longer the laboratory's responsibility but that of the operator.

THE FUTURE

There is no doubt that in the future, biochemical testing of patients outside the laboratory will become practical for many of the analytes currently measured in the laboratory. There is, however, likely to be much debate about costs and the clinical usefulness of such non-laboratory based analyses.

Case history 3

At a village fete, a local charity group was fundraising by performing certain side-room tests. An 11-year-old boy was found to have a blood glucose of 14.4 mmol/l. His family was concerned, and an hour later his cousin, a recently diagnosed diabetic, confirmed the hyperglycaemia with his home monitoring equipment, and found glycosuria +++.

- What is the significance of these findings?

Comment on page 152.

Biochemical testing outside the laboratory

- Many biochemical tests are performed outwith the normal laboratory setting, for the convenience of patient and clinician.
- Although apparently simple, such tests may yield erroneous results because of operator errors.
- It is important that advice be readily available to interpret each result in the clinical context.

REFERENCE RANGES

The list below does not include reference ranges for all tests performed in the clinical biochemistry laboratory, and it is provided for **guidance only** in answering the cases and examples in this book. These reference ranges are in use at the Institute of Biochemistry, Royal Infirmary, Glasgow. Each clinical biochemistry laboratory will issue ranges specific for the services and tests it provides. *In practice, always use the reference ranges of the laboratory performing the test. These will either be printed on the report form or will be readily available from the local laboratory.*

CORE BIOCHEMISTRY

The urea and electrolyte profile (U & E's)

Na^+	K^+	Cl^-	HCO_3^-	Urea	Creatinine
mmol/l					*µmol/l*
135–145	3.4–4.9	95–105	21–28	2.5–8.0	40–130

Arterial blood gases

H^+	PCO_2	HCO_3^-	PO_2
nmol/l	*kPa*	*mmol/l*	*kPa*
35–45	4.4–5.6	21–28	12–15

Liver function tests (LFTs)

Bilirubin	AST	ALT	Alkaline phosphatase
µmol/l	*U/l*		
3–22	12–48	3–55	80–280

Calcium group of tests

Calcium	Phosphate	Albumin	Calcium (adj)
mmol/l		*g/l*	*mmol/l*
2.2–2.6	0.7–1.4	40–52	2.2–2.6

Alphabetical list of reference values

All reference ranges listed are for serum measurements in adults unless otherwise stated:

Alanine aminotransferase (ALT)	3–55 U/l
Albumin	40–52 g/l
Alkaline phosphatase (ALP)	80-280 U/l
Aspartate aminotransferase (AST)	12–48 U/l
Amylase	70–300 U/l
Bicarbonate	21–28 mmol/l
Bilirubin (total)	3–22 µmol/l
Calcium (adjusted)	2.2–2.6 mmol/l
Chloride	95–105 mmol/l
Cholesterol, total (plasma)[1]	should be < 6.5 mmol/l
Cortisol	280–720 nmol/l (07.00–09.00 h) 60–340 nmol/l (21.00–24.00 h)
Creatine kinase (CK)	<150 U/l
Creatinine	40–130 µmol/l
Creatinine (urine)	9–18 mmol/24h
Creatinine clearance	80–130 ml/min
Digoxin (plasma)[2]	0.7–2.5 nmol/l
Ferritin	15–300 µgl/l
FSH	3–13 U/l follicular phase 9–18 U/l mid cycle 1–10 U/l luteal phase 1–12 U/l adult men
γ-glutamyl transpeptidase (γGT)	<36 U/l
Glucose (blood)	4.0–5.5 mmol/l
Growth hormone (GH)	< 10mU/l
Iron	18–45 µmol/l (males), 14–32 µmol/l (females)
Lactate dehydrogenase (LDH)	230–525 U/l
LH	2–15 U/l follicular phase 22–90 U/l mid cycle 1–19 U/l luteal phase 2–12 U/l adult men
Magnesium	0.7–1.0 mmol/l
Osmolality	275–295 mmol/kg
Osmolality (urine)	up to 1400 mmol/kg
Oestradiol	200–1500 pmol/l (female)
Phosphate	0.7–1.4 mmol/l
Potassium	3.4–4.9 mmol/l
Potassium (urine)[3]	40–90 mmol/24h
Progesterone	> 20 nmol/l confirm ovulation
Prolactin	60–500 mU/l (females) 60–360 mU/l (males)
Protein, total	62–82 g/l
Salicylate[2]	up to 2.5 mmol/l
Sodium	135–145 mmol/l
Sodium (urine)[3]	130–250 mmol/24h
Testosterone	1.0–3.2 nmol/l (female) 11–36 nmol/l (male)
Thyroxine (T4)	55–144 nmol/l
Thyroid stimulating hormone (TSH)	0.35–5.0 mU/l (adults) <25 mU/l (infants <15 days)
Triglyceride, fasting (plasma)[1]	should be < 2.5 mmol/l
Urea	2.5–8.0 mmol/l

Notes

[1]It is preferable to consider 'action limits' rather than reference ranges for lipid analyses. Individuals with concentrations outside these limits should be considered for intervention.

[2]The reference interval given is a therapeutic range, i.e., a range of steady state plasma drug concentrations achieved not less than 6 hours after the last oral dose, which will result in desirable therapeutic effect without signs and symptoms of toxicity.

[3]The urinary electrolyte range is given only as a guide. Under physiological conditions a wide range of urinary sodium and potassium concentrations are possible, depending on intake.

CORE BIOCHEMISTRY

FLUID AND ELECTROLYTE BALANCE: Concepts and Vocabulary

INTRODUCTION

Fluid and electrolyte balance is central to the management of any patient who is seriously ill. Measurement of serum sodium, potassium, urea and creatinine, frequently with chloride and bicarbonate, is the most commonly requested biochemical profile and yields a great deal of information about a patient's fluid and electrolyte status and renal function. A typical report is shown in Figure 1.

How should these results be interpreted? They represent concentrations of some of the major constituents of plasma, but the results can only be discussed if other clinical information about the patient is available. The clinician needs to know if the patient has lost fluid or is fluid overloaded. That information can only be obtained by taking a careful history and performing a clinical examination.

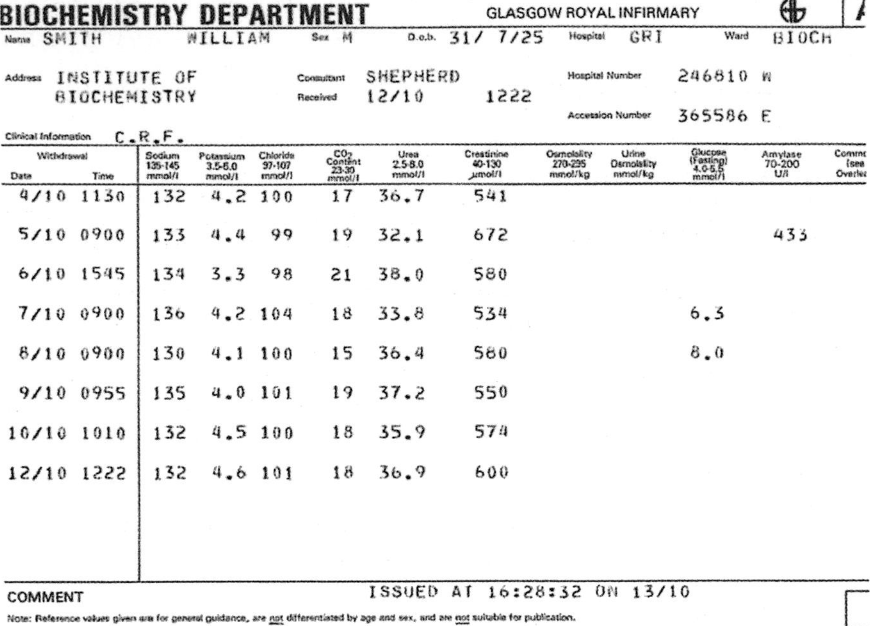

BIOCHEMISTRY DEPARTMENT GLASGOW ROYAL INFIRMARY

Name SMITH WILLIAM Sex M D.o.b. 31/ 7/25 Hospital GRI Ward BIOCH

Address INSTITUTE OF BIOCHEMISTRY Consultant SHEPHERD Received 12/10 1222 Hospital Number 246810 W Accession Number 365586 E

Clinical Information C.R.F.

Withdrawal Date	Time	Sodium 135-145 mmol/l	Potassium 3.5-5.0 mmol/l	Chloride 97-107 mmol/l	CO_2 Content 23-30 mmol/l	Urea 2.5-8.0 mmol/l	Creatinine 40-130 µmol/l	Osmolality 270-295 mmol/kg	Urine Osmolality mmol/kg	Glucose (Fasting) 4.0-5.5 mmol/l	Amylase 70-200 U/l	Comment (see Overleaf)
4/10	1130	132	4.2	100	17	36.7	541					
5/10	0900	133	4.4	99	19	32.1	672				433	
6/10	1545	134	3.3	98	21	38.0	580					
7/10	0900	136	4.2	104	18	33.8	534			6.3		
8/10	0900	130	4.1	100	15	36.4	560			8.0		
9/10	0955	135	4.0	101	19	37.2	550					
10/10	1010	132	4.5	100	18	35.9	574					
12/10	1222	132	4.6	101	18	36.9	600					

COMMENT ISSUED AT 16:28:32 ON 13/10

Note: Reference values given are for general guidance, are not differentiated by age and sex, and are not suitable for publication.

Fig. 1 **A cumulative report form showing electrolyte results in a patient with chronic renal failure.**

BODY FLUID COMPARTMENTS

The major body constituent is water. An 'average' person, weighing 70 kg, contains about 42 litres of water in total. The intracellular fluid compartment (ICF) is the volume of fluid inside the cells (28 l), and the extracellular fluid compartment (ECF) is that volume of fluid which lies outside cells (14 l). The ECF can be further subdivided into plasma (3.5 l) and interstitial fluid (10.5 l).

A schematic way of representing fluid balance is a water tank model which has a partition and an inlet and outlet (Fig. 2). The inlet supply represents fluids taken orally or by intravenous infusion, while the outlet is normally the urinary tract. Insensible loss can be thought of as surface evaporation.

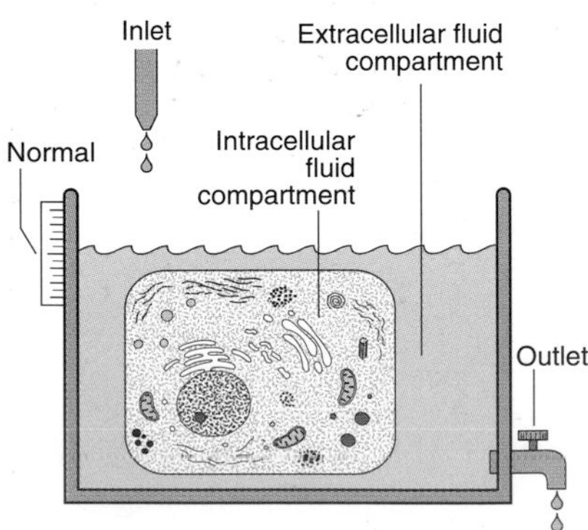

Fig. 2 **Water tank model of body fluid compartments.**

Selective loss of fluid from each of these compartments gives rise to distinct signs and symptoms. Intracellular fluid loss, for example, causes cellular dysfunction which is most notably evident as lethargy, confusion and coma. Loss of blood, an ECF fluid, leads to circulatory collapse, renal shutdown and shock. Loss of total body water will eventually produce similar effects. However, the signs of fluid depletion are not seen at first since the water loss, albeit substantial, is spread across both ECF and ICF compartments.

The water tank model illustrates the relative volumes of each of these compartments and can be used to help visualise some of the clinical disorders of fluid and electrolyte balance. It is important to realize that the assessment of the *volume* of body fluid compartments is not the undertaking of the biochemistry laboratory. The patient's state of hydration, i.e. the volume of the body fluid compartments, is assessed on clinical grounds. The term 'dehydration' simply means that fluid loss has occurred from body compartments. Over-hydration occurs when fluid accumulates in body compartments. Figure 3 illustrates dehydration and overhydration by reference to the water tank model. When interpreting electrolyte results it may be useful to construct this 'biochemist's picture' to visualize what is wrong with the patient's fluid balance and what needs to be done to correct it. The principal features of disordered hydration are shown in Table 1. Clinical assessments of skin turgor, eyeball tension and the mucous membranes are not always reliable. Ageing affects skin elasticity and the oral mucous membranes may appear dry in patients breathing through their mouths.

Table 1 **The principal clinical features of severe hydration disorders**

Feature	Dehydration	Overhydration
Pulse	Increased	Normal
BP	Decreased	Normal or increased
Skin turgor	Decreased	Increased
Eyeballs	Soft / sunken	Normal
Mucous membranes	Dry	Normal
Urine output	Decreased	May be normal or decreased
Consciousness	Decreased	Decreased

ELECTROLYTES

Electrolytes are positively and negatively charged ions which are in solution in all body fluids. Sodium (Na^+) is the principal extracellular cation, and potassium (K^+), the principal intracellular cation. Inside cells the main anions are protein and phosphate, whereas in the ECF chloride (Cl^-) and bicarbonate (HCO_3^-) predominate.

A request for measurement of serum 'electrolytes' usually generates values for the concentration of sodium and potassium ions, together with chloride and bicarbonate ions. Sodium ions are present at the highest concentration and hence make the largest contribution to the total plasma osmolality (see later). Although potassium ion concentrations in the ECF are small compared with the high concentrations inside cells, changes in plasma concentrations are very important and may have life threatening consequences (see pp. 22 - 23).

Urea and creatinine concentrations are frequently measured with the serum electrolytes and provide an indication of renal function, increased concentrations indicating a decreased glomerular filtration rate (see pp. 26 – 27).

CONCENTRATION

Remember that a concentration is a ratio of two variables: the amount of solute (e.g. sodium), and the amount of solvent, the volume of water. A concentration can change because either or both variables have changed. For example, a sodium concentration of 140 mmol/l may become 130 mmol/l because the amount of sodium in the solution has fallen or because the amount of water has increased (see page 6).

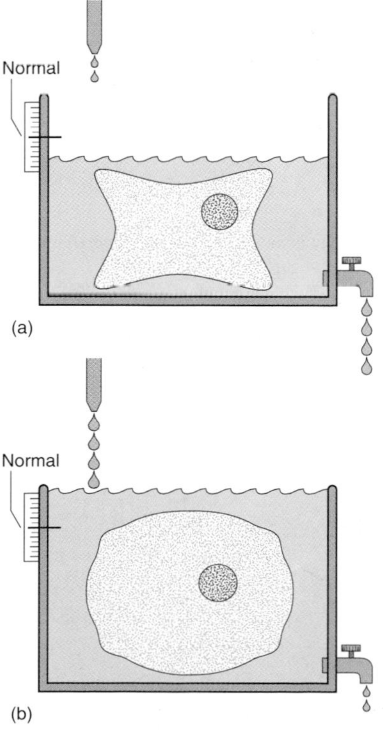

Fig. 3 **The effect of volume depletion and volume expansion on the water tank model of body compartments.**
(a) Dehydration: loss of fluid in ICF and ECF due to increased urinary losses.
(b) Overhydration: increased fluid in ICF and ECF due to increased intake.

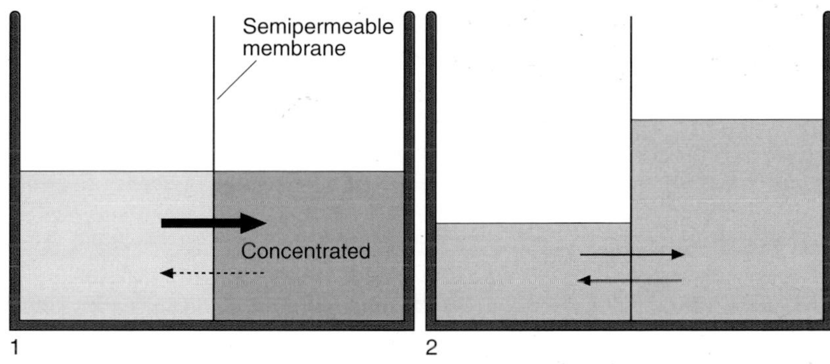

Fig. 4 **Osmolality changes and water movement in body fluid compartments.** The osmolality in different body compartments must be equal. This is achieved by the movement of water across semipermeable membranes in response to concentration changes.

OSMOLALITY

Body fluids vary greatly in their composition. However, while the concentration of substances may vary in the different body fluids, the overall number of solute particles, the osmolality, is identical. Body compartments are separated by semipermeable membranes through which water moves easily. Osmotic pressure must always be the same on both sides of a cell membrane, and water moves to keep the osmolality the same, even if this water movement causes cells to shrink or expand in volume (Fig. 4). The osmolality of the ICF is *always the same as the osmolality of the ECF*. The two compartments contain isotonic solutions.

The osmolality of a solution is expressed in mmol solute per kilogram of solvent which is usually water. In man, the osmolality of serum (and all other body fluids except urine) is around 285 mmol/kg.

Osmolality of a serum or plasma sample can be measured directly, or it may be calculated if the concentrations of the major solutes are already known. There are many formulae used to calculate the serum osmolality. Clinically, the simplest is:

Serum osmolality = 2 x serum [sodium]
(mmol/kg) (mmol/l)

This simple formula only holds if the serum concentration of urea and glucose are within the reference ranges. If either or both are abnormally high, the concentration of either or both (in mmol/l) must be added in to give the calculated osmolality. Sometimes there is an apparent difference between the measured and calculated osmolality. This is known as the *osmolal gap* (p. 17).

Clinical note

Although biochemical testing is important in the assessment and management of a patient with a fluid and electrolyte disorder, it is no substitute for keeping accurate fluid balance charts. Documentation of a patient's fluid intake and output throughout the day gives the clinician valuable information about the patient's state of hydration.

Fluid and electrolyte balance: concepts and vocabulary

- The body has two main fluid compartments, the intracellular fluid and the extracellular fluid.
- The ICF is twice as large as the ECF.
- Water retention will cause an increase in the volume of both ECF and ICF.
- Water loss (dehydration) will result in a decreased volume of both ECF and ICF.
- Sodium ions are the main ECF cations.
- Potassium ions are the main ICF cations.
- The volumes of the ECF and ICF are estimated from knowledge of the patient's history and by clinical examination.
- Serum osmolality can be measured directly or calculated from the serum sodium, urea and glucose concentrations.

WATER AND SODIUM BALANCE

Body water and the electrolytes it contains are in a state of constant flux. We drink, we eat, we pass urine and we sweat; during all this it is important that we maintain a steady state. A motor car's petrol tank might hold about 42 litres, similar to the total body water content of the average 70 kg male. If 2 litres were lost quickly from the tank it would hardly register on the fuel indicator. However, if we were to lose the same volume from our intravascular compartment we would be in serious trouble. We are vulnerable to changes in our fluid compartments, and a number of important homeostatic mechanisms exist to prevent or minimize these. Changes to the electrolyte concentration are also kept to a minimum.

To survive, multicellular organisms must maintain their ECF volume. Humans deprived of fluids die after a few days, from circulatory collapse as a result of the reduction in the total body water. Failure to maintain ECF volume, with the consequence of impaired blood circulation, rapidly leads to tissue death due to lack of oxygen and nutrients, and failure to remove waste products.

WATER

Normal water balance is illustrated in Figure 1. *Water intake* largely depends on social habits and is very variable. Some people drink less than half a litre each day, and others may imbibe more than five litres in 24 hours without harm. Thirst is rarely an overriding factor in determining intake in Western societies.

Water losses are equally variable and are normally seen as changes in the volume of urine produced. The kidneys can respond quickly to meet the body's need to get rid of water. The urine flow rate can vary widely in a very short time. However, even when there is need to conserve water, man cannot completely shut down urine production. Total body water remains remarkably constant in health despite massive fluctuations in intake. Water excretion by the kidney is very tightly controlled by arginine vasopressin (AVP; also called antidiuretic hormone, ADH).

The body is also continually losing water through the skin as perspiration, and from the lungs during respiration. This is called the 'insensible' loss. This water loss is unregulated and amounts to between 500–850 ml/day. Water may also be lost in disease from fistulae, or in diarrhoea, or because of prolonged vomiting.

AVP AND THE REGULATION OF OSMOLALITY

Specialized cells in the hypothalamus sense differences between their intracellular osmolality and that of the extracellular fluid, and adjust the secretion of AVP from the posterior pituitary gland. A rising osmolality promotes the secretion of AVP, a declining osmolality switches the secretion off (Fig. 2). AVP causes water to be retained by the kidneys. Fluid deprivation results in the stimulation of endogenous AVP secretion which reduces the urine flow rate to as little as 0.5 ml/min in order to conserve body water. However, within an hour of drinking 2 litres of water, the urine flow rate may rise to 15 ml/min as AVP secretion is shut down. Thus, by regulating water excretion or retention, AVP maintains normal electrolyte concentrations within the body.

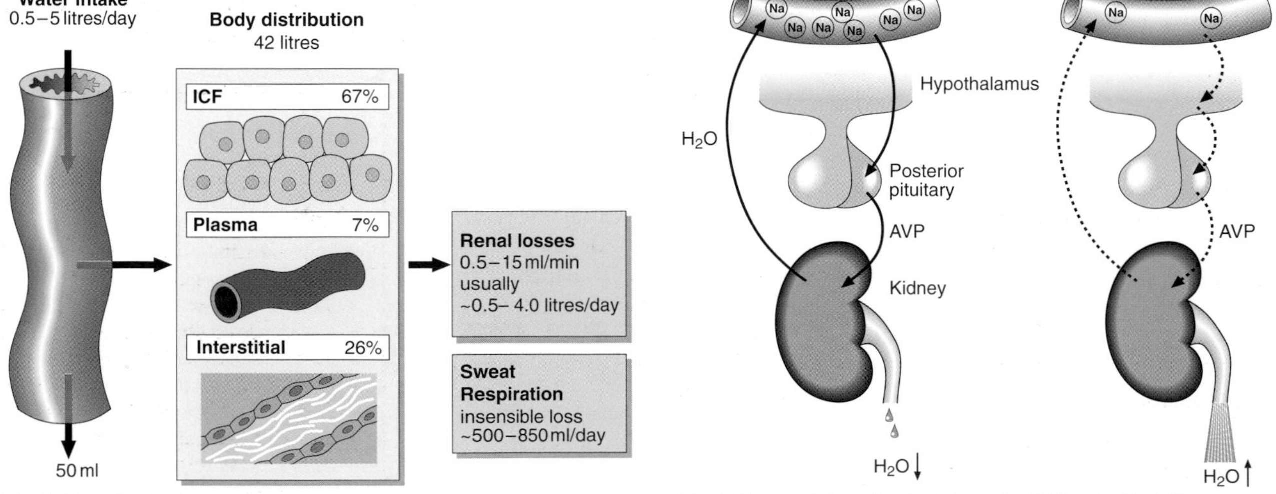

Fig. 1 **Normal water balance.**

Fig. 2 **The regulation of water balance by AVP and osmolality.**

SODIUM

The total body sodium of the average 70 kg man is approximately 3700 mmol, of which approximately 75% is exchangeable (Fig. 3). A quarter of the body sodium is termed non-exchangeable which means it is incorporated into tissues such as bone and has a slow turnover rate. Most of the exchangeable sodium is in the extracellular fluid. In the ECF, which comprises both the plasma and the interstitial fluid, the sodium concentration is tightly regulated around 140 mmol/l.

Sodium intake is variable, a range of less than 100 mmol/day to more than 300 mmol/day being encountered in Western

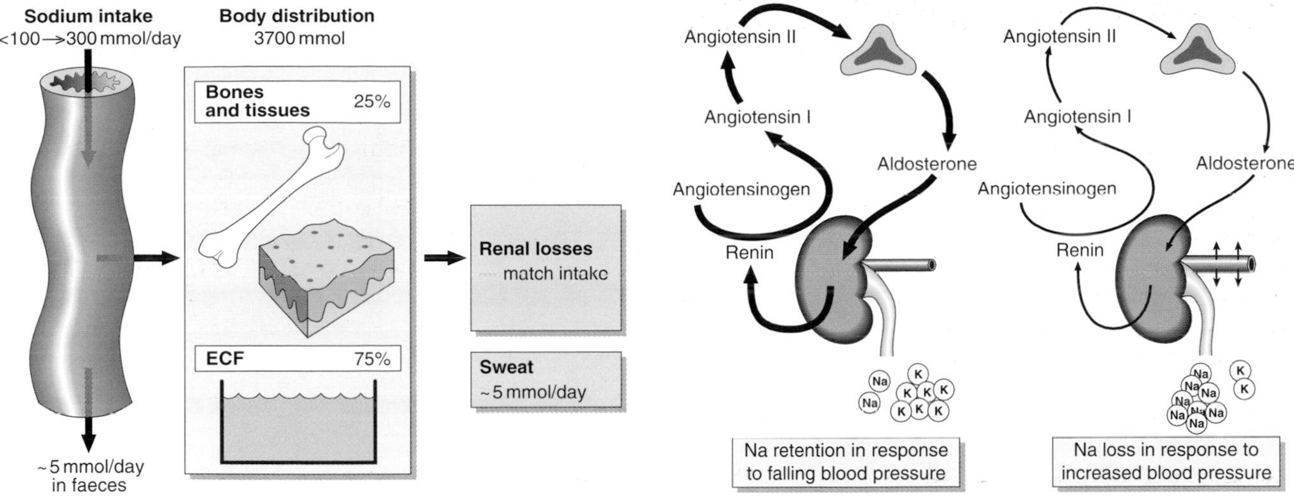

Fig. 3 **Normal sodium balance.**

Fig. 4 **The regulation of sodium balance by aldosterone.**

societies. In health, total body sodium does not change even if intake falls to as little as 5 mmol/day or is greater than 750 mmol/day.

Sodium losses are just as variable. In practical terms, urinary sodium excretion matches sodium intake. Most sodium excretion is via the kidneys. Some sodium is lost in sweat (approximately 5 mmol/day) and in the faeces (approximately 5 mmol/day). In disease the gastrointestinal tract is often the major route of sodium loss. This is a very important clinical point, especially in paediatric practice, as infantile diarrhoea may result in death from salt and water depletion.

Urinary sodium output is regulated by two hormones:

- aldosterone
- atrial natriuretic peptide.

Aldosterone

Aldosterone decreases urinary sodium excretion by increasing sodium reabsorption in the renal tubules at the expense of potassium and hydrogen ions. Aldosterone also stimulates sodium conservation by the sweat glands and the mucosal cells of the colon, but in normal circumstances these effects are trivial. A major stimulus to aldosterone secretion is the volume of the ECF. Specialized cells in the juxtaglomerular apparatus of the nephron sense decreases in blood pressure and secrete renin, the first step in a sequence of events which leads to the secretion of aldosterone by the glomerular zone of the adrenal cortex (Fig. 4).

Atrial natriuretic peptide

Atrial natriuretic peptide is a polypeptide hormone predominantly secreted by the cardiocytes of the right atrium of the heart. It increases urinary sodium excretion. The physiological role, if any, of this hormone is unclear, but it probably only plays a minor role in the regulation of ECF volume and sodium concentration. To date no disease state can be attributed to a primary disorder in the secretion of atrial natriuretic peptide.

REGULATION OF VOLUME

It is important to realize that water will only remain in the extracellular compartment if it is held there by the osmotic effect of ions. As sodium (and accompanying anions, mainly chloride) are largely restricted to the extracellular compartment, the *amount* of sodium in the ECF determines what the volume of the compartment will be. This is an important concept.

Aldosterone and AVP interact to maintain normal volume and concentration of the ECF. Consider a patient who has been vomiting and has diarrhoea from a gastrointestinal infection. With no intake the patient becomes fluid depleted. Water and sodium have been lost. Because the ECF volume is low, aldosterone secretion is high. Thus, as the patient begins to take fluids orally, any salt ingested is maximally retained. As this raises the ECF osmolality, AVP action then ensures that water is retained too. Thus, aldosterone and AVP interaction continues until ECF fluid volume and composition return to normal.

Case history 4

A man is trapped in a collapsed building after an earthquake. He has sustained no serious injuries or blood loss. He has no access to food or water until he is rescued after 72 hrs.

- What will have happened to his body fluid compartments?

Comment on page 152.

Clinical note

Assessment of the volumes of body fluid compartments is not carried out in the clinical biochemistry laboratory. This must be done clinically by history taking and examination.

Water and sodium balance

- Water is lost from the body as urine and as obligatory 'insensible' losses from the skin and lungs.
- Sodium may be lost from the body in prolonged vomiting, diarrhoea and intestinal fistulae.
- Arginine vasopressin (AVP) regulates renal water loss and thus causes changes in the osmolality of body fluid compartments.
- Aldosterone regulates renal sodium loss and controls the sodium content of the ECF.
- Changes in sodium content of the ECF cause changes in volume of this compartment because of the combined actions of AVP and aldosterone.

HYPERNATRAEMIA

Hypernatraemia is an increase in serum sodium concentration above the reference range of 135 – 145 mmol/l. Before considering in detail the implications of a high sodium concentration in a patient's serum specimen, clinical factors which may have contributed to the patient's electrolyte disturbance should be examined. Remember that the volume of body fluid compartments is assessed on clinical grounds, not in the laboratory. The following questions should be asked:

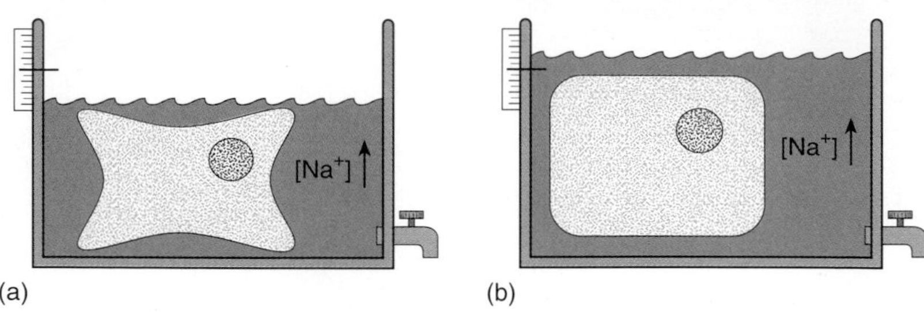

Fig. 1 **Hypernatraemia is commonly associated with a contracted ECF volume, and less commonly with an expanded compartment.**
(a) Volumes of ECF and ICF are reduced.
(b) ECF volume is shown here to be slightly expanded; ICF volume is normal.

- Is there evidence that the patient has lost fluid?
- On clinical examination, is the volume of the ECF reduced?
- If there has been fluid loss, was this predominantly water, or both water and sodium?
- Has the patient been given inappropriate fluid therapy, or ingested sodium salts?

Only when these questions have been addressed is it possible to interpret whether the hypernatraemia is associated with a decreased ECF volume, or a normal or even expanded compartment (Fig. 1). The patient's treatment depends on this knowledge.

ASSESSING THE CAUSE OF THE HYPERNATRAEMIA

A patient may become hypernatraemic because of:

- water depletion
- water and sodium depletion
- excessive sodium intake or retention in the ECF
- very rarely renal failure with an inability to excrete sodium.

Water depletion

Water depletion may arise from a decreased intake or excessive loss. A decreased water intake over a period of time when insensible losses have continued leads to decreased ECF and ICF volumes. The failure of intake to match the insensible water loss is the cause of the hypernatraemia. The total sodium content of the ECF is unchanged. This is the most common reason for hypernatraemia. A frequently encountered example is the elderly person who becomes ill and is unable to get something to drink.

Water loss resulting in hypernatraemia can also be caused by a breakdown of the normal homeostatic mechanisms which regulate water balance. AVP secretion is impaired in diabetes insipidus; consequently the renal tubules do not conserve water and hypernatraemia follows. In addition, AVP action is compromised in nephrogenic diabetes insipidus, where renal tubular cells do not respond to the hormone.

Water and sodium depletion

In situations where both sodium and water are lost from the ECF, hypernatraemia will occur only if more water than sodium is lost. An osmotic diuresis, as seen in the patient with diabetes mellitus, causes a deficit of both water and sodium ions and may result in hypernatraemia with decreased ECF volume. Excessive sweating or diarrhoea, especially in children, may also give this picture.

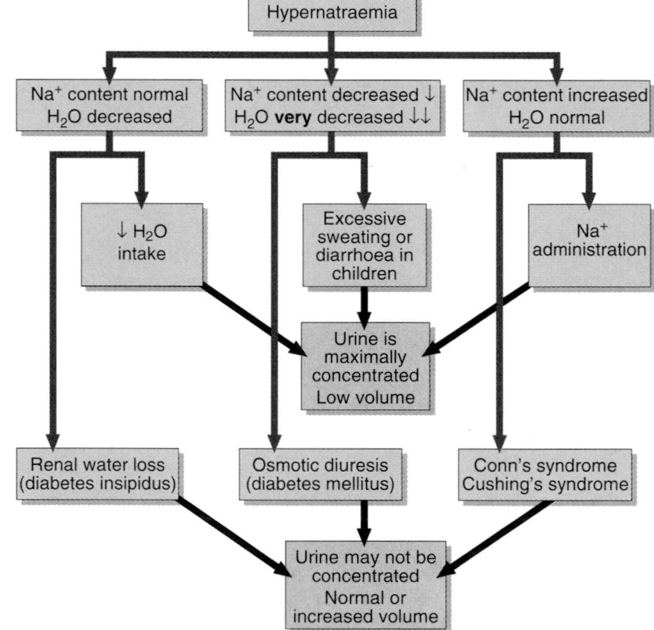

Fig. 2 **The causes of hypernatraemia.**

Loss of body fluids because of vomiting, diarrhoea or from a fistula usually results in *hyponatraemia* rather than hypernatraemia (pp. 20–21). Sodium chloride is lost, but is replaced by water, resulting in hyponatraemia.

Increase in sodium content of the ECF

Hypernatraemia may be a consequence of increased ECF sodium content. The administration of sodium bicarbonate for the correction of an acidosis is a practice which should be performed with caution, in the extreme situations when such therapy is needed. It is sometimes not appreciated that bicarbonate solutions may contain sodium at a concentration greatly in excess of the physiological (8.4% sodium bicarbonate is 1000 mmol/l), and administering too much can give rise to hypernatraemia. A less concentrated solution (1.26%, 150 mmol/l) is available and is preferred.

The pathophysiological parallel to the administration of sodium is the rare condition of primary hyperaldosteronism (Conn's syndrome), where there is excessive aldosterone secretion and consequent sodium retention by the renal tubules. Similar findings may be made in the patient with Cushing's syndrome, where there is excess cortisol production. Cortisol has weak mineralocorticoid activity. However, in these two conditions the serum sodium concentration rarely rises above 150 mmol/l.

Urine osmolality and sodium concentration may sometimes be of value in the differential diagnosis of hypernatraemia. In practice, hypernatraemia due to excess sodium intake and that due to water loss should be easily distinguished from the patient's clinical history.

The causes of hypernatraemia are summarized in Figure 2.

CLINICAL FEATURES

The clinical features associated with the hypernatraemic patient are variable. If there has been fluid loss, then the features of dehydration may be present (p. 12, and Fig. 3). In the case of salt gain, there may be indications of fluid overload such as raised jugular venous pressure and pulmonary oedema.

TREATMENT

Hypernatraemia is less common than hyponatraemia, but is usually of much more clinical significance. It is important not to correct hypernatraemia due to water loss too quickly. The patient should be given water orally if possible; if not, then 5% dextrose is given intravenously (pp. 24–25).

OTHER OSMOLALITY DISORDERS

A high plasma osmolality may sometimes be encountered for reasons other than hypernatraemia. Causes include:

- increased urea in renal disease
- hyperglycaemia in diabetes mellitus
- the presence of ethanol or some other ingested substance.

A large discrepancy between the measured osmolality and the calculated osmolality is called the osmolal gap (see p. 13) and suggests the presence of a significant contributor to the osmolality unaccounted for in the calculation. In practice, this is almost always due to the presence of ethanol in the blood. Very occasionally, however, it may be due to other substances such as methanol or ethylene glycol from the ingestion of antifreeze. The calculation of the osmolal gap can be clinically very useful in the assessment of comatose patients.

Hypo-osmolality is synonymous with hyponatraemia because sodium is the only ion present in the ECF in sufficient amount such that a decrease in concentration would significantly affect the osmolality.

The consequences of disordered osmolality are due to the changes in volume which arise as water moves in or out of cells to maintain osmotic balance. Note that of the three examples above, only glucose causes significant fluid movement. Glucose cannot freely enter cells, and an increasing ECF concentration causes water to move out of cells and leads to intracellular dehydration. Urea and ethanol permeate cells and do not cause such fluid shifts, as long as concentration changes occur slowly.

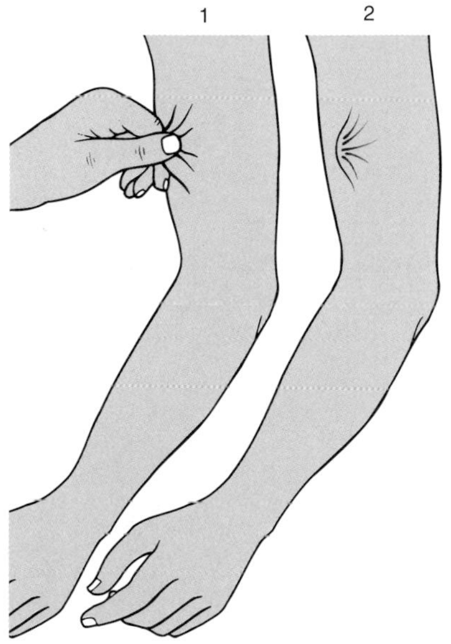

Fig. 3 **Decreased skin turgor.** This sign is frequently unreliable in the elderly, who have reduced skin elasticity. In the young it is a sign of severe dehydration with fluid loss from the ECF.

Clinical note

Patients often become hypernatraemic because they are unable to complain of being thirsty. The comatose patient is a good example. He or she will be unable to communicate his/her needs, yet insensible losses of water will continue from lungs/skin and need to be replaced.

Case history 5

A 76-year-old man with depression and very severe incapacitating disease was admitted as an acute emergency. He was clinically dehydrated. His skin was lax and his lips and tongue were dry and shrivelled looking. His pulse was 104/min, and his blood pressure was 95/65 mmHg. The following biochemical results were obtained on admission:

Na^+	K^+	Cl^-	HCO_3^-	Urea	Creatinine
mmol/l					*µmol/l*
162	3.6	132	18	22.9	155

- Comment on these biochemical findings.
- What is the diagnosis?

Comment on page 152.

Hypernatraemia

- Hypernatraemia is most commonly due to water loss (e.g. because of continuing insensible losses in the patient who is unable to drink).
- Failure to retain water as a result of impaired AVP secretion or action may cause hypernatraemia.
- Hypernatraemia may be the result of a loss of both sodium and water as a consequence of an osmotic diuresis e.g. in diabetic ketoacidosis.
- Excessive sodium intake, particularly from the use of intravenous solutions, may cause hypernatraemia. Rarely, primary hyperaldosteronism (Conn's syndrome) may be the cause.
- A high plasma osmolality may be due to the presence of glucose, urea or ethanol, rather than sodium.

HYPONATRAEMIA (1)

Hyponatraemia is a significant fall in serum sodium concentration below the reference range of 135–145 mmol/l. A patient may become hyponatraemic because of:

- *Retention of water*. More water than normal is retained in the body compartments and dilutes the constituents of the extracellular space causing hyponatraemia.
- *Loss of sodium*. Sodium is the main extracellular cation. Where loss of sodium ions exceeds loss of water, hyponatraemia may result. This is particularly likely if sodium-containing body fluids (e.g. from vomiting or from fistulae) are replaced simply by water.

These different conditions may be visualized in Figure 1. This figure emphasizes that the biochemical observation of hyponatraemia gives no information about the volume of the ECF compartment, that information only being obtained from the patient's history and by clinical examination.

Hyponatraemia with water retention is considered here; hyponatraemia due to sodium loss is discussed on pages 20–21.

HYPONATRAEMIA WITH WATER RETENTION

The causes of hyponatraemia due to water retention are shown in Figure 2. If fluid loss is not apparent from the patient's clinical history, the reason for the hyponatraemia is usually water retention.

Hyponatraemia due to water overload without a decrease in total body sodium is the commonest biochemical disturbance encountered in clinical practice. Further consideration of hyponatraemia of this type, and its treatment, depends on whether the patient has oedema or not. Oedema is an accumulation of fluid in the interstitial compartment. It is readily diagnosed by looking for pitting in the lower extremities of ambulant patients (Fig. 3) or in the sacral area of recumbent patients.

NON-OEDEMATOUS HYPONATRAEMIA

Patients with non-oedematous hyponatraemia have a normal total body sodium and exhibit the features of the so-called syndrome of inappropriate antidiuresis (the SIAD). The patients are hyponatraemic, normotensive, have a normal glomerular filtration rate and a normal serum urea and creatinine concentration. Their urine flow rate is usually less than 1.5 l/day.

This syndrome is encountered in many conditions:

- infections, e.g. pneumonia, subphrenic abscess
- malignancy, e.g. carcinoma of the bowel or the lung
- trauma, e.g. abdominal surgery
- drug-induced, e.g. thiazide diuretics, chlorpropamide.

Patients suffering from any of the above have non-osmotic AVP stimulation and, if they are exposed to excessive water loads, in the form of oral drinks or intravenous glucose solutions, they will become hyponatraemic.

In health, AVP secretion is regulated by changes in the concentration of sodium in the ECF. AVP concentration fluctuates by between 0 and 5 pmol/l and these small changes in hormone concentration regulate water reabsorption in the kidney tubules and, hence, urine flow. However, non-osmotic stimuli can cause huge increases in AVP concentration of up to 500 pmol/l. These stimuli include:

- reduction in circulating blood volume and/or hypotension

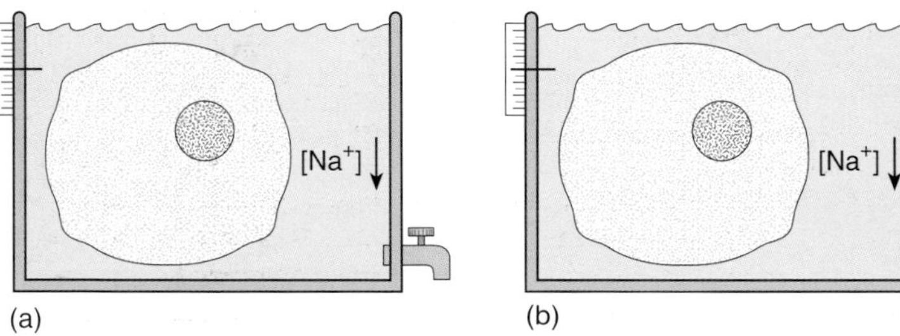

Fig. 1 **Water tank models of hyponatraemia.**
(a) Water retention throughout ECF and ICF. **(b)** Sodium loss.

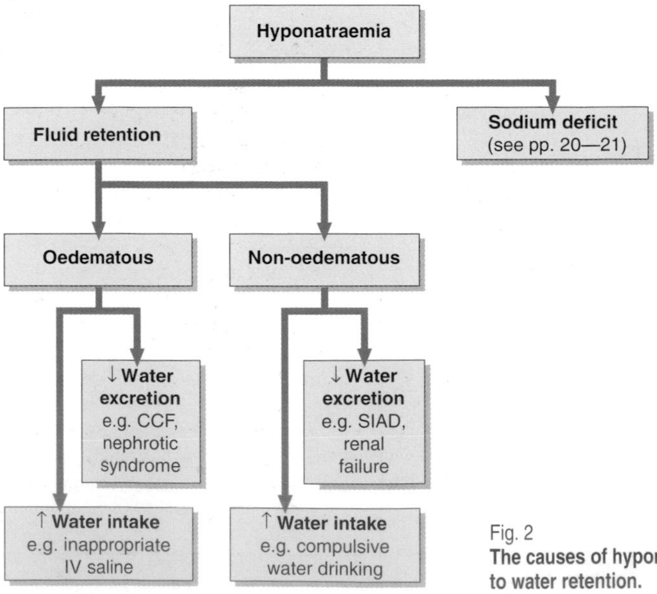

Hyponatraemia

Fluid retention

Sodium deficit (see pp. 20—21)

Oedematous

Non-oedematous

↓ Water excretion e.g. CCF, nephrotic syndrome

↓ Water excretion e.g. SIAD, renal failure

↑ Water intake e.g. inappropriate IV saline

↑ Water intake e.g. compulsive water drinking

Fig. 2
The causes of hyponatraemia due to water retention.

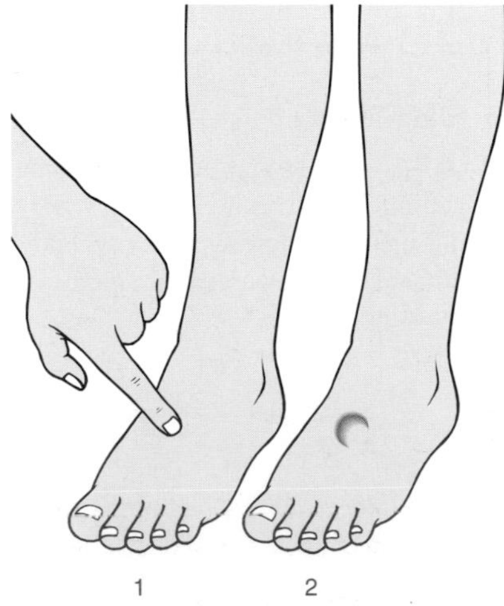

Fig. 3 **Pitting oedema.**
After depressing the skin firmly for a few seconds an indentation or pit is seen.

- nausea and vomiting
- hypoglycaemia
- pain.

The non-osmotic regulation of AVP overrides the osmotic regulatory mechanism and this results in water retention which is a nonspecific feature of illness. This is illustrated by the finding that while only 4% of the healthy population have a serum sodium concentration less than 138 mmol/l, more than 40% of hospital in-patients have hyponatraemia to this extent.

AVP has other effects in the body aside from regulating renal water handling. These are outlined in Table 1 and will not be considered further here.

Table 1 **Actions of AVP, other than renal water regulation**

Potent vasoconstrictor
Potent hormonal stimulator of hepatic glycogenolysis
Increases the plasma concentration of Factor VIII — hence the use of the AVP analogue DDAVP in mild haemophilia
Augments ACTH secretion from the anterior pituitary thus increasing cortisol production

Treatment

In these patients the water load is distributed iso-osmotically between the intracellular fluid and the extracellular fluid, and thus the clinical signs of water overload may be absent or very mild. Usually patients are asymptomatic as the syndrome develops over a period of days to weeks and the body adapts during this time. Treatment is therefore simply the reduction of fluid intake to less than 750 ml/day.

Very rarely a rapid increase in body water results in neurological symptoms such as confusion, convulsions and coma. Only in such circumstances should the cautious use of hypertonic saline be considered in an attempt to correct the hyponatraemia.

OEDEMATOUS HYPONATRAEMIA

Patients who have generalized oedema have an increase in both total body sodium and water. The principal causes of oedema are heart failure and hypoalbuminaemia, and in both these conditions patients have a reduced effective blood volume.

- *Heart failure.* The effective blood volume is reduced because the pumping action of the heart is unable to maintain a satisfactory circulation of the blood and ECF.
- *Hypoalbuminaemia.* The effective blood volume is reduced because the hypoalbuminaemia lowers the plasma oncotic pressure. This disrupts the normal exchange of solutes and fluid in the capillary bed resulting in unsatisfactory circulation of the blood and ECF. Hypoalbuminaemia occurs when synthesis is inadequate due to liver disease (pp. 50–51) or when losses exceed the liver's synthetic capacity as occurs in the nephrotic syndrome (p. 44).

In response to the reduced effective blood volume, aldosterone is secreted and causes sodium retention to allow the ECF volume to expand. The reduction in the effective blood volume is one of the non-osmotic stimuli for AVP secretion and consequently water is retained. The retention of relatively more water than sodium in the ECF results in hyponatraemia. The sequence of events in the development of hyponatraemia in the patient with oedema is shown in Figure 4.

Treatment

Treatment of oedematous hyponatraemia is based upon two principles. The underlying condition should be treated, whether that be, for example, heart failure, glomerulonephritis or alcoholic cirrhosis. Excess sodium and water should be reduced by means of a diuretic to induce a natriuresis, and by fluid restriction.

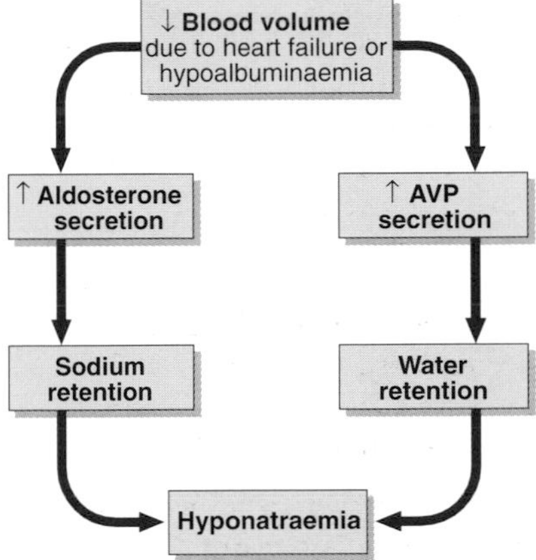

Fig. 4 **The development of hyponatraemia in the oedematous patient.**

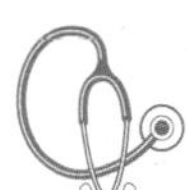

Clinical note

Oedema is not just a consequence of secondary hyperaldosteronism. In some situations, the factors which cause the expansion of the ECF compartment (such as inflammation or restricted venous return) are localized.

Case history 6

A 64-year-old woman was admitted with anorexia, weight loss and anaemia. Carcinoma of the colon was diagnosed. She was normotensive and did not have oedema. The following biochemical results were obtained shortly after admission.

Na^+	K^+	Cl^-	HCO_3^-	Urea	Creatinine
mmol/l					*µmol/l*
123	3.9	86	22	6.2	115

Serum osmolality was measured as 247 mmol/kg; urine osmolality was 178 mmol/kg.

- How may this patient's hyponatraemia be explained?
- What contribution does the urine osmolality make to the diagnosis?

Comment on page 152.

Hyponatraemia: water retention

- Hyponatraemia because of water retention is the commonest biochemical disturbance encountered in clinical practice. In many patients the non-osmotic regulation of AVP overrides the osmotic regulatory mechanism and this results in water retention which is a non-specific feature of illness.
- Hyponatraemic patients without oedema, who have normal serum urea and creatinine and blood pressure, have water overload. This may be treated by fluid restriction.
- Hyponatraemic patients with oedema are likely to have both water and sodium overload. These patients may be treated with diuretics and fluid restriction.

HYPONATRAEMIA (2)

HYPONATRAEMIA DUE TO SODIUM LOSS

Although hyponatraemia commonly results from water retention, it may also be associated with sodium depletion. This occurs only when there is pathological sodium loss. Such losses may be from the gastrointestinal tract or in urine.

Gastrointestinal losses (Table 1) include those from:

- vomiting, especially if this is severe and protracted as occurs in pyloric stenosis.
- diarrhoea
- fistula.

Urinary loss may be due to:

- aldosterone deficiency as a consequence of a failure of the adrenal glands (Addison's disease)
- drugs which antagonize aldosterone action such as spironolactone.

Initially in all of the above, sodium loss is accompanied by water loss and the serum sodium concentration remains normal. As sodium loss proceeds, the reduction in ECF and blood volume stimulates arginine vasopressin secretion. Remember that the non-osmotic control of AVP secretion overrides the osmotic control mechanism. The increased AVP secretion causes water retention and thus patients become hyponatraemic.

Patients become hyponatraemic because a deficit of isotonic sodium-containing fluid is replaced only by water, either orally or intravenously.

Hyponatraemia due to a decreased intake of sodium ions is an extremely rare occurrence. The causes of hyponatraemia associated with sodium deficit are summarized in Figure 1.

Table 1 **A guide to the electrolyte composition of gastrointestinal fluids.**

Fluid	Concentration Na^+ (mmol/l)	K^+	Cl^-
Gastric juice	70	10	110
Small intestinal fluid	120	10	100
Diarrhoea	50	30	50
Rectal mucus	100	40	100
Bile, pleural and peritoneal fluids	140	5	100

DIAGNOSIS

The diagnosis of sodium depletion is usually made on the basis of the patient's history. Of the clinical signs of ECF depletion (Fig. 2), the most important are hypotension and tachycardia. If these signs are present in the recumbent state severe life-threatening sodium depletion is indicated and immediate treatment is needed. In the early phases of sodium depletion postural hypotension may be the only sign.

TREATMENT

Treatment is based upon two principles:

- correction of the sodium loss
- treatment of the underlying disorder.

Correction of the sodium loss is a priority and may be very satisfactorily achieved orally even in severe cases, with gastrointestinal losses, though intravenous infusions of 0.9% NaCl are frequently required. Treatment of the underlying disorder may involve steroid therapy for Addison's disease or medical or surgical treatment of gastrointestinal disorders.

Individuals, unaccustomed to very hot conditions, may lose considerable amounts of sodium in sweat during the first few days in a tropical climate.

These fluid losses are usually replaced by drinking sodium-free fluids, and this results in a hyponatraemia. The process of acclimatization includes a re-setting of sodium excretion of the sweat glands, leading to increased heat tolerance. The preventive treatment of this hyponatraemia is with oral salt tablets.

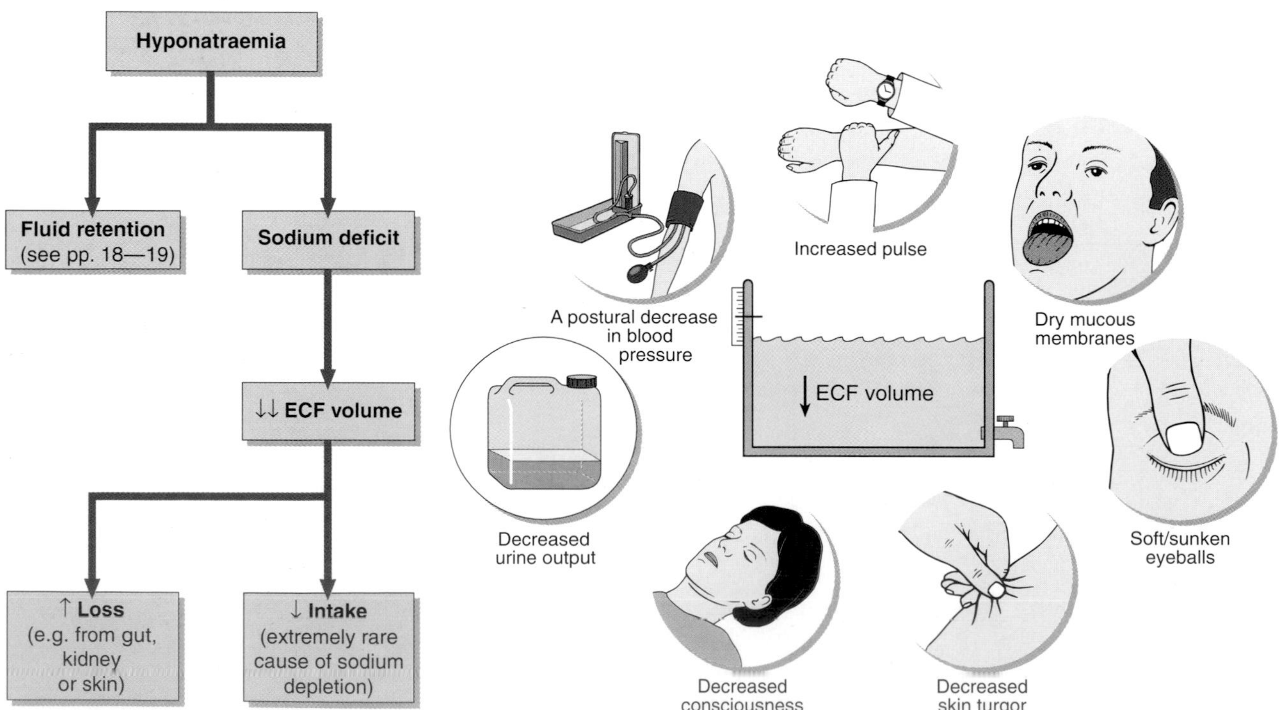

Fig. 1 **The causes of hyponatraemia with sodium loss.**

Fig. 2 **The clinical features of ECF compartment depletion.**

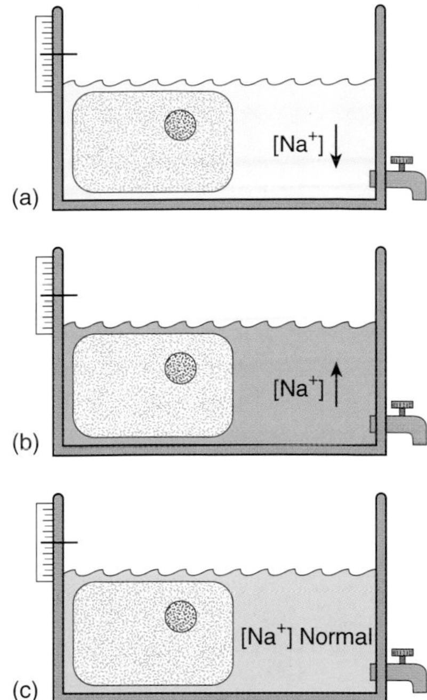

Fig. 3 **Water tank models showing that reduced ECF volume may be associated with reduced, increased or normal serum [Na+].**

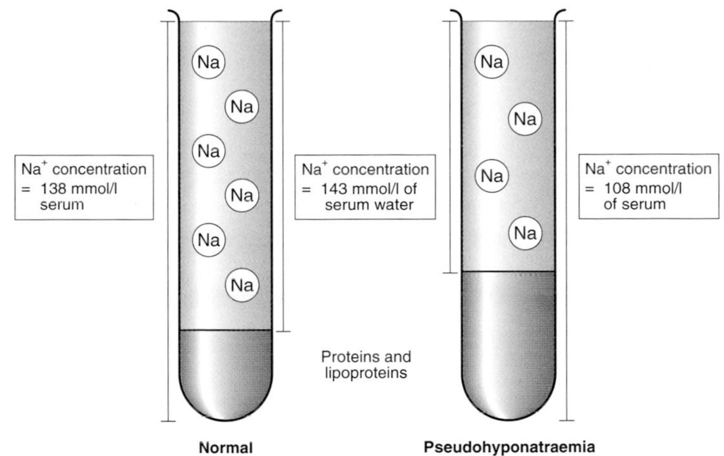

Fig. 4 **Pseudohyponatraemia.**

SODIUM DEPLETION— A NOTE OF CAUTION

In this section we have indicated that hyponatraemia may commonly be encountered in patients who have lost sodium-containing fluids and whose ECF volumes are reduced. On pages 16 and 17 it was noted that some patients with sodium loss may become hypernatraemic. It is also possible that patients with life-threatening sodium depletion may present with a normal serum sodium concentration (Fig. 3). This illustrates clearly that the clinician must always pay more attention to the patient's history, signs and symptoms than to the biochemical results.

PSEUDOHYPONATRAEMIA

A low sodium concentration is sometimes reported in patients with severe hyperproteinaemia or hyperlipoproteinaemia. This is an artefact caused by the method used to measure sodium concentration by some analytical instruments. These patients have in fact a normal sodium concentration in their plasma water. The increased amounts of protein or lipoprotein occupy a larger fraction of the plasma volume than usual, and the water a smaller fraction. The analyser measures the amount of sodium in a small volume and assumes that the water content of that sample is normal. The result is an apparently reduced sodium concentration (Fig. 4). This so-called pseudohyponatraemia can be detected by measuring the serum osmolality which will be normal.

If a low sodium concentration is suspicious, measure the serum osmolality. Knowing the glucose and urea concentration, the *calculated* osmolality can also be obtained. If the two results differ (that is, if there is a significant osmolal gap), the measured sodium concentration is likely to be the misleading result.

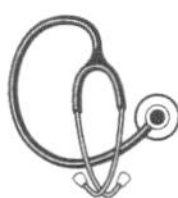

Clinical note

The use of oral glucose and salt solution to correct sodium depletion in infective diarrhoea is one of the major therapeutic advances of the century and is life saving, particularly in developing countries. Sachets of oral rehydration glucose and salt to be mixed with a fixed volume of drinking water are readily available from pharmacies.

Family practitioners, nurses and even parents are able to treat sodium depletion using these oral salt solutions, without making biochemical measurements.

Case history 7

A 42-year-old man was admitted with a two-day history of severe diarrhoea with some nausea and vomiting. During this period his only intake was water. He was weak, unable to stand and when recumbent his pulse was 104/min and blood pressure was 100/55 mmHg. On admission, his biochemistry results were:

Na^+	K^+	Cl^-	HCO_3^-	Urea	Creatinine
		mmol/l			*μmol/l*
131	3.0	86	19	17.8	150

- What is the most appropriate treatment for this patient?

Comment on page 152.

Hyponatraemia: sodium loss

- Hyponatraemia may occur in the patient with gastrointestinal or renal fluid losses which have caused sodium depletion. The low sodium concentration in serum occurs because water retention is stimulated by increased AVP secretion.
- Patients with hyponatraemia because of sodium depletion show clinical signs of fluid loss such as hypotension. They do not have oedema.
- Treatment of hyponatraemia, due to sodium depletion, should be with sodium and water replacement, preferably orally.

POTASSIUM DISORDERS

POTASSIUM METABOLISM

The total body potassium of the average 70 kg man is approximately 3600 mmol. Almost all is inside cells (Fig. 1). *Potassium intake* is variable, 30–100 mmol/day in the UK, but much higher in other countries. *Potassium losses* are equally variable. The kidney excretes the bulk of ingested potassium. Urinary potassium excretion rises in response to increased intake. Potassium excretion by the kidney is primarily dependent upon glomerular filtration. The most important factor which regulates potassium excretion in the urine is the plasma potassium concentration.

Some potassium is lost in the faeces (approximately 5 mmol/day). In pathological states, gastrointestinal losses can be greatly increased. Only small amounts of potassium are lost via the skin in sweat.

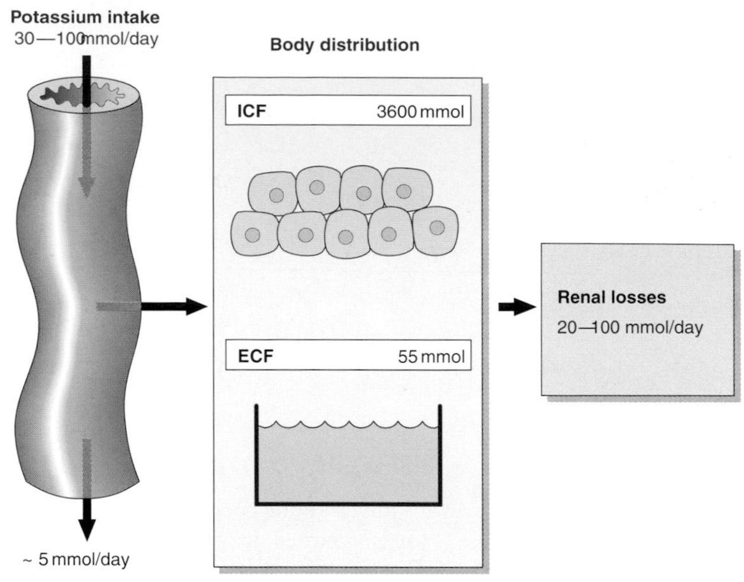

Fig. 1 **Potassium balance.**

SERUM POTASSIUM

The small fraction (2%) of the total body potassium which is in the extracellular compartment is distributed proportionately between the interstitial and plasma spaces. The concentration in serum is around 4.5 mmol/l. Whereas serum potassium concentration does not vary appreciably in response to water loss or retention, factors which cause even a small or sudden shift of intracellular potassium will cause a big change in the ECF potassium content and concentration. Cellular uptake of potassium is stimulated by insulin. Of particular importance is the reciprocal relationship between potassium and hydrogen ions. Many hydrogen ions are buffered inside cells. As the concentration of hydrogen ions increases with the development of acidosis, potassium ions are displaced from the cell in order to maintain electroneutrality (Fig. 2). The opposite can occur in a metabolic alkalosis. These hydrogen ion changes cause marked alterations in serum potassium concentration.

Serum potassium concentrations say little about the total body potassium content, although in practice where acid–base status is normal, hypokalaemic patients are usually potassium depleted.

Despite its low concentration in the ECF, potassium determines the resting membrane potential of cells. Changes in plasma potassium concentration means that 'excitable' cells, such as nerve and muscle, may respond differently to stimuli. In particular, because the heart is largely muscle and nerve, too high or too low a plasma potassium concentration may have life-threatening consequences.

HYPERKALAEMIA

Hyperkalaemia is the commonest and most serious electrolyte emergency encountered in clinical practice. Hyperkalaemia causes muscle weakness which may be preceded by paraesthesiae. However, the first manifestation is often cardiac arrest. The cardiac signs are heralded by the development of tall or peaked T-waves on the ECG (Fig. 3). Above 7.0 mmol/l there is a serious risk of cardiac arrest. However, the ECG changes in hyperkalaemia may mimic other conditions such as myocardial infarction. Thus, it is important to check the serum potassium concentration in patients after cardiac arrest.

The causes of hyperkalaemia include:

- *Renal failure*. The kidneys may not be able to excrete a potassium load when the glomerular filtration rate is very low. The acidosis associated with renal failure contributes to the problem.
- *Mineralocorticoid deficiency*. This is most frequently seen in Addison's Disease or in patients receiving aldosterone antagonists. In these patients there is an increase in the total body potassium.
- *Acidosis*. Hyperkalaemia results from a redistribution of potassium from the intracellular to the extracellular fluid space (Fig. 2).
- *Potassium release from damaged cells*. Because of the very high potassium concentration inside cells, cell damage can give rise to a very high serum potassium as occurs in rhabdomyolysis (pp. 136–137), trauma and malignancy.

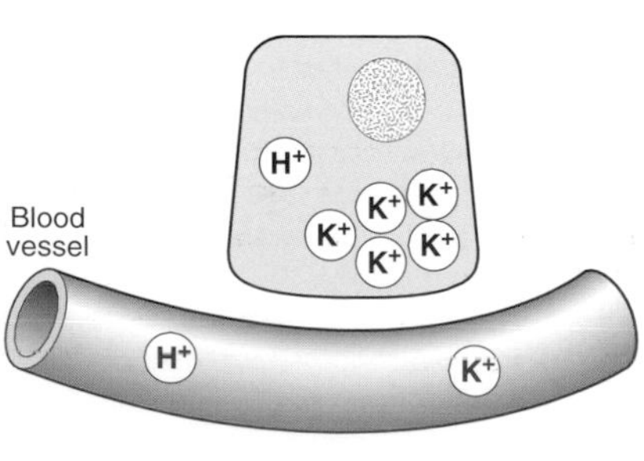

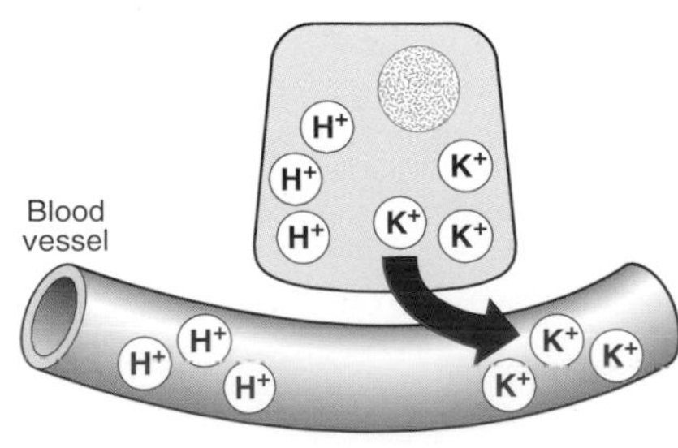

Fig. 2 **Hyperkalaemia is associated with acidosis.**

(a)

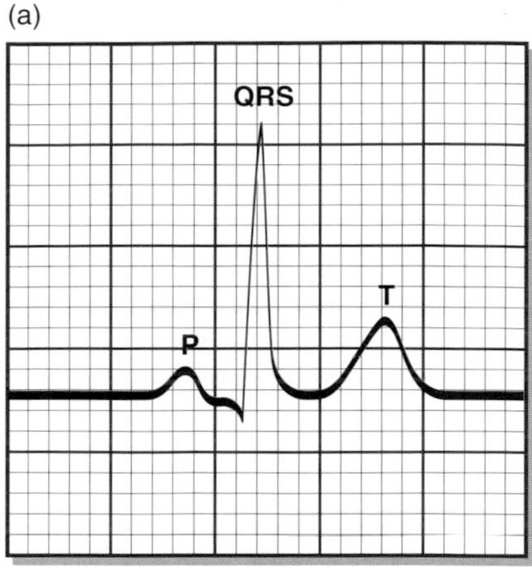

(b)

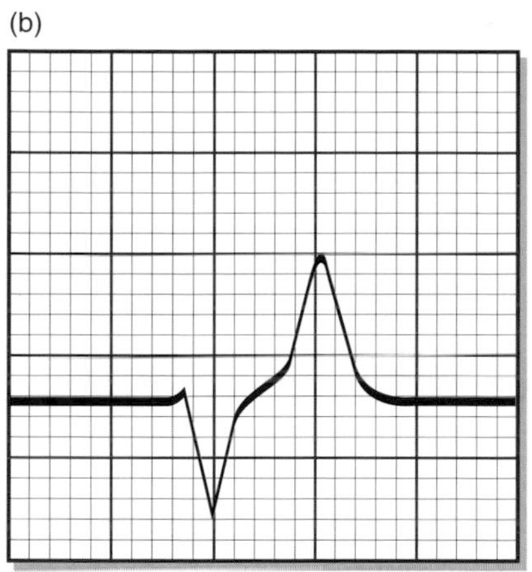

(c)

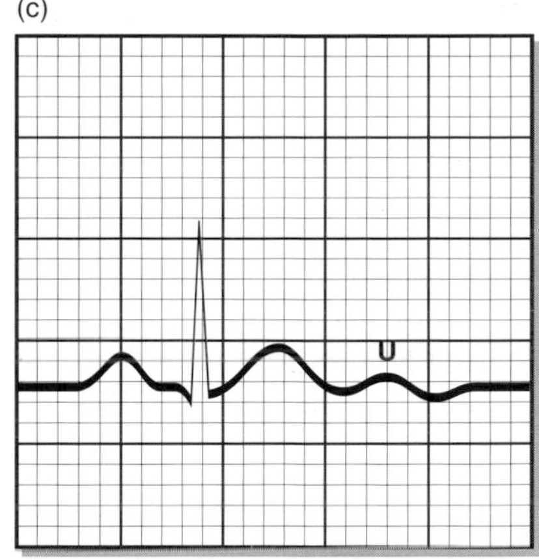

Fig. 3 **Typical ECG changes associated with hyperkalaemia and hypokalaemia. (a)** Normal ECG (lead II). **(b)** Patient with hyperkalaemia: note peaked T-wave and widening of the QRS complex. **(c)** Patient with hypokalaemia: note flattened T-wave. U-waves are prominent in all leads.

An artefactually high potassium is commonly seen if haemolysis has occurred in collecting the sample, or there has been delay in separating the serum from the clotted blood sample.

Treatment

The commonest form of treatment for acute hyperkalaemia is the infusion of insulin and glucose to move potassium ions into cells. An infusion of calcium gluconate may also be given to counteract the effects of hyperkalaemia. Dialysis is frequently necessary to treat severe hyperkalaemia. When there is a slow rise in the plasma potassium this may be stopped or reversed by oral administration of a cation exchange resin such as Resonium A.

HYPOKALAEMIA

The main clinical effects of hypokalaemia are severe weakness, hyporeflexia and cardiac arrhythmias. Typical ECG changes are seen (Fig. 3) and there is increased sensitivity to digoxin. Severe hypokalaemia may be asymptomatic if it develops slowly.

The causes of hypokalaemia include:

- *Gastrointestinal losses.* Potassium may be lost from the intestine due to vomiting, diarrhoea or a surgical fistula.
- *Renal losses.* These may be from the kidney due to renal disease, administration of diuretics or increased aldosterone production.
- *Drug-induced.* Thiazide diuretics and corticosteroids are the most important. Carbenoxolone has mineralocorticoid activity.
- *Alkalosis.* An alkalosis may cause a shift of potassium from the ECF to the ICF.

Treatment

Potassium salts are unpleasant to take orally and are usually given prophylactically in an enteric coating. Severe potassium depletion often has to be treated by intravenous potassium as patients may have a deficit of well over 500 mmol.

Intravenous potassium should not be given faster than 20 mmol/h except in extreme cases and under ECG monitoring.

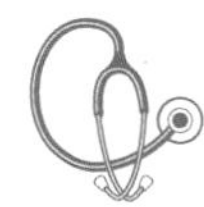

Clinical note

Thiazide diuretic therapy often causes potassium depletion which may turn out to be the reason for an unexplained metabolic alkalosis.

Case history 8

AB, a 55-year-old man, was trapped for 7 hours in a railway accident. He sustained severe multiple injuries including crush injuries to both thighs, fractures of the pelvis and scalp lacerations. On arrival at Accident & Emergency he was still conscious and breathing spontaneously. His pulse was 130/min and his BP was 60/40 mmHg. A set of U & Es showed the following:

Na^+	K^+	Cl^-	HCO_3^-	Urea	Creatinine
		mmol/l			*μmol/l*
141	8.1	108	9	6.9	107

- What are the priorities in managing this patient?

Comment on page 152.

Potassium disorders

- Potassium is the main intracellular cation, but the small amount in the ECF is important in maintaining the membrane potential of muscle and nerve cells.
- Changes in serum potassium concentration may reflect gains or losses in whole body potassium content, or shifts of potassium in and out of cells.
- Hyperkalaemia is potentially life-threatening, and death may occur with no clinical warning signs. A high serum potassium is associated with a decreased renal function.
- Hypokalaemia is usually caused by excessive gastrointestinal or renal loss of potassium.

INTRAVENOUS FLUID THERAPY

Treating disorders of fluid and electrolyte balance is an everyday occurrence in clinical practice, yet it is often a neglected area of good patient care. With a little thought, problems can be anticipated if some general guidelines are followed.

PLANNING FLUID THERAPY: ASSESSING THE PATIENT

History

As always, any clinical exercise begins by speaking to the patient, if possible. Important points to note are cardiac or renal disease and a history of fluid loss such as vomiting or diarrhoea. Nausea, headache or confusion are also important as discussed below.

Examination

The various fluid compartment volumes can be assessed clinically to some extent. An indication of plasma volume can be obtained from blood pressure (BP), pulse, jugular venous pressure (JVP) and central venous pressure (CVP). The interstitial volume can be assessed by looking for oedema. The intracellular fluid compartment is the most difficult to assess clinically, but evidence of disordered cerebral function may be important.

Other important factors leading to potential fluid and electrolyte imbalance include the presence of fever, nasogastric suction, surgical drains and fistulae or artificial ventilation.

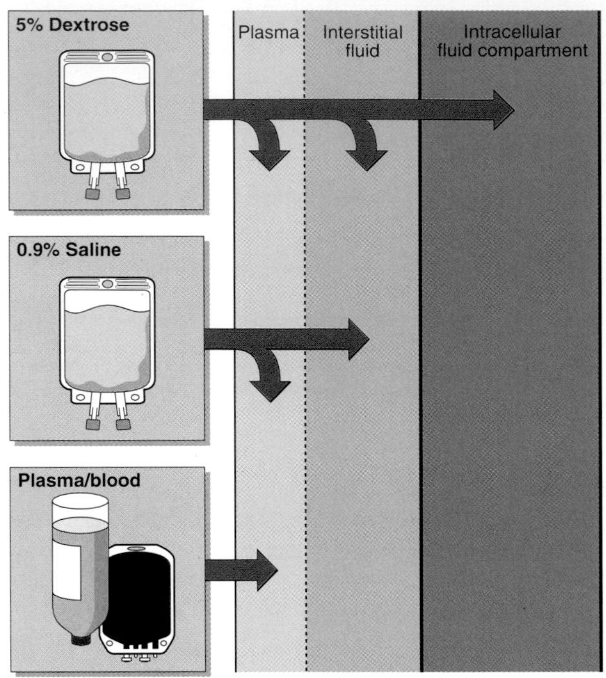

Fig. 1 **The three types of fluid usually used in fluid therapy are shown here with the different contributions they make to the body fluid compartments.**

Biochemical results

The measurement of serum electrolytes (Na^+, K^+, Cl^- and HCO_3^-) may add useful information to that obtained clinically, but should never be regarded in isolation from the full clinical picture. The serum sodium concentration is often thought of as an indicator of ECF water content rather than ECF sodium content. Profound ECF volume depletion may be associated with hyponatraemia, hypernatraemia or may occur with a normal serum sodium concentration because body fluids lost by many routes are isotonic, that is sodium and water are lost together. The serum potassium concentration may change either as a result of changes in total body potassium or of shifts into, or out of, the cells. Because of the latter, serum potassium concentration often reflects changes in serum hydrogen ion concentration, rather than gains or losses of body potassium.

HOW TO GIVE FLUIDS

The easiest and best way to effect fluid replacement is by the normal physiological route, that is orally. In practice this is often impossible or undesirable, especially if patients have an established electrolyte deficit. Salts, particularly potassium salts, are very unpleasant to take orally and often cause gastrointestinal upset.

WHAT FLUIDS TO GIVE

When intravenous fluid therapy has been decided upon, certain general principles determine which fluid to be used (Fig. 1).

- *Water* should be given in the form of 5% dextrose (glucose), since pure water if infused will haemolyze blood cells as it enters the vein. The addition of dextrose renders the water isotonic, but the dextrose is rapidly metabolized. The water which remains will be distributed evenly through all body compartments and will contribute to both ECF and ICF. This fluid is therefore designed to replace deficits in total body water rather than specifically ECF volume deficits.
- *Isotonic sodium chloride* (0.9% NaCl) will be distributed throughout the ECF. Such a solution is therefore designed to replace deficits in ECF volume and it will contribute to both plasma volume and interstitial fluid volume.
- *Plasma, whole blood, or plasma expanders*, replace deficits in the volume of the plasma compartment only.

These three, together with 1.26% sodium bicarbonate and potassium supplements, are all that is needed in the repertoire of intravenous fluids. While many other solutions are available, they should only be used after careful thought and appropriate clinical experience.

HOW MUCH TO GIVE

In prescribing fluid therapy there are two main objectives:

- to make up the losses that have already occurred of both fluid and electrolytes.
- to keep up with the anticipated losses which will occur in the next 24 h.

In trying to achieve this it is essential to consider:

- What are the insensible losses?
- What are the measured losses?

Insensible losses

The insensible losses are those which occur in all individuals from the skin, respiration and normal faeces. These are not normally measured and amount to around 800 ml/day. Of course, this volume may increase greatly in abnormal states, e.g. in excessive sweating or artificial ventilation.

Measured losses

Measured losses include urine, surgical drains and fistulae, vomit and diarrhoea. These volumes should be carefully recorded on the patients' fluid balance charts and will be important in assessing future requirements. Electrolyte composition of these fluids may also be important, e.g. gastrointestinal fluid may contain a lot of potassium or bicarbonate.

Intravenous fluids normally come in units of 500 ml. Estimated losses and deficits are only rough guides. It is rarely possible to make a closer estimate than ± 500 ml of water and ± 75 mmol of sodium. Potassium deficits cannot be accurately measured. However, if a patient has a clinically apparent potassium deficit in the absence of an acid–base disturbance, then the total body potassium loss will be in excess of 500 mmol.

The margin of safety is usually wide because the body can manipulate almost any parenteral load provided the kidneys and heart function normally. However, in patients with known cardiac and renal disease, or in the elderly or the very young, much more care must be taken with the prescription of intravenous fluids.

Clinical note

Assessing a patient's fluid and electrolyte status has as much, if not more, to do with clinical skill than biochemical interpretation. Look at the patient in Figure 2 and think about what information is available. Your answer may include consideration of the following:

- case records (details of patient history, examination)
- examination of patient (JVP, CVP, Pulse, BP, presence of oedema, chest sounds, skin turgor)
- fluid balance, and nursing charts (BP, pulse, temp, fluid-input and output)
- nasogastric and surgical wound drainage in addition to urinary catheter bag
- presence of intravenous fluid therapy (type, volume)
- ambient temperature (wall thermometer).

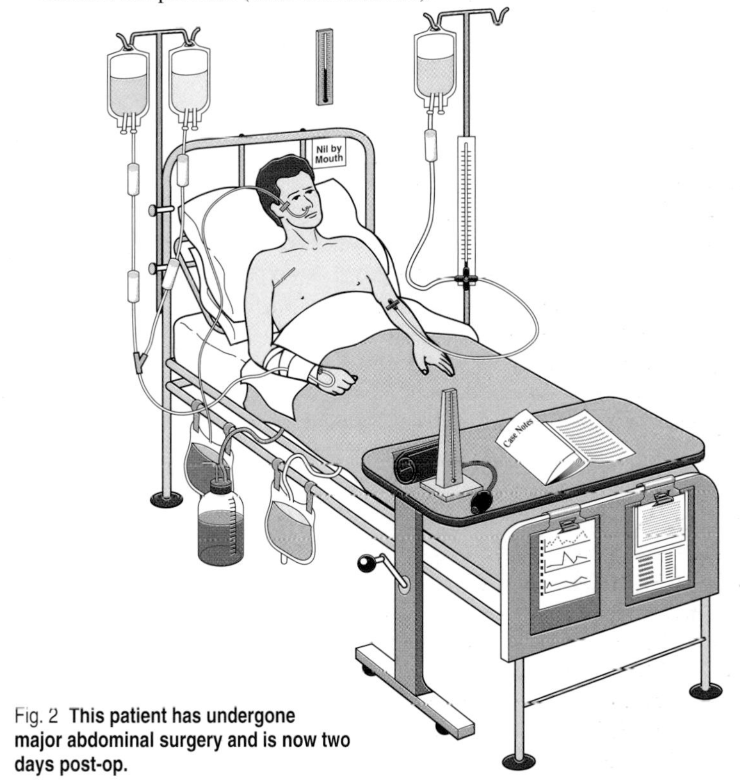

Fig. 2 **This patient has undergone major abdominal surgery and is now two days post-op.**

MONITORING INTRAVENOUS FLUID THERAPY

The use of intravenous fluids may fail to correct the fluid – electrolyte balance, and the therapy may give rise to further problems if it is not monitored closely. This should include:

- clinical assessment
- pulse, BP, JVP and CVP if appropriate
- body weight
- good fluid balance charts
- serum electrolytes.

Case History 9

Postoperatively, a 62-year-old woman was noted to be getting progressively weaker. There was no evidence of fever, bleeding or infection. Blood pressure was 120/80 mmHg. Before the operation her serum electrolytes were normal, as were her renal function and cardiovascular system. Three days after the operation her electrolytes were repeated.

Na^+	K^+	Cl^-	HCO_3^-	Urea	Creatinine
mmol/l					*µmol/l*
125	4.2	77	32	21.4	145

Random urine osmolality = 920 mmol/kg
Urine $[Na^+]$ < 10 mmol/l
Urine $[K^+]$ = 15 mmol/l

- What is the pathophysiology behind these findings?
- What other information do you require in order to prescribe the appropriate fluid therapy?

Comment on page 152.

Intravenous fluid therapy

- Intravenous fluid therapy is commonly used to correct fluid and electrolyte imbalance.
- The simple guidelines for i.v. fluid therapy are:
  - First assess patient clinically, then biochemically paying particular attention to cardiac and renal function.
  - Use simple solutions.
  - In prescribing fluids, attempt to make up deficits and anticipate future losses.
  - Monitor patient closely at all times during fluid therapy.

INVESTIGATION OF RENAL FUNCTION (1)

FUNCTIONS OF THE KIDNEY

The functional unit in the kidney is the nephron, shown in Figure 1. The kidneys regulate ECF volume and electrolyte composition to compensate for wide daily variations in water and electrolyte intake. They form urine in which the potentially toxic waste products of metabolism are excreted. The functions of the kidneys therefore include:

- regulation of water, electrolyte and acid–base balance
- excretion of the products of protein and nucleic acid metabolism: urea, creatinine, creatine, uric acid, sulphate and phosphate.

The kidneys are also endocrine organs, producing a number of hormones, and are subject to control by others (Fig. 2). Arginine vasopressin (AVP) acts to influence water balance, and aldosterone affects sodium reabsorption in the nephron. Parathyroid hormone promotes tubular reabsorption of calcium, phosphate excretion and the synthesis of 1,25 dihydroxy-cholecalciferol, which regulates calcium absorption by the gut. Renin, an enzyme, is made by the juxtaglomerular cells and catalyzes the formation of angiotensin I from angiotensinogen. Angiotensin converting enzyme (ACE) converts angiotensin I into angiotensin II which stimulates aldosterone synthesis. Erythropoietin, a peptide hormone, promotes haemoglobin synthesis. The endocrine functions of the kidney remain clinically intact until the end stages of renal failure.

It is convenient to discuss renal function in terms of the assessment of *glomerular* and *tubular* function.

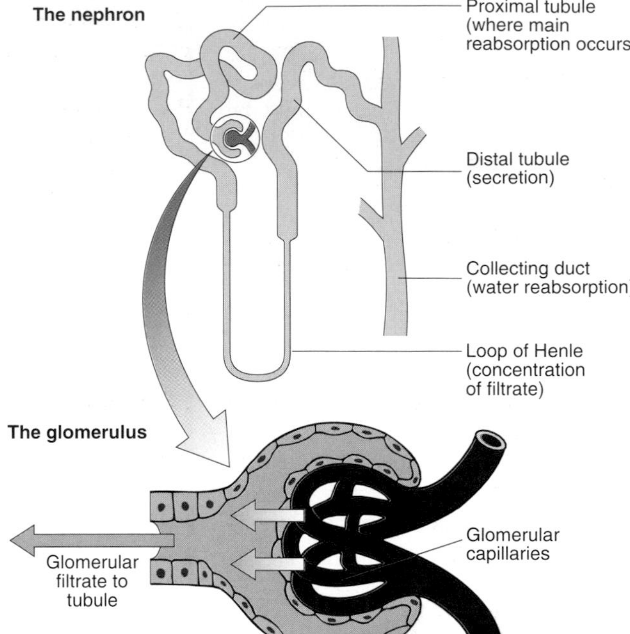

Fig. 1 **Diagrammatic representation of a nephron.**

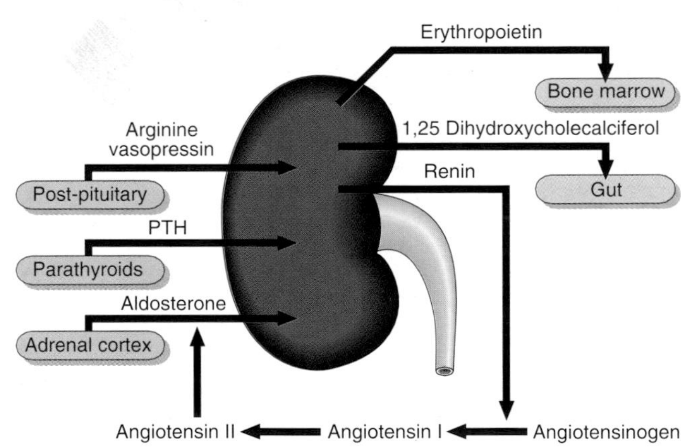

Fig. 2 **Endocrine links in the kidney.**

TESTS OF GLOMERULAR FUNCTION

The glomerular filtrate is an ultrafiltrate of plasma, and has the same composition as plasma without most of the proteins. Plasma is filtered by the glomeruli at a rate of approximately 140 ml/minute. A normal glomerular filtration rate (GFR) will depend on there being normal renal blood flow and pressure. GFR is directly related to body size, and consequently is higher in men than women. It is also affected by age, declining in the elderly.

If the GFR falls due to restriction of the renal blood supply, or as a result of destruction of nephrons by renal disease, there is retention of the waste products of metabolism in the blood. In chronic disease, a new 'steady state' is reached with a constant elevation in the serum concentration of substances such as urea and creatinine. As the renal disease progresses, urea and creatinine concentrations may increase slowly over many months.

Clearance

The problem is how to measure the GFR. It helps to consider firstly the concept of 'clearance'. Consider any plasma constituent which is also present in urine. The amount excreted can be calculated by measuring the urinary concentration (U, say mmoles per litre) and multiplying that by the volume of urine collected in a given time (V, say litres in a 24h period). Thus, the amount excreted in urine is $U \times V$. The volume of plasma which would have contained that amount can be worked out by dividing the amount excreted ($U \times V$) by the plasma concentration of the substance (P),

$$\textit{Volume of plasma} = \frac{U \times V}{P}$$

This is the volume of plasma which would have to be completely 'cleared' of the substance in the time specified to give the amount seen in urine. This is the 'clearance' for that substance.

The maximum rate that the plasma can be 'cleared' of any substance is equal to the GFR. This could be calculated from the clearance of some plasma constituent which is freely filtered at the glomerulus, and is neither reabsorbed nor secreted in the tubule. ^{51}Cr-EDTA or inulin (a plant carbohydrate) can be infused and used to measure GFR, but in practice creatinine, which is already present in blood as a normal product of muscle metabolism, comes close to fulfilling the above requirements.

Creatinine clearance

An estimate of the GFR can be calculated from the creatinine content of a 24-hour urine collection, and the plasma concentration within this period. The 'clearance' of creatinine from plasma is directly related to the GFR provided that:

- the urine volume is collected accurately
- there are no ketones or heavy proteinuria

present to interfere with the creatinine determination.

The GFR is calculated as follows:

$$GFR = \frac{U \times V}{P}$$

U = urine concentration of creatinine
P = serum or plasma concentration of creatinine

Note that these should be in the *same units*. Urine creatinine is usually reported as mmol/l, and serum creatinine as µmol/l, so the former should be multiplied by 1000, or the latter divided by 1000, in the calculation.

V = urine flow in ml/min

A common mistake is to consider *V* as urine volume, which it is not. It is the urine volume collected in 24 hours, and this figure is divided by 24 x 60 to give the volume produced per minute, the way GFR is usually expressed.

Serum creatinine and urea

The concentrations of creatinine and urea in serum samples are used as convenient, but insensitive, measures of glomerular function.

Figure 3 shows how the GFR must fall to about half its normal value before a significant increase in serum creatinine becomes apparent. Hence, a 'normal' serum creatinine (i.e. within the reference range) does not necessarily mean all is well. The reference intervals will vary with age and body size. For example, consider an asymptomatic person who shows a serum creatinine of 130 µmol/l:

- In a young adult female this might well be abnormal and requires follow up to exclude renal disease.
- In a muscular young male this is the expected result.
- In an elderly person this is a reflection of the physiological decline of GFR with age.

Serum urea concentration is less useful as a measure of glomerular function. Dietary protein intake affects serum urea concentration. Gastrointestinal bleeding will cause serum urea to be elevated, and this does not indicate that glomerular filtration is compromised.

Urea is reabsorbed in the tubules. This reabsorption increases at low urine flow rates.

Most laboratories will measure both serum creatinine and urea. The ratio of the two is of value in the investigation of renal disorders (pp. 30–33).

Proteinuria

The glomerular basement membrane does not usually allow passage of albumin and large proteins. A small amount of albumin, usually less than 25 mg/24h, is found in urine. When larger amounts, in excess of 250 mg/24h, are detected, significant damage to the glomerular membrane has occurred. Quantitative urine protein measurements should always be made on complete 24-hour urine collections.

Albumin excretion in the range 25–300 mg/24h is termed microalbuminuria (p. 59). Tubular proteinuria is discussed on pages 28–29.

URINE COLLECTIONS

It is not widely appreciated that the biggest error in the determination of creatinine clearance, or indeed in the measurement of the daily excretion of any metabolite, lies in *the collection of the timed urine sample*. The most sophisticated technology is at the mercy of patients' and staff's abilities to ensure that an accurate urine collection is obtained. This is how it should be done.

At a given time, say 8.00am, the patient should be asked to empty the bladder. *The urine passed here is discarded.* All urine produced for the remainder of that day and overnight is added to the specimen container. At 8.00am the next morning, the bladder is emptied again, and the urine is added to the container to make up a complete 24 h collection.

Case History 10

A male aged 35 presenting with loin pain has a serum creatinine of 150 µmol/l. A 24-hour urine of 2160 ml is collected and found to have a creatinine concentration of 7.5 mmol/l.

- Calculate the creatinine clearance and comment on the results.

An error in the timed collection was subsequently reported by the nursing staff, and the collection time was reported to be 17 hours.

- How does this affect the result and its interpretation?

Comment on page 153.

Clinical note

The glomerular filtration rate, like the heart and respiration rates, fluctuates throughout the day. A change in the GFR of up to 20% between two consecutive creatinine clearances may not indicate any change in renal function.

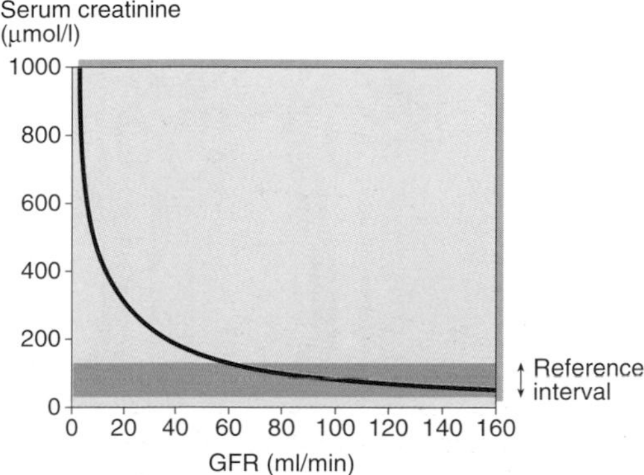

Fig. 3 **The relationship between glomerular filtration rate and serum creatinine concentration.** Glomerular filtration rate may fall considerably before serum creatinine is significantly increased.

Assessing glomerular function

- The capacity of the kidneys to filter plasma at the glomeruli can be assessed by measuring the creatinine clearance, which approximates to the glomerular filtration rate.
- Serum creatinine concentration is an insensitive index of renal function, as it may not appear to be elevated until the GFR has fallen below 50% of normal. Once the serum creatinine is found to be abnormal, changes in concentration reflect changes in GFR.
- Large amounts of protein in a urine specimen may indicate glomerular damage.
- The biggest error in measuring any metabolite in a timed urine collection lies in the collection of the urine.

INVESTIGATION OF RENAL FUNCTION (2)

RENAL TUBULAR FUNCTION

The glomeruli provide an efficient filtration mechanism for ridding the body of waste products and toxic substances. To ensure that important constituents such as water, sodium, glucose and amino acids are not lost from the body, tubular reabsorption must be equally efficient. For example, 180 litres of fluid pass into the glomerular filtrate each day, and more than 99% of this is recovered. Compared with the GFR as an assessment of glomerular function, there are no easily performed tests which measure tubular function in a quantitative manner.

TUBULAR DYSFUNCTION

Some disorders of tubular function are inherited, for example, some patients are unable to reduce their urine pH below 6.5, because of a specific failure of hydrogen ion secretion. Renal tubular damage is often secondary to other conditions such as exposure to heavy metals or nephrotoxic drugs, or amyloidosis.

INVESTIGATION OF TUBULAR FUNCTION

Osmolality measurements in plasma and urine

Of all the tubular functions, the one most frequently affected by disease is the ability to concentrate the urine. If the tubules and collecting ducts are working efficiently, and if AVP is present, they will be able to reabsorb water. Just how well can be assessed by measuring urine concentration. This is conveniently done by determining the osmolality, and then comparing this to the plasma. In normal individuals on an average fluid intake the urine:plasma osmolality ratio is usually between 1.0 and 3.0. In other words, the urine is more concentrated than the plasma. When the urine: plasma osmolality ratio is 1.0 or less, the renal tubules are not reabsorbing water.

The water deprivation test

The causes of polyuria are summarized in Table 1. Occasionally it may be necessary to deprive a patient of water in an effort to find the cause of excessive polyuria. The water deprivation test involves complete fluid deprivation during a 24-hour period, with measurement of the osmolality of all the urine specimens passed during the second 12 hours of the test. An osmolality of greater than 700 mmol/kg should be attained and the urine:plasma osmolality ratio should be 2.0 or above. In polyuria of diabetes insipidus, where the hormone AVP is lacking, the ratio will remain between 0.2 and 0.7 even after fluid restriction. In the polyuria associated with so-called 'compulsive water drinkers', the ratio may be normal without fluid restriction but increases after fluid restriction. In some hospitals this form of concentration test involves fluid restriction overnight (8 pm–10 am) and measuring the osmolality of urine voided in the morning.

In practice, the water deprivation test is extremely unpleasant for the patient. It is potentially dangerous if there is severe inability to retain water. The test must be terminated if weight loss exceeds 3 kg or if more than 3 litres of urine is passed.

Administration of AVP as the synthetic analogue DDAVP will result in increased urinary concentration (osmolality greater than 700 mmol/kg) if the failure to concentrate is due to diabetes insipidus. No response will be obtained if the AVP receptors cannot respond to the hormone. This is called 'nephrogenic' diabetes insipidus.

Table 1 **Causes of polyuria**

Cause	Urine osmolality (mmol/kg)	Plasma osmolality (mmol/kg)
Increased osmotic load e.g. due to glucose	~500	~310
Increased water ingestion	<200	~280
Diabetes insipidus	<200	~300
Nephrogenic diabetes insipidus	<200	~300

The acid load test

The acid load test is occasionally used for the diagnosis of renal tubular acidosis, conditions in which metabolic acidosis arises from diminished tubular secretion of hydrogen ions. Ammonium chloride is administered orally in gelatin capsules. Urine samples are collected for the following 8 hours. With normal renal function, the pH of at least one sample should be less than 5.3. If necessary in a difficult diagnosis, the excretion rates of titratable acid and ammonium ion, and serum bicarbonate concentration, are all measured. This test should not be performed on patients who are already acidotic or who have liver disease.

Renal tubular acidosis may be characterized as follows:

- *Type I.* There is a defective hydrogen ion secretion in the distal tubule which may be inherited or acquired.
- *Type II.* The capacity to reabsorb bicarbonate in the proximal tubule is reduced.
- *Type IV.* Bicarbonate reabsorption by the renal tubule is impaired as a consequence of aldosterone deficiency, aldosterone receptor defects, or drugs which block aldosterone action.

There is no separate type III renal tubular acidosis.

Specific proteinuria

Causes of proteinuria are summarized in Figure 1. Mention has already been made of protein in urine as an indicator of leaky glomeruli (pp. 26–27). β_2 microglobulin and α_1 microglobulin are small proteins which are filtered at the glomeruli and are usually reabsorbed by the tubular cells.

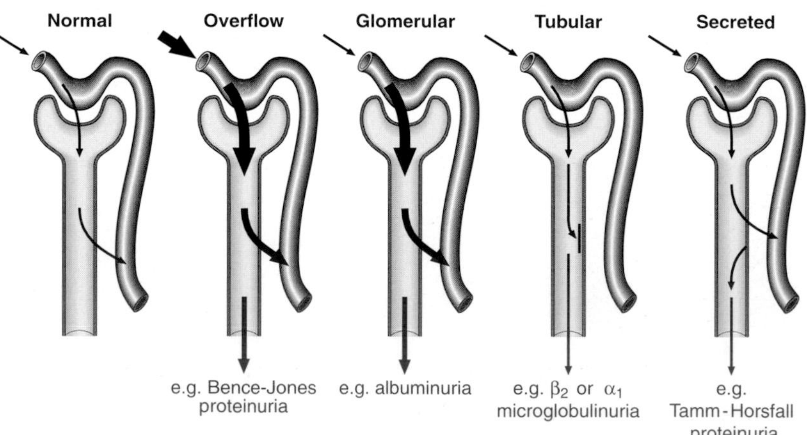

Fig. 1 **The classification of proteinuria.**

An increased concentration of these proteins in urine is a sensitive indicator of renal tubular cell damage.

Glycosuria

The presence of glucose in urine when blood glucose is *normal* usually reflects the inability of the tubules to reabsorb glucose because of a specific tubular lesion. Here, the renal threshold (the capacity for the tubules to reabsorb the substance in question) has been reached. This is called renal glycosuria and is a benign condition. Glycosuria can also present in association with other disorders of tubular function - the Fanconi syndrome.

Aminoaciduria

Normally, amino acids in the glomerular filtrate are reabsorbed in the proximal tubules. They may be present in urine in excessive amount because the plasma concentration exceeds the renal threshold, or because there is specific failure of normal tubular reabsorptive mechanisms, such as in the inherited metabolic disorder, cystinuria, or more commonly because of acquired renal tubular damage.

SPECIFIC TUBULAR DEFECTS

The Fanconi syndrome

The Fanconi syndrome is used to describe the occurrence of generalized tubular defects such as renal tubular acidosis, aminoaciduria and tubular proteinuria. It can occur as a result of heavy metal poisoning, or from the effects of toxins and inherited metabolic diseases such as cystinosis.

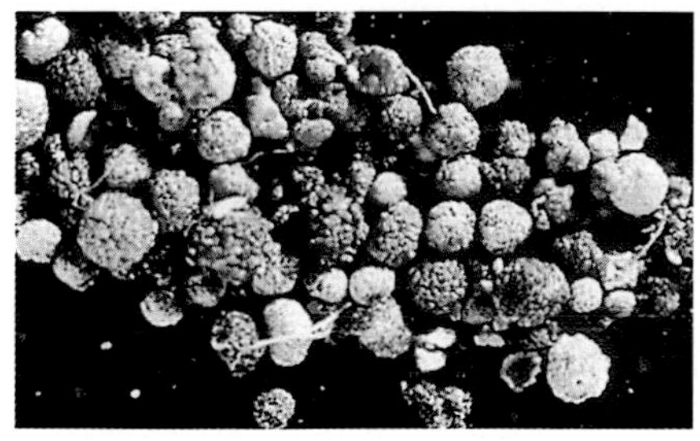

Fig. 2 **Renal calculi.**

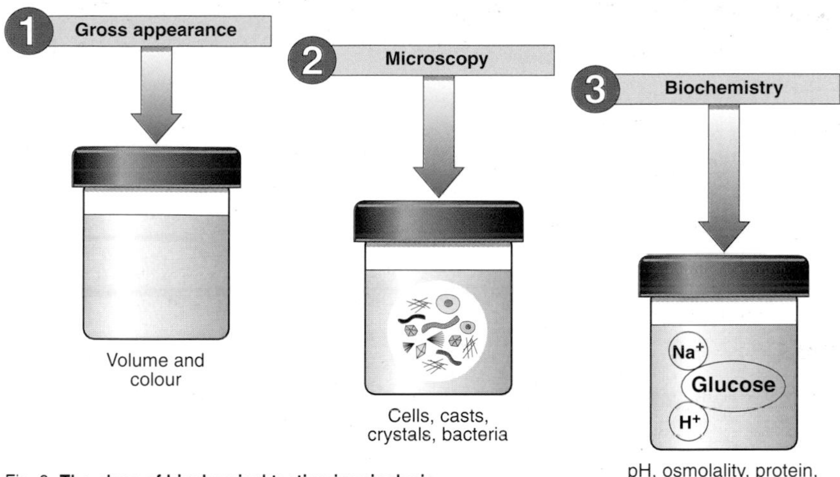

Fig. 3 **The place of biochemical testing in urinalysis.**

Renal stones

Renal stones (calculi) produce severe pain and discomfort, and are common causes of obstruction in the urinary tract (Fig. 2). Chemical analysis of renal stones is important in the investigation of why they have formed. Types of stone include:

- *Calcium phosphate*: may be a consequence of primary hyperparathyroidism or renal tubular acidosis.
- *Magnesium, ammonium and phosphate*: these are often associated with urinary tract infections.
- *Oxalate*: may be a consequence of hyperoxaluria.
- *Uric acid*: may be a consequence of hyperuricaemia (see pp. 134–135).
- *Cystine*: these are rare and a feature of the inherited metabolic disorder cystinuria (see pp. 146–147).

URINALYSIS

Examination of a patient's urine should not be restricted to biochemical tests. Figure 3 summarizes the ways urine may be examined to assist in the assessment of the patient with renal disease.

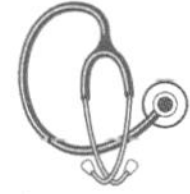

Clinical note

Orthostatic, or postural, proteinuria is common in teenagers. It is a benign condition in which proteinuria occurs only when the subjects are standing upright, and is a result of an increase in the hydrostatic pressure in the renal veins.

Case history 11

RS, a 30-year-old woman, fractured her skull in an accident. She had no other major injuries, no significant blood loss, and her cardiovascular system was stable. She was unconscious for two days after the accident. On the fourth day of her admission to hospital she was noted to be producing large volumes of urine and complaining of thirst. Biochemical findings were:

Na^+	K^+	Cl^-	HCO_3^-	Urea	Creatinine	Glucose
mmol/l					*µmol/l*	*mmol/l*
150	3.6	106	25	5.5	80	5.4

Serum osmolality = 310 mmol/kg
Urine osmolality = 110 mmol/kg
Urine volume = 8 litres/24h

- Is a water deprivation test required to make the diagnosis in this patient?

Comment on page 153.

Assessing tubular function

- Chemical examination of urine is just one aspect of urinalysis.
- A comparison of urine and serum osmolality measurements will indicate if a patient has the ability to concentrate urine.
- Specific tests are available to measure urinary concentrating ability and the ability to excrete an acid load.
- The presence of specific small proteins in urine indicates tubular damage.
- Chemical analysis of renal stones is important in the investigation of their aetiology.

ACUTE RENAL FAILURE

Renal failure is the cessation of kidney function. In acute renal failure (ARF), the kidneys fail over a period of hours or days. Chronic renal failure (CRF) develops over months or years and leads eventually to end stage renal failure (ESRF). ARF may be reversed and normal renal function regained, whereas CRF is irreversible.

AETIOLOGY

ARF arises from a variety of problems affecting the kidneys and/or their circulation. It usually presents as a sudden deterioration of renal function indicated by rapidly rising serum urea and creatinine concentrations. As acute renal failure is common in the severely ill, sequential monitoring of kidney function is important for early detection in this group of patients.

Usually, urine output falls to less than 400 ml/24 h, and the patient is said to be oliguric. The patient may pass no urine at all, and be anuric. Occasionally urine flow remains high when tubular dysfunction predominates.

Kidney failure or uraemia can be classified as (Fig. 1):

- *Pre-renal*: the kidney fails to receive a proper blood supply.
- *Post-renal:* the urinary drainage of the kidneys is impaired because of an obstruction.
- *Renal*: intrinsic damage to the kidney tissue. This may be due to a variety of diseases, or the renal damage may be a consequence of prolonged pre-renal or post-renal problems.

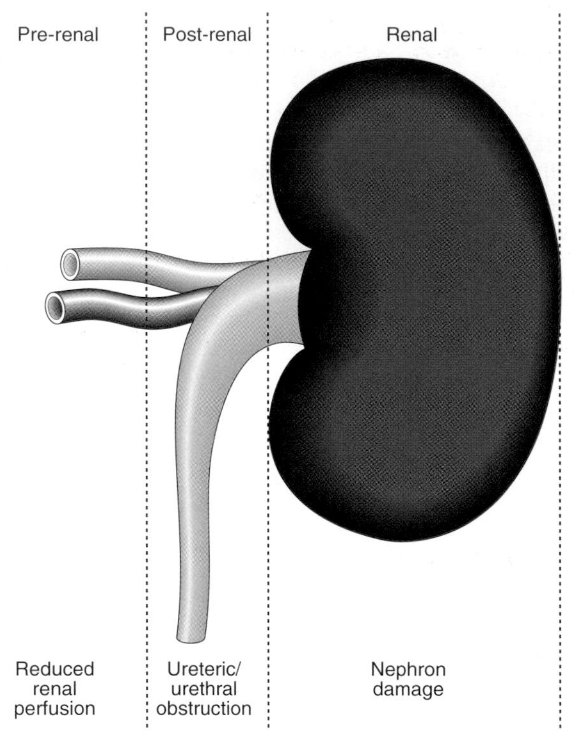

Fig. 1 **The classification of acute renal falure.**

DIAGNOSIS

In nearly all cases the clinical history and presentation will indicate that a patient has, or may develop, ARF. The first step in assessing the patient with ARF is to identify any pre- or post-renal factors which could be readily corrected and allow recovery of renal function. The history and examination of the patient, including the presence of other severe illness, drug history and time course of the onset of the ARF, may well provide important clues. It is important to note that in the first 24 hrs of ARF the serum and urine tests may not reveal any abnormality. Factors which precipitate pre-renal uraemia are usually associated with a reduced effective ECF volume and include:

- decreased plasma volume because of blood loss, burns, prolonged vomiting, or diarrhoea
- diminished cardiac output
- local factors such as an occlusion of the renal artery.

Pre-renal factors lead to decreased renal perfusion and reduction in GFR. Both AVP and aldosterone are secreted maximally and a small volume of concentrated urine is produced.

Biochemical findings in pre-renal uraemia include the following:

- *Serum urea and creatinine are increased.* Urea is increased proportionally more than creatinine because of its reabsorption by the tubular cells, particularly at low urine flow rates. This leads to a relatively higher serum urea concentration than creatinine which is not so reabsorbed.
- *Metabolic acidosis*: because of the inability of the kidney to excrete hydrogen ions.
- *Hyperkalaemia*: because of the decreased glomerular filtration rate and acidosis.
- *A high urine osmolality.*

Post-renal factors cause decreased renal function, because the effective filtration pressure at the glomeruli is reduced due to the back pressure caused by the blockage. Causes include:

- renal stones
- carcinoma of cervix, prostate, or occasionally bladder.

If these pre- or post-renal factors are not corrected, patients will develop intrinsic renal damage (acute tubular necrosis).

Acute tubular necrosis

Acute tubular necrosis may develop in the absence of pre-existing pre-renal or post-renal failure. The causes include:

- acute blood loss in severe trauma
- septic shock
- specific renal disease such as glomerulonephritis
- nephrotoxins such as the aminoglycosides, or analgesics

Patients in the early stages of acute tubular necrosis may have only a modestly increased serum urea and creatinine which then rise rapidly over a period of days, in contrast to the slow increase over months and years seen in chronic renal failure.

It may be difficult to decide the reason for a patient's oliguria. The biochemical features which distinguish pre-renal uraemia from intrinsic renal damage are shown in Table 1.

Table 1 **Biochemical features in the differential diagnosis of the oliguric patient**

Biochemical feature	Pre-renal failure	Intrinsic renal damage
Urine sodium	<20 mmol/l	>40 mmol/l
Urine/serum urea	>10:1	<3:1
Urine/plasma osmolality	>1.5:1	<1.1:1

MANAGEMENT

Important issues in the management of the patient with ARF include:

- *Correction of pre-renal factors, if present, by replacement of any ECF volume deficit.* Care should be taken that the patient does not become fluid overloaded. In cardiac failure, inotropic agents may be indicated.
- *Treatment of the underlying disease* (e.g. to control infection).
- *Biochemical monitoring.* Daily fluid balance charts provide an assessment of body fluid volume. Serum creatinine indicates the degree of impairment of the GFR and the rate of deterioration or improvement. Serum potassium should be monitored closely.
- *Dialysis.* Indications for dialysis include a rapidly rising serum potassium concentration, severe acidosis, and fluid overload.

RECOVERY

There may be three distinct phases in the resolving clinical course of a patient with acute renal failure (Fig. 2). An initial oliguric phase, where glomerular impairment predominates. This is followed by a diuretic phase when urine output is high, as glomerular function improves but tubular function remains impaired. During a recovery phase, complete renal function may return. Careful clinical and biochemical monitoring is necessary throughout the course of the patient's illness.

It should be noted that initially the urea and creatinine may be normal in ARF. The serum potassium usually rises very quickly in catabolic patients, with or without tissue damage, and falls quickly once the urine flow rate increases. The urine volume cannot be related to the GFR. The serum urea and creatinine remain high during the diuretic phase, because the GFR is still low and the large urine volumes reflect tubular damage. In the recovery phase the serum urea and creatinine fall as the GFR improves and the serum potassium concentration returns to normal, as the tubular mechanisms recover.

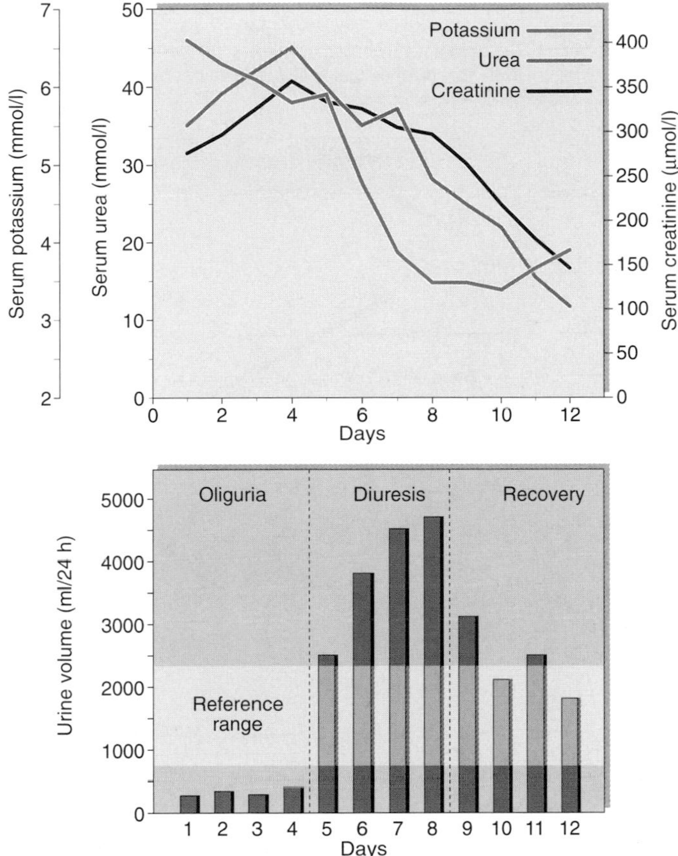

Fig. 2 **The biochemical course of a typical patient with acute renal failure.**

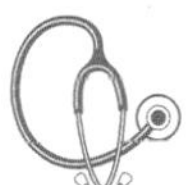

Clinical note

Acute tubular necrosis is the commonest cause of severe life-threatening hyperkalaemia. The rapidly increasing serum potassium is usually the indication to start the patient on dialysis.

Case history 12

A male, aged 50, presented with pyrexia. He was clinically dehydrated and oliguric.

Na^+	K^+	Cl^-	HCO_3^-	Urea	Creatinine
		mmol/l			*µmol/l*
140	5.9	112	16	22.9	155

Serum osmolality = 305 mmol/kg
Urine osmolality = 629 mmol/kg.

- What do these biochemistry results indicate about the patient's condition?

Comment on page 153.

Acute renal failure

- ARF is the failure of renal function over a period of hours or days identified by a rising serum urea and creatinine.
- Acute renal failure may be classified as pre-renal, renal or post-renal.
- Prompt identification of pre- or post-renal factors may allow correction of the problem before damage to nephrons occurs.
- Management of a patient with intrinsic renal damage will include sequential measurement of creatinine, sodium, potassium and bicarbonate in serum, and urine sodium and potassium excretion and osmolality.
- Care should be taken to prevent fluid overload in the treatment of patients with renal disease.
- Life threatening hyperkalaemia may be a consequence of ARF.

CHRONIC RENAL FAILURE

Chronic renal failure (CRF) is the progressive irreversible destruction of kidney tissue by disease which, if not treated by dialysis or transplant, will result in the death of the patient. The aetiology of CRF encompasses the spectrum of known kidney diseases. The end result of progressive renal damage is the same no matter what the cause of the disease may have been. The major effects of renal failure all occur because of the loss of functioning nephrons. It is a feature of CRF that patients may have few if any symptoms until the glomerular filtration rate falls below 15 ml/min (i.e. to 10% of normal function), and the disease is far advanced.

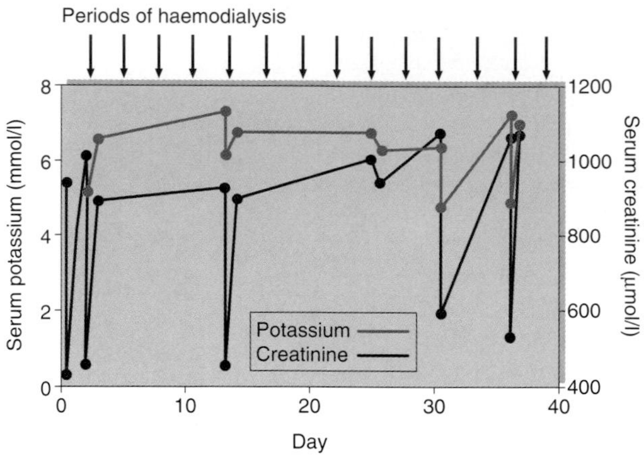

Fig. 1 **The biochemical course of a typical patient with chronic renal failure. Note that biochemical analyses have not been performed before and after all periods of dialysis.**

CONSEQUENCES OF CRF

All of the activities of the kidneys are affected in end stage renal failure, with important metabolic consequences. The areas involved and the clinical biochemical features are described below.

Sodium and water metabolism

Most CRF patients retain the ability to reabsorb sodium ions, but the renal tubules may lose their ability to reabsorb water and so concentrate urine. Polyuria, although present, may not be excessive because the GFR is so low. Because of their impaired ability to regulate water balance, patients in renal failure may become fluid overloaded or fluid depleted very easily.

Potassium metabolism

Hyperkalaemia is a feature of advanced CRF and poses a threat to life (Fig.1). The ability to excrete potassium decreases as the GFR falls, but hyperkalaemia may not be a major problem in CRF until the GFR falls to very low levels. Then, a sudden deterioration of renal function may precipitate a rapid rise in serum potassium concentration. An unexpectedly high serum potassium concentration in an outpatient should always be investigated with urgency.

Acid–base balance

As CRF develops, the ability of the kidneys to regenerate bicarbonate and excrete hydrogen ions in the urine becomes impaired. The retention of hydrogen ions causes a metabolic acidosis.

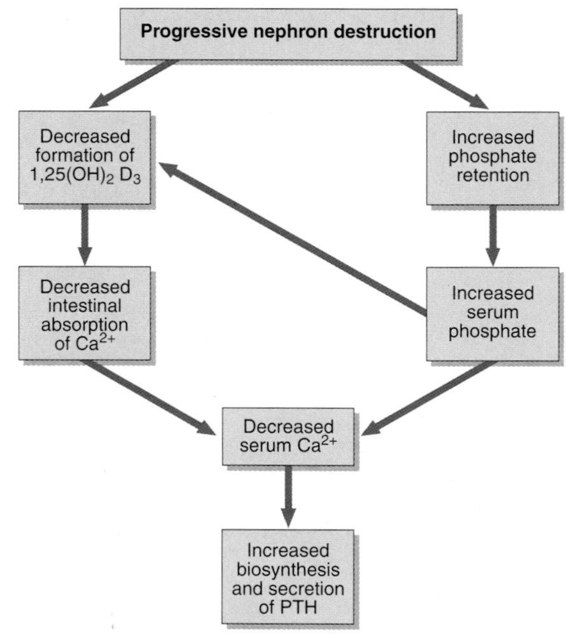

Fig. 2 **How hypocalcaemia and secondary hyperparathyroidism develop in renal disease.**

Calcium and phosphate metabolism

The ability of the renal cells to make 1,25 dihydroxycholecalciferol falls as the renal tubular damage progresses. Calcium absorption is reduced and there is a tendency towards hypocalcaemia. Parathyroid hormone is stimulated in an attempt to restore plasma calcium to normal, and high circulating PTH may have adverse effects on bone if this is allowed to continue (Fig. 2). Secondary hyperparathyroidism causes the changes in bone which are characteristic of renal osteodystrophy.

Erythropoietin synthesis

Anaemia is often associated with chronic renal disease. The normochromic normocytic anaemia is due primarily to failure of erythropoietin production. Biosynthesised human erythropoietin may be used to treat the anaemia of CRF.

CLINICAL FEATURES

The clinical features of chronic renal failure reflect the impairment of the above systems. The inability to rid the body of other toxic metabolites may be responsible for the occurrence of many of the features of CRF which are illustrated in Figure 3. Early in chronic renal failure the normal reduction in urine formation when the patient is recumbent and asleep is lost. Patients who do not experience daytime polyuria may nevertheless have nocturia as their presenting symptom.

MANAGEMENT

In some cases it may be possible to treat the cause of the CRF and at least delay the progression of the disease. Conservative measures may be used to alleviate symptoms before dialysis becomes necessary, and these involve much use of the biochemical laboratory. Important considerations are:

- Water and sodium intake should be carefully matched to the losses. Dietary sodium restriction and diuretics may be required to prevent sodium overload.
- Hyperkalaemia may be controlled by

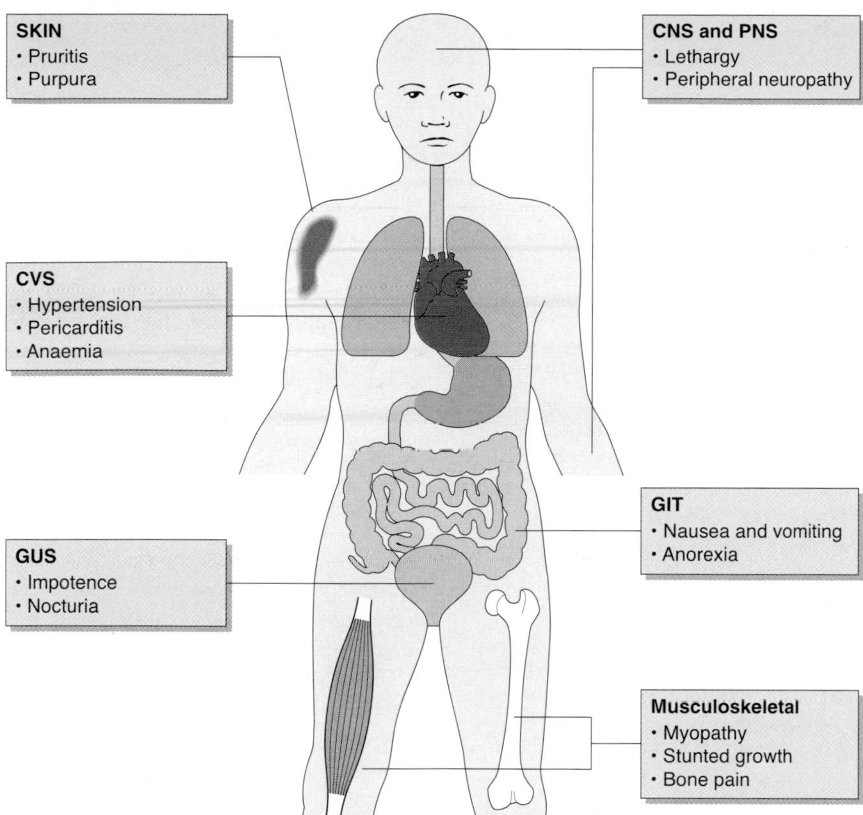

Fig. 3 **The clinical consequences of CRF.**

oral ion-exchange resins (Resonium A).

- Hyperphosphataemia may be controlled by oral aluminium or magnesium salts which act by sequestering ingested phosphate in the gut.
- The administration of hydroxylated vitamin D metabolites may prevent the development of secondary hyperparathyroidism. There is a risk of hypercalcaemia with this treatment.
- Dietary restriction of protein, to reduce the formation of nitrogenous waste products, may give symptomatic improvement. A negative nitrogen balance should, however, be avoided.

Most patients with CRF will eventually require dialysis, in which case these conservative measures must be continued. In contrast, after a successful kidney transplant, normal renal function is re-established.

Dialysis

Haemodialysis and peritoneal dialysis will sustain life when other measures can no longer maintain fluid, electrolyte and acid–base balance. The key to dialysis is the provision of a semipermeable membrane through which ions and small molecules, present in plasma at high concentration, can diffuse into the low concentrations of a rinsing fluid. In haemodialysis, an artificial membrane is used. In peritoneal dialysis, the dialysis fluid is placed in the peritoneal cavity, and molecules move out of the blood vessels of the peritoneal wall. Continuous ambulatory peritoneal dialysis (CAPD) is an effective way of removing waste products. The dialysis fluid is replaced every six hours.

Note that haemodialysis and peritoneal dialysis may relieve many of the symptoms of chronic renal failure and rectify abnormal fluid and electrolyte and acid–base balance. These treatments do not, however, reverse the other metabolic, endocrine or haematological consequences of chronic renal failure.

Renal transplant

Although transplant of a kidney restores almost all of the renal functions, patients require long-term immunosuppression. Cyclosporine is nephrotoxic at high concentrations and monitoring of both creatinine and cyclosporine is necessary to balance the fine line between rejection and renal damage due to the drug.

Clinical note

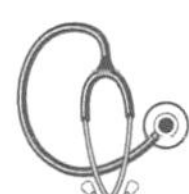

Hypertension is both a common cause and a consequence of renal disease. Good blood pressure control is an essential part of treatment and delays the progression of chronic renal failure.

Case history 13

MH is a 40-year-old female with chronic renal failure who is being treated by haemodialysis. Her serum biochemistry just prior to her last dialysis showed:

Na^+	K^+	Cl^-	HCO_3^-	Urea	Creatinine
mmol/l					*μmol/l*
130	5.7	100	16	25.5	1430

- What is the significance of these results?
- What other biochemical tests should be performed, and how might the results influence treatment?

Comment on page 153.

Chronic renal failure

- Chronic renal failure is the progressive irreversible destruction of kidney tissue by disease which, if not treated by dialysis or transplant, will result in the death of the patient.
- Patients with CRF may be without symptoms until the GFR falls to very low values.
- Consequences of chronic renal failure include disordered water and sodium metabolism, hyperkalaemia, abnormal calcium and phosphate metabolism, and anaemia.

ACID–BASE: Concepts and Vocabulary

HYDROGEN ION CONCENTRATION

Blood hydrogen ion concentration $[H^+]$ is maintained within tight limits in health. Normal levels lie between 35–45 nmol/l. Values greater than 120 nmol/l or less than 20 nmol/l are usually incompatible with life. In the past, $[H^+]$ in blood was described as pH, but now it is more usual for results to be reported in molar concentration units, as nmol/l (Fig. 1).

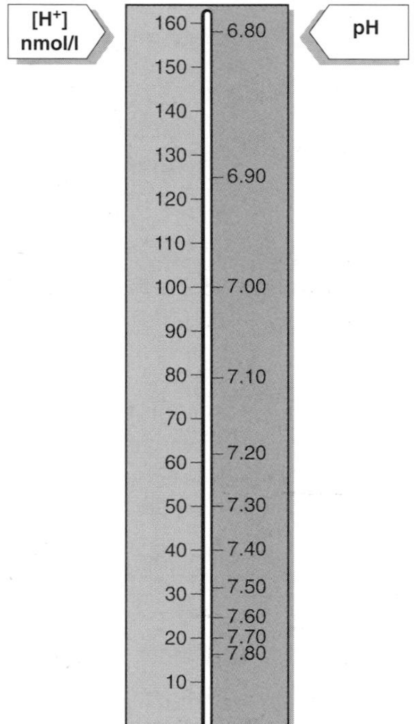

Fig. 1 **The negative logarithmic relationship between $[H^+]$ and pH.**

Hydrogen ions are produced in the body as a result of metabolism, particularly from the oxidation of the sulphur-containing amino acids of protein ingested as food. The total amount of hydrogen ion produced each day in this way is of the order of 60 mmoles. If all of this was to be diluted in the extracellular fluid (≈14 litres), $[H^+]$ would be 4 mmol/l, or 100 000 times more acid than normal! This just does not happen, as all the hydrogen ions produced are efficiently excreted in urine. Everyone who eats a diet rich in animal protein passes a urine which is profoundly acid.

Metabolism also produces carbon dioxide. In solution this gas forms a weak acid. Large amounts of CO_2 are produced by cellular activity each day with the potential to upset acid–base balance, but under normal circumstances all of this CO_2 is excreted via the lungs, having been transported in the blood. Only when respiratory function is impaired do problems occur.

BUFFERING

A buffer is a solution of the salt of a weak acid which is able to bind hydrogen ions. Buffering does not remove hydrogen ions from the body. Rather, buffers temporarily mop up any excess hydrogen ions which are produced, in the same way that a sponge soaks up water. Buffering is only a short term solution to the problem of excess hydrogen ion. Ultimately, the body must get rid of the hydrogen ions by renal excretion.

The body contains a number of buffers to even out sudden changes in hydrogen ion production. Proteins can act as buffers, and the haemoglobin in the erythrocytes has a high capacity for binding hydrogen ion. In the ECF, bicarbonate buffer is the most important. In this buffer system, bicarbonate (HCO_3^-) combines with hydrogen ion to form carbonic acid (H_2CO_3). This buffer system is unique in that the H_2CO_3 can dissociate to water and carbon dioxide.

Whereas simple buffers rapidly become ineffective as the association of the hydrogen ion and the anion of the weak acid reaches equilibrium, the bicarbonate system keeps working because the carbonic acid is removed as carbon dioxide. The limit to the effectiveness of the bicarbonate system is the initial concentration of bicarbonate. Only when all the bicarbonate is used up does the system have no further buffering capacity. The acid–base status of patients is assessed by consideration of the bicarbonate system of plasma.

The association of hydrogen ion with bicarbonate occurs rapidly, but the breakdown of carbonic acid to carbon dioxide and water happens relatively slowly. The reaction is accelerated by an enzyme, carbonic anhydrase, which is present particularly where this reaction is most needed, in the erythrocytes and in the kidneys. Buffering by the bicarbonate system effectively removes hydrogen ion from the ECF at the expense of bicarbonate. The carbon dioxide which is formed can be blown off in the lungs, and the water mixes with the large body water pool. The extracellular fluid contains a large amount of bicarbonate, around 24 mmol/l. If hydrogen ions begin to build up for any reason, the bicarbonate concentration falls as the buffering system comes into play.

HYDROGEN ION EXCRETION IN THE KIDNEY

All the hydrogen ion which is buffered must eventually be excreted from the body via the kidneys, regenerating the bicarbonate used up in the buffering process and maintaining the plasma bicarbonate concentration within normal limits (Fig. 2). Secretion of hydrogen ion by the tubular cells serves initially to reclaim bicarbonate from the glomerular filtrate so that this is not lost from the body. When all the bicarbonate has been recovered, any deficit due to the buffering process is regenerated. The mechanisms for bicarbonate *recovery* and for bicarbonate *regeneration* are very similar and are sometimes confused (Fig. 2).

The excreted hydrogen ions must be buffered in urine or the $[H^+]$ would rise to very high levels. Phosphate acts as one such buffer, while ammonia is another (Fig. 3).

ASSESSING ACID–BASE STATUS

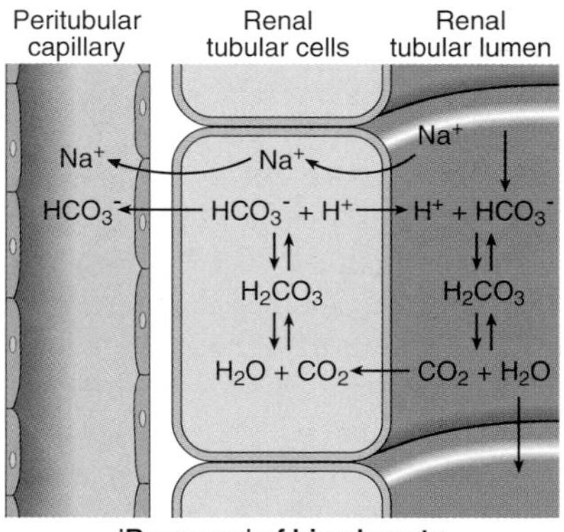

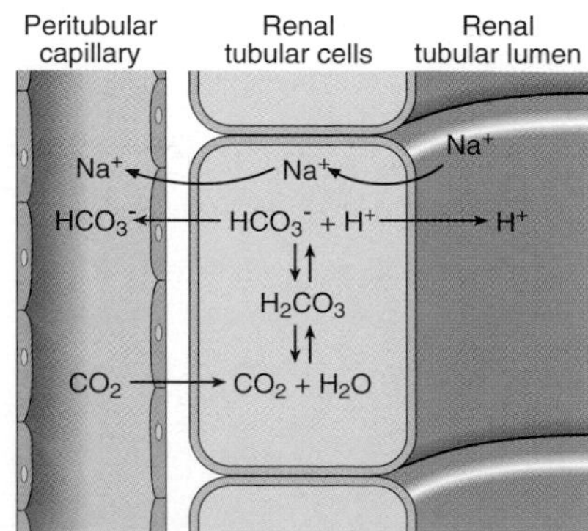

Fig. 2 **The recovery and regeneration of bicarbonate by excretion of H^+ in the renal tubular cell. Note that H^+ is actively secreted into the urine while CO_2 diffuses along its concentration gradient.**

An indication of the acid–base status of the patient can be obtained by measuring the components of the bicarbonate buffer system. In chemical terms, the bicarbonate buffer system can be considered in the same way as any other chemical dissociation.

$$[H^+] + [HCO_3^-] \rightleftharpoons [H_2CO_3]$$

By the Law of Mass Action:

$$[H^+] = \frac{K\,[H_2CO_3]}{[HCO_3^-]}$$

(Where K is the first dissociation constant of carbonic acid)

But the carbonic acid component is related to the dissolved carbon dioxide. The dissolved CO_2 is proportional to the partial pressure of the CO_2. Indeed, Henry's Law shows that $[CO_2]$ in solution = s.PCO_2, where *s* is the solubility of the gas in water.

$[H_2CO_3]$ can therefore be replaced in the mass action equation by PCO_2. At this point, an understanding of the role of the bicarbonate buffer system in assessing clinical acid–base disorders can be achieved simply by reference to the relationship:

$$[H^+] \text{ is proportional to } \frac{PCO_2}{[HCO_3^-]}$$

which shows that the hydrogen ion concentration in blood varies as the bicarbonate concentration and PCO_2 change. If everything else remains constant:

- Adding hydrogen ion, removing bicarbonate or increasing the PCO_2 will all have the same effect; that is, an increase in $[H^+]$.
- Removing hydrogen ions, adding bicarbonate or lowering PCO_2 will all cause the $[H^+]$ to fall.

Blood $[H^+]$ is 40 nmol/l and is controlled by our normal pattern of respiration and the functioning of our kidneys.

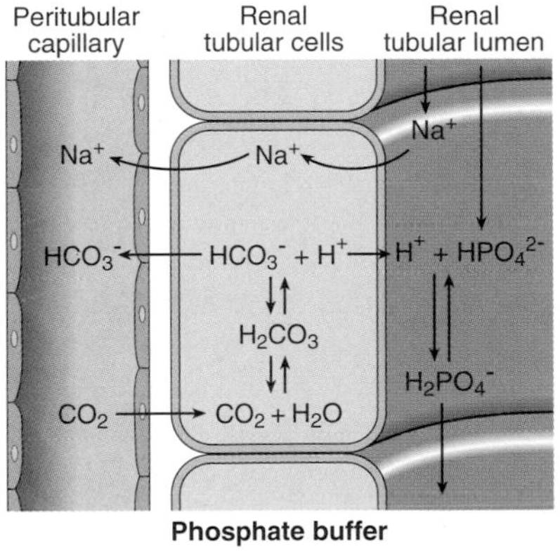

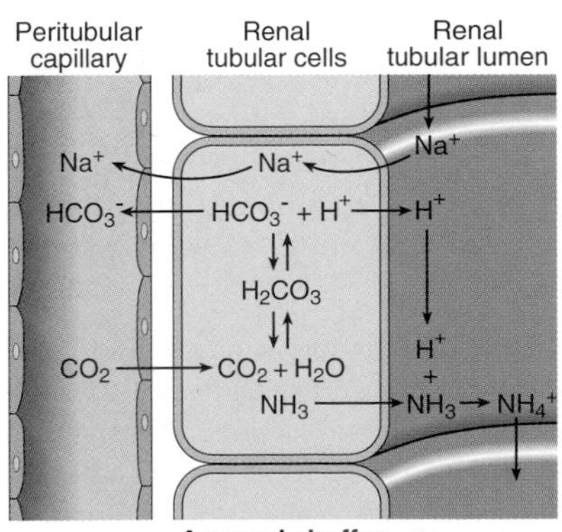

Fig. 3 **Buffering of hydrogen ions in urine.**

ACID–BASE DISORDERS

'Metabolic' acid–base disorders are those which directly cause a change in the bicarbonate concentration. Examples include diabetes mellitus, where altered intermediary metabolism in the absence of insulin causes a build up of hydrogen ion from the ionization of acetoacetic and β-hydroxybutyric acids, or loss of bicarbonate from the extracellular fluid, e.g. from a duodenal fistula.

'Respiratory' acid–base disorders affect directly the PCO_2. Impaired respiratory function causes a build up of CO_2 in blood, whereas, less commonly, hyperventilation can cause a decreased PCO_2.

Compensation

The simple relationships of the bicarbonate buffer system are complicated by physiological mechanisms which have evolved to try to return a disordered $[H^+]$ to normal. Where lung function is compromised, the body attempts to increase the excretion of hydrogen ion via the renal route. This is known as *renal compensation* for the primary respiratory disorder. Renal compensation is slow to take effect.

Where there are metabolic disorders, some compensation is possible by the lungs. This is known as *respiratory compensation* for the primary metabolic disorder. Respiratory compensation is quick to take effect.

If compensation is complete, the $[H^+]$ returns to within reference limits, although the PCO_2 and $[HCO_3^-]$ remain grossly abnormal. The acid–base disorder is said to be 'fully compensated'. Compensation is often partial, in which case the $[H^+]$ has not been brought within the reference limits.

The actual blood $[H^+]$ at any time in the course of an acid–base disorder is a consequence of the severity of the primary disturbance and the amount of compensation which has occurred.

Terminology

Acidosis and alkalosis are clinical terms which define the primary acid–base disturbance. They can be used even when the $[H^+]$ is within the normal range, i.e. when the disorders are fully compensated. The definitions are:

- *Metabolic acidosis*. The primary disorder is a decrease in bicarbonate concentration.
- *Metabolic alkalosis*. The primary disorder is an increased bicarbonate.
- *Respiratory acidosis*. The primary disorder is an increased PCO_2.
- *Respiratory alkalosis*. The primary disorder is a decreased PCO_2.

'Acidaemia' and 'alkalaemia' refer simply to whether the $[H^+]$ in blood is higher or lower than normal, and the terms are not frequently used.

Acid–base: concepts and vocabulary

- The assessment of acid–base status is carried out by measuring $[H^+]$, $[HCO_3^-]$ and PCO_2, the components of the bicarbonate buffer system in plasma.
- Adding hydrogen ions, removing bicarbonate or increasing the PCO_2 will all have the same effect, an increase in $[H^+]$.
- Removing hydrogen ions, adding bicarbonate or lowering PCO_2 will all cause the $[H^+]$ to fall.
- Primary problems with hydrogen ion production or excretion are reflected in the $[HCO_3^-]$; and these are called 'metabolic' acid–base disorders.
- Primary problems with CO_2 excretion are reflected in PCO_2; these are called 'respiratory' acid–base disorders.
- The body has physiological mechanisms which try to restore $[H^+]$ to normal. These processes are called 'compensation'.
- The observed $[H^+]$ in any acid–base disorder reflects the balance between the primary disturbance and the amount of compensation.

METABOLIC ACID–BASE DISORDERS

Metabolic acid–base disorders are reflected in changes in the ECF bicarbonate concentration which commonly occur because of a build-up or loss of hydrogen ion. Direct loss or gain of bicarbonate will also cause metabolic acid–base disorders. Primary metabolic acid–base disorders are recognized by inspecting the bicarbonate concentration (Fig. 1). Respiratory compensation takes place quickly, so patients with metabolic acid–base disorders will usually show some change in blood PCO_2 because of hyperventilation or hypoventilation (Fig. 2).

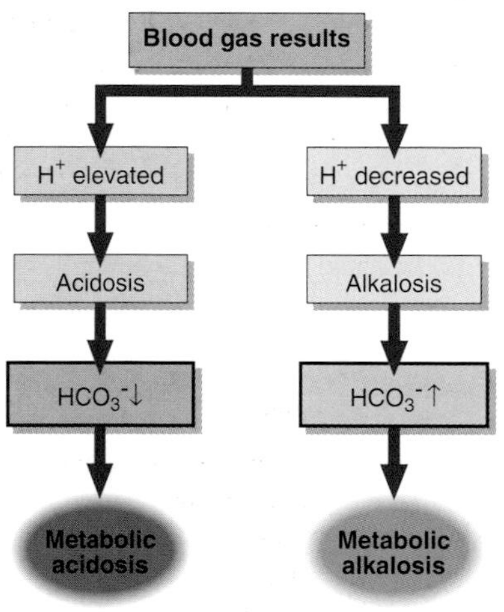

Fig. 1 **Recognizing primary metabolic acid base disorders by inspecting the HCO_3^- concentration.**

METABOLIC ACIDOSIS

In a metabolic acidosis the primary problem is a reduction in the bicarbonate concentration of the extracellular fluid. The main causes of a metabolic acidosis are shown in Figure 3. These are:

- increased production of hydrogen ions
- ingestion of hydrogen ions, or of drugs which are metabolized to acids
- impaired excretion of hydrogen ions by the kidneys
- loss of bicarbonate from the gastro-intestinal tract or in the urine.

The anion gap

The cause of a metabolic acidosis will nearly always be apparent from the clinical history of the patient, but occasionally knowledge of the anion gap may be helpful. This can be assessed by looking at the serum electrolyte results and calculating the difference between the sum of the two main cations, sodium and potassium, and the sum of the two main anions, chloride and bicarbonate. There is no real gap, of course, as plasma proteins are negatively charged at normal $[H^+]$. These negatively charged amino acid side chains on the proteins account for most of the apparent discrepancy when the measured electrolytes are compared. *The anion gap is thus a biochemical tool which is sometimes of help in assessing acid–base problems. It is not a physiological reality.*

In practice, because the potassium concentration is so small and will vary by so little, it is generally excluded when calculating the anion gap. Thus:

$$Anion\ gap = [Na^+] - ([Cl^-] + [HCO_3^-])$$

In a healthy person, the anion gap has a value of between 6–18 mmol/l. When the bicarbonate concentration rises or falls, other ions must take its place to maintain electrochemical neutrality. If chloride substitutes for bicarbonate, the anion gap does not change. However, the anion gap value will increase in metabolic conditions in which acids, such as sulphuric, lactic or acetoacetic, are produced, or when salicylate is present.

Causes of metabolic acidosis

Metabolic acidosis with an *elevated* anion gap occurs in:

- *Renal disease.* Hydrogen ions are retained along with anions such as sulphate and phosphate.
- *Diabetic ketoacidosis.* Altered metabolism of fatty acids, as a consequence of the lack of insulin, causes endogenous production of acetoacetic and β-hydroxybutyric acids.
- *Lactic acidosis.* This results from a number of causes, particularly tissue anoxia. *In acute hypoxic states such as respiratory failure or cardiac arrest lactic acidosis develops within minutes and is life-threatening.* Lactic acidosis may also be caused by liver disease. The presence of a lactic acidosis can be confirmed, if necessary, by the measurement of plasma lactate concentration.
- *Certain cases of overdosage or poisoning.* The mechanism common to all of these is the production of acid metabolites, for example in salicylate overdose where build-up of lactate occurs, or methanol poisoning when formate accumulates, or ethylene glycol poisoning where oxalate is formed.

Metabolic acidosis with a *normal* anion gap is sometimes referred to as a 'hyperchloraemic acidosis' because a reduced HCO_3^- concentration is balanced by increased Cl^- concentration. It is seen in:

- *Chronic diarrhoea or intestinal fistula.* Fluids containing bicarbonate are lost from the body.

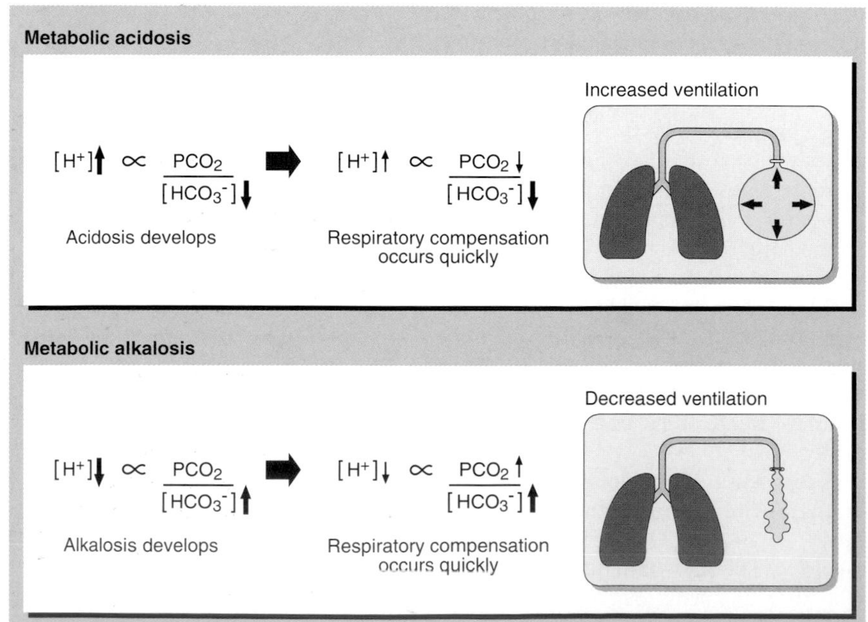

Fig. 2 **Compensation in primary metabolic disorders.**

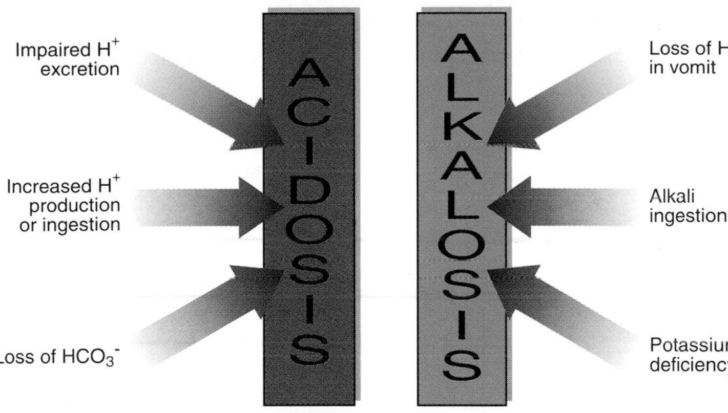

Fig. 3 **Reasons for metabolic acidosis and alkalosis.**

- *Renal tubular acidosis.* Renal tubular cells are unable to excrete hydrogen ions efficiently, and bicarbonate is lost in the urine.

Clinical effects of acidosis

The compensatory response to metabolic acidosis is hyperventilation, since the increased [H^+] acts as a powerful stimulant of the respiratory centre. The deep, rapid and gasping respiratory pattern is known as Kussmaul breathing. Hyperventilation is the appropriate physiological response to acidosis and it occurs rapidly.

A raised [H^+] leads to increased neuromuscular irritability. There is a hazard of arrhythmias progressing to cardiac arrest, and this is made more likely by the presence of hyperkalaemia which will accompany the acidosis (pp. 22–23). Depression of consciousness can progress to coma and death.

METABOLIC ALKALOSIS

The causes of a metabolic alkalosis are shown in Figure 3. The condition may be due to:

- *Loss of hydrogen ion in gastric fluid during vomiting.* This is especially seen when there is pyloric stenosis preventing parallel loss of bicarbonate-rich secretions from the duodenum.
- *Ingestion of an absorbable alkali such as sodium bicarbonate.* Very large doses are required to cause a metabolic alkalosis unless there is renal impairment.
- *Potassium deficiency.* In severe potassium depletion, often a consequence of diuretic therapy, hydrogen ions are retained inside cells to replace the missing potassium ions. In the renal tubule more hydrogen ions, rather than potassium, are exchanged for reabsorbed sodium. So, despite there being an alkalosis, the patient passes an acid urine. This is often referred to as a 'paradoxical' acid urine, because in other causes of metabolic alkalosis urinary [H^+] usually falls.

Clinical effects of alkalosis

The clinical effects of alkalosis include hypoventilation, confusion and eventually coma. Muscle cramps, tetany and paraesthesia may be a consequence of a decrease in the unbound plasma calcium concentration which is a consequence of the alkalosis.

Clinical note

A patient who has had prolonged nasogastric suction following surgery will lose gastric fluid in large quantities and may develop a metabolic alkalosis.

Case history 14

A 28–year–old man is admitted to hospital with a week–long history of severe vomiting. He confessed to self–medication of his chronic dyspepsia. He was clinically severely dehydrated and had shallow respiration. Initial biochemical results were:

Arterial blood gases:

H^+	PCO_2	HCO_3^-	PO_2
nmol/l	*kPa*	*mmol/l*	*kPa*
28	7.2	43	15

Serum:

Na^+	K^+	Cl^-	HCO_3^-	Urea	Creatinine
mmol/l					*µmol/l*
146	2.8	83	41	31	126

A random urine sample was obtained, and had the following biochemical results: osmolality 630 mmol/kg, Na^+ < 20 mmol/l, K^+ 35 mmol/l, pH 5.

- What is the acid–base disorder and how has it arisen?
- How might the urine results help in the diagnosis?

Comment on page 153.

Metabolic acid–base disorders

- In metabolic acidosis, the blood [H^+] may be high or normal, but the [HCO_3^-] is always low. In compensated conditions, PCO_2 is lowered.
- The commonest causes of metabolic acidosis are renal disease, diabetic ketoacidosis and lactic acidosis.
- Consideration of the anion gap may sometime be helpful in establishing the cause of a metabolic acidosis.
- In metabolic alkalosis, the [H^+] is depressed and the [HCO_3^-] is always raised. Respiratory compensation results in an elevated PCO_2.
- The commonest cause of a metabolic alkalosis is prolonged vomiting.

RESPIRATORY AND MIXED ACID–BASE DISORDERS

In respiratory acid–base disorders the primary disturbance is caused by changes in arterial blood PCO_2 (Fig. 1). Respiratory disorders are related to changes either in the amount of air moving in or moving out of the lungs (ventilation), or of the ability of gases to diffuse across the alveolar membrane (gas exchange). In both cases PCO_2 changes and the carbonic acid concentration rises or falls.

It may appear confusing that carbonic acid can cause an acidosis, since for each hydrogen ion produced, a bicarbonate molecule is also generated. However, the effect of adding one hydrogen ion to a concentration of 40 nanomoles/l is much greater than adding one bicarbonate molecule to a concentration of 26 millimoles/l.

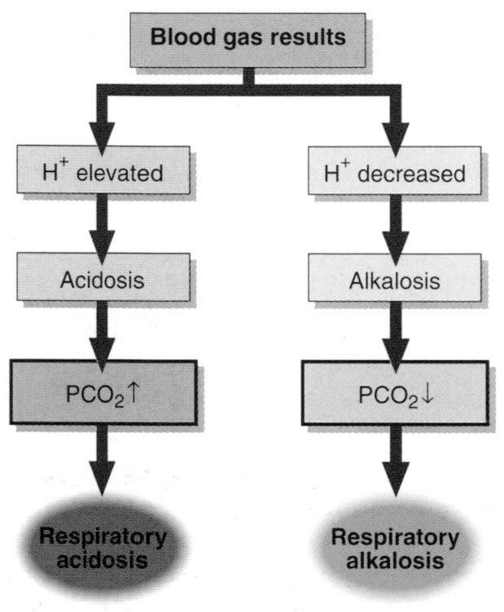

Fig. 1 **Primary respiratory disorders are recognized by inspecting the PCO_2.**

RESPIRATORY ACIDOSIS

Respiratory acidosis may be acute or chronic. Acute conditions occur within minutes or hours. They are uncompensated. Renal compensation has no time to develop as the mechanisms which adjust bicarbonate reabsorption take 48–72 h to become fully effective. The primary problem in acute respiratory acidosis is alveolar hypoventilation. If airflow is completely or partially reduced, the PCO_2 in the blood will rise immediately and the $[H^+]$ will rise quickly (Fig. 2). A resulting low PO_2 and high PCO_2 causes coma. If this is not relieved rapidly, death results.

Examples of acute, and hence uncompensated, respiratory acidosis are:

- choking
- bronchopneumonia
- acute exacerbation of asthma.

Chronic respiratory acidosis is usually a long-standing condition, and is accompanied by maximal renal compensation. In a chronic respiratory acidosis the primary problem again is usually impaired alveolar ventilation, but renal compensation contributes markedly to the acid–base picture. Compensation may be partial or complete. The kidney increases hydrogen ion excretion and ECF bicarbonate levels rise. Blood $[H^+]$ tends back towards normal (Fig. 3).

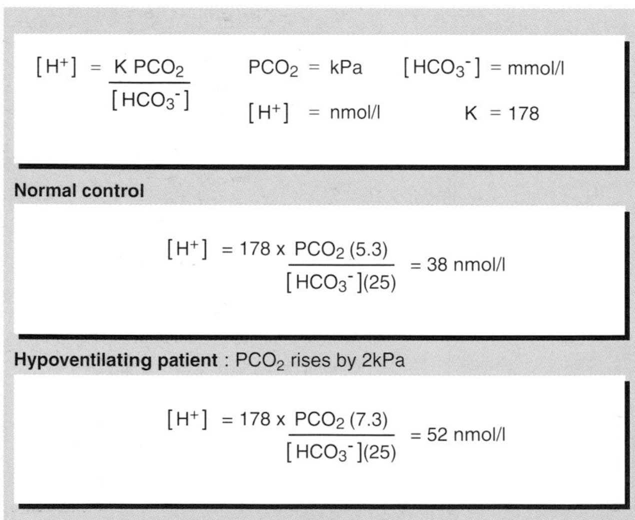

Fig. 2 **Why an increased PCO_2 causes an acidosis.**

It takes some time for the kidneys to respond to a high PCO_2 and a high $[H^+]$, and therefore compensation will only be maximal some days after the onset of the clinical problem. In many patients with chronic respiratory conditions, extensive renal compensation will keep the blood $[H^+]$ near normal, despite grossly impaired ventilation. In stable chronic bronchitis the $[H^+]$ may be within the reference range despite a very high PCO_2. This is achieved only by maintaining a plasma bicarbonate concentration twice that of normal. The PO_2 is usually depressed, and becomes more so as lung damage increases with time (pp. 40–41). Examples of chronic respiratory disorders are:

- chronic bronchitis
- emphysema.

The causes of respiratory acidosis are summarized in Figure 4.

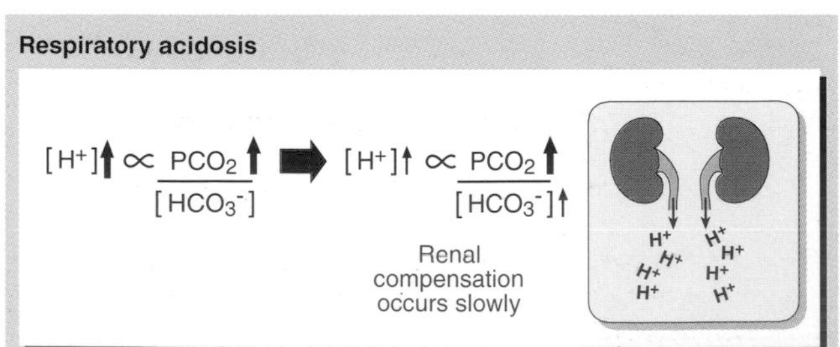

Fig. 3 **Renal compensation in primary respiratory acidosis.**

RESPIRATORY ALKALOSIS

Respiratory alkalosis is much less common than acidosis but can occur when respiration is stimulated or is no longer subject to feedback control (Fig. 4). Usually these are acute conditions, and there is no renal compensation. The treatment is to inhibit or remove the cause of the hyperventilation, and the acid–base balance should return to normal. Examples are:

- hysterical overbreathing
- mechanical over-ventilation
- raised intracranial pressure, or hypoxia, both of which may stimulate the respiratory centre.

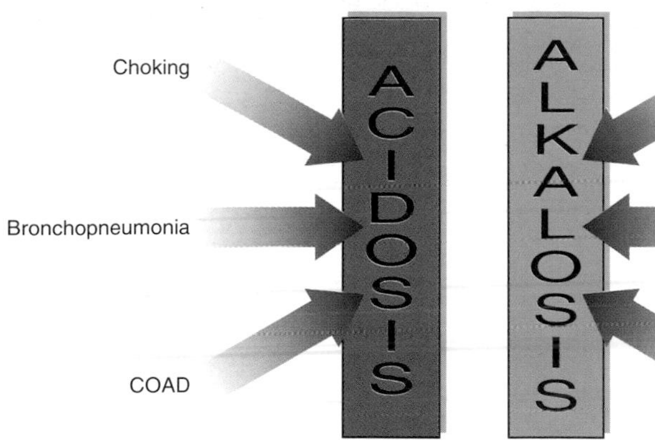

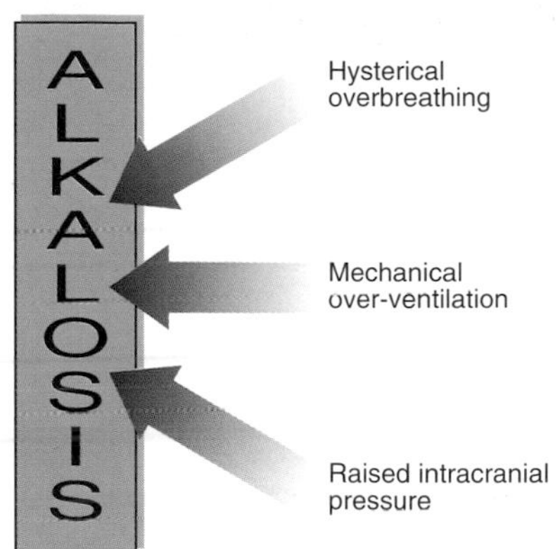

Fig. 4 **Causes of respiratory acidosis and alkalosis.**

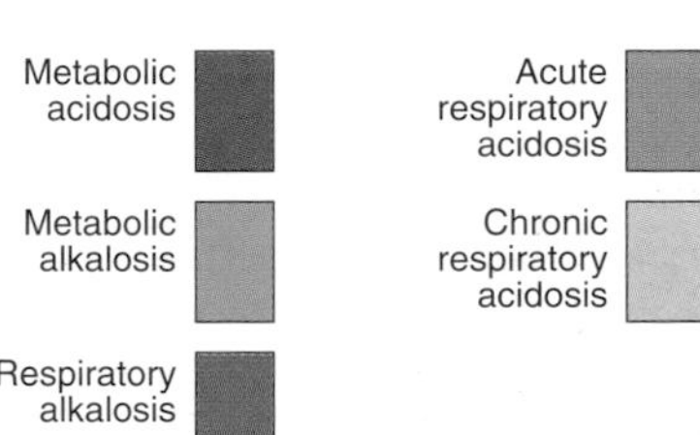

Fig. 5 **The 95% confidence intervals for arterial blood gases in primary acid-base disorders.** Arterial [H^+] is plotted against PCO_2 with lines of equal [$HCO3^-$] radiating from origin. The hatched box shows normal values. Graphs such as these may be used to chart the progress of a patient under treatment to correct an acid–base disorder.

MIXED ACID–BASE DISORDERS

It is not uncommon for patients to have more than one acid–base disorder. A patient may have both a metabolic and respiratory acidosis, such as the chronic bronchitic patient who develops renal impairment. In such a patient with a raised [H^+], the PCO_2 will be increased and the bicarbonate concentration will be low, both expected findings in primary respiratory and primary metabolic acidosis.

Where the two acid–base conditions are antagonistic in the way they affect the [H^+], one of the disorders may mimic the compensatory response. A patient may present with a metabolic acidosis and a co-existent respiratory alkalosis, as occurs commonly in salicylate overdose. The respiratory disorder may appear, at first sight, to be simply the compensatory response.

Other examples of mixed acid–base disorders commonly encountered are:

- a patient with chronic obstructive airways disease, causing a respiratory acidosis, with thiazide-induced potassium depletion and consequent metabolic alkalosis
- hyperventilation causing a respiratory alkalosis, with prolonged nasogastric suction which causes a metabolic alkalosis
- salicylate poisoning in which respiratory alkalosis occurs due to stimulation of the respiratory centre, together with metabolic acidosis due to the effects of the poison on metabolism.

Care must be taken in the interpretation of the blood gas results in these patients. Knowledge of the clinical picture is essential. Theoretically, the limits of the compensatory responses in simple primary acid–base disorders are known (Fig. 5). When compensation apparently falls outside of these expected limits, it is likely that a second acid–base disorder is present.

There is further discussion on the interpretation of blood gas results on pages 42-43.

Case history 15

Miss AM was admitted to hospital with a crushed chest. On admission her arterial blood gases were:

H^+	HCO_3^-	PCO_2	PO_2
nmol/l	*mmol/l*	*kPa*	*kPa*
63	29	10.1	6.4

- What do these results indicate?

Comment on page 153.

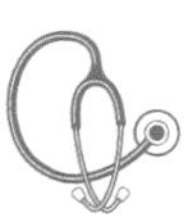

Clinical note

When interpreting acid–base results, the patient's clinical history is the most important factor in determining the nature of the disorder, or indeed in deciding if more than one disorder might be present. Biochemical measurements are the only means of quantifying the severity of the disorder(s) and the degree of compensation.

Respiratory and mixed acid–base disorders

- In respiratory acidosis the blood [H^+] is usually high, but may be within the reference range. The PCO_2 is always raised. In compensated conditions, [HCO_3^-] is also raised.
- Acute respiratory acidosis is a medical emergency and needs to be dealt with by removing the source of the respiratory problem.
- In contrast to respiratory compensation in metabolic disorders, the renal compensating mechanisms are much slower to take effect.
- In chronic respiratory disorders the [H^+] often settles at a new steady state, within the reference range, at which compensation is maximal.
- Respiratory alkalosis is uncommon and can be a result of mechanical overventilation or hysterical overbreathing.
- The interpretation of mixed acid–base disorders may be confusing if one of the disorders mimics the expected compensation. Knowledge of the clinical picture is important if the correct interpretation is to be placed on the results.

OXYGEN TRANSPORT

NORMAL OXYGEN TRANSPORT

Only a small fraction (2%) of the total oxygen in blood is in solution, and this dissolved oxygen is directly proportional to the arterial PO_2. The arterial PO_2 is also an important factor affecting the amount of oxygen which is bound to haemoglobin, as oxyhaemoglobin. The relationship is shown in the oxygen–haemoglobin dissociation curve (Fig. 1).

The total blood oxygen content is the sum of the dissolved oxygen and that bound to haemoglobin. Measurement of blood *oxygen saturation*, the percentage of the total haemoglobin present as oxyhaemoglobin, may be used to assess the ability of blood to carry oxygen to the tissues. This clearly depends on the relative amounts of both oxygen and haemoglobin, as well as their ability to bind together. Delivery of oxygen to the tissues also depends on blood flow, which is in turn influenced by other factors (Table 1).

When arterial PO_2 is high (above 10 kPa), the blood haemoglobin is almost fully saturated with oxygen and measurements of oxygen saturation are not normally required. Indeed, measurements of oxygen saturation are not widely available outside of intensive therapy units. However, in patients who have anaemia or whose haemoglobin function is abnormal or impaired, measurement of PO_2, oxygen saturation and haemoglobin may all be necessary. For example, in patients exposed to carbon monoxide following smoke inhalation, the PO_2 may give a misleading indication of the amount of oxygen being carried in the blood. PO_2 may be within normal limits but oxygen saturation will be severely reduced because carbon monoxide binds to haemoglobin with greater affinity than does oxygen (Fig. 1). Smokers may have carboxyhaemoglobin concentrations of up to 10% all of the time, which reduces the supply of oxygen available to the tissues.

When metabolic needs exceed the supply of oxygen, cells switch to anaerobic glycolysis to provide ATP, and produce lactic acid. Measurement of serum lactate concentration can provide additional evidence of the adequacy of tissue oxygenation.

In practice, tissue perfusion is more important than blood oxygen content in ensuring that aerobic metabolism can continue.

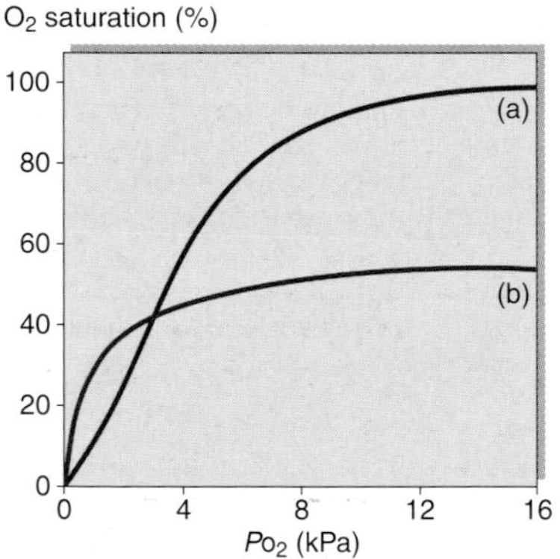

Fig. 1 **Dissociation curves—the relationship between PO_2 and oxygen binding to haemoglobin. (a)** The normal oxygen–haemoglobin dissociation curve. **(b)** The effect of 50% CO.

Table 1 **Factors affecting the delivery of oxygen to the tissues**

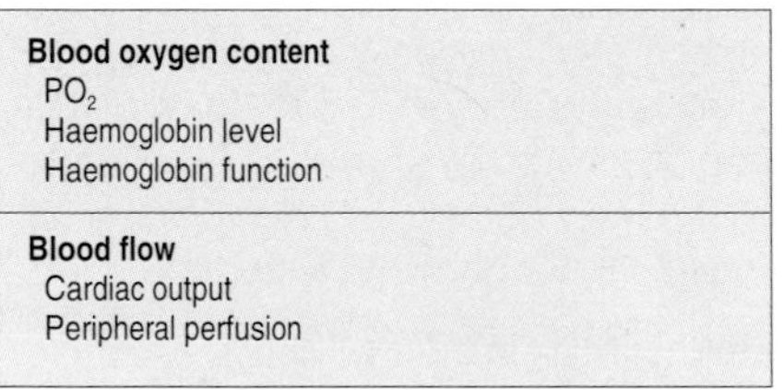

Blood oxygen content PO_2 Haemoglobin level Haemoglobin function
Blood flow Cardiac output Peripheral perfusion

Table 2 **Chemical stimuli to ventilation**

• Carbon dioxide: an increased PCO_2 is the most important stimulus
• [H^+]: a rise in hydrogen ion concentration stimulates ventilation; in respiratory disease [H^+] and PCO_2 rise together.
• Oxygen: a decreased PO_2 increases ventilation, but is of less importance unless PO_2 falls below 8 kPa

RESPIRATORY FAILURE

Figure 2 shows how the partial pressures of oxygen and carbon dioxide change as blood flows to the tissues and returns to the lungs. The mechanical process of moving air into and out of the respiratory tract is called ventilation. Carbon dioxide diffuses through alveolar membranes much more efficiently than oxygen, even though there is only a small pressure gradient. The PCO_2 of arterial blood is thus identical to the PCO_2 within the alveoli, and the arterial PCO_2 is therefore a measure of alveolar ventilation. If ventilation is impaired, alveolar PO_2 falls and alveolar PCO_2 rises. Arterial blood reflects these changes. The main chemical stimuli to ventilation are shown in Table 2.

It is possible to calculate the alveolar–arterial PO_2 gradient to determine the extent of defective gas exchange (Fig. 3), but in practice it is rarely necessary to do this.

A low arterial PO_2 is termed hypoxia and indicates respiratory impairment. A value less than 8.0 kPa in a patient breathing air at rest is known as 'respiratory failure'. Classically, hypoxia with carbon dioxide retention is called type 2 respiratory failure. Hypoxia without carbon dioxide retention is type 1 respiratory failure, but these biochemical definitions are not helpful in understanding the pathophysiology of respiratory disease.

Two processes contribute to the blood gas pattern in those patients with hypoxia, where PCO_2 is not elevated (type 1 respiratory failure). These are:

- impaired diffusion
- ventilation/perfusion imbalance.

Impaired diffusion

Here the presence of fluid, as in pulmonary oedema, or thickened alveolar walls, such as occurs in pulmonary fibrosis, inhibits

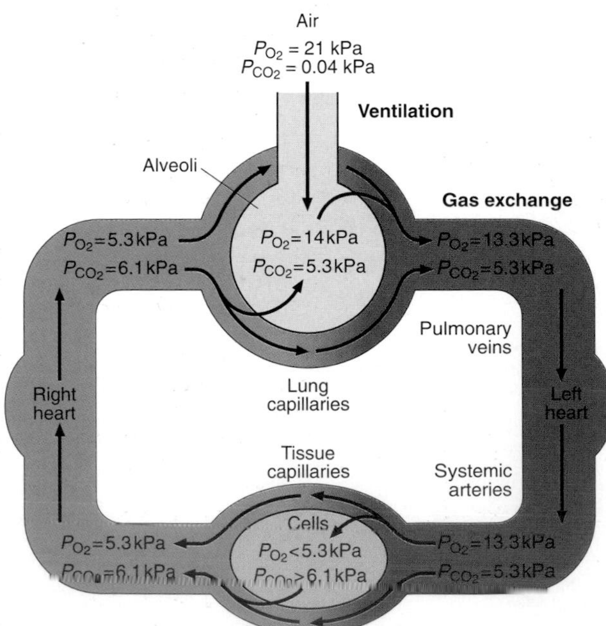

Fig. 2 **Normal gas pressures are maintained by ventilation and gas exchange.**

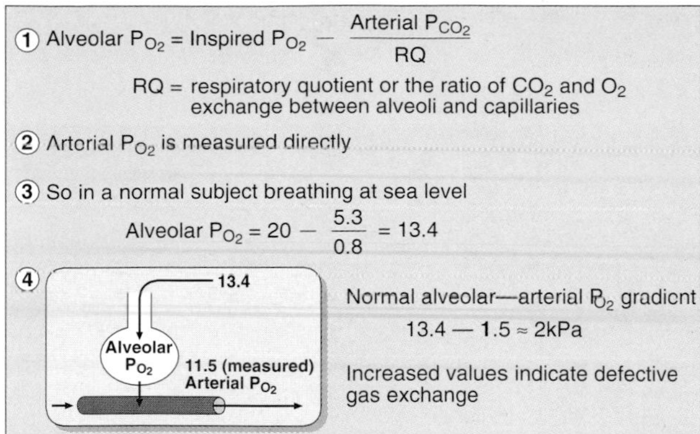

Fig. 3 **How to calculate the alveolar–arterial PO_2 difference.**

Clinical note

Pulse oximetry is an accurate non-invasive way of assessing oxygen saturation. Oxygenated and reduced haemoglobin absorb light at different wavelengths. If light of these wavelengths is passed through a blood vessel, the proportion of oxygenated haemoglobin can be calculated. Pulse oximetry allows these measurements in 'pulsing' blood only, producing results that approximate to arterial values.

oxygen diffusion, although carbon dioxide passage is more readily accomplished. PO_2 is low but PCO_2 may be within reference limits.

Ventilation/perfusion imbalance

Ventilation/perfusion imbalance can be a cause of hypoxia in patients with certain types of disease. In patients with a *lobar* pneumonia, some of the blood perfusing the lungs does not come into contact with functional alveoli and retains its carbon dioxide, and is not oxygenated. In blood reaching other parts of the lungs, gas exchange takes place efficiently. Arterial blood is a mixture of that exiting both regions. The increased PCO_2 stimulates ventilation and ensures that the functioning alveoli are worked harder to restore PCO_2 to normal. The blood gas results will show normal or even low PCO_2 as a result of this hyperventilation (Fig. 4). But increased ventilation cannot dramatically raise alveolar PO_2 as long as the patient is breathing air. The arterial blood will always have a low PO_2 because the mix includes blood with an even lower PO_2 from the non-functioning region of the lung.

Blood passing from the right side of the heart directly to the arterial circulation without being exposed to the inspired gas in the ventilated alveoli is an extreme example of ventilation/perfusion imbalance. This right to left 'shunting' occurs in cyanotic congenital heart disease. Again, these patients have some normal alveolar function and hyperventilate, which may prevent the PCO_2 from rising.

Hypoxia with raised PCO_2 (type 2 respiratory failure) indicates diminished ventilation and impaired gas exchange, and may be seen in patients with bronchial pneumonia or chronic bronchitis.

(a) Uniform ventilation
P_{CO_2}=6.1 kPa
P_{O_2}=5.3 kPa
Mixed venous blood
Arterial blood flow
Uniform blood flow
P_{CO_2}=5.3 kPa
P_{O_2}=13.3 kPa

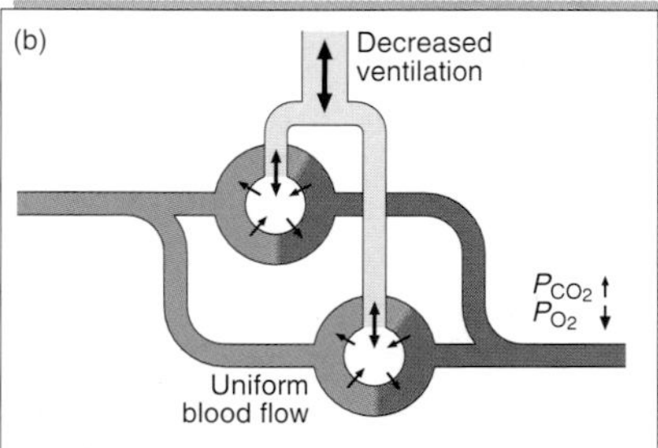

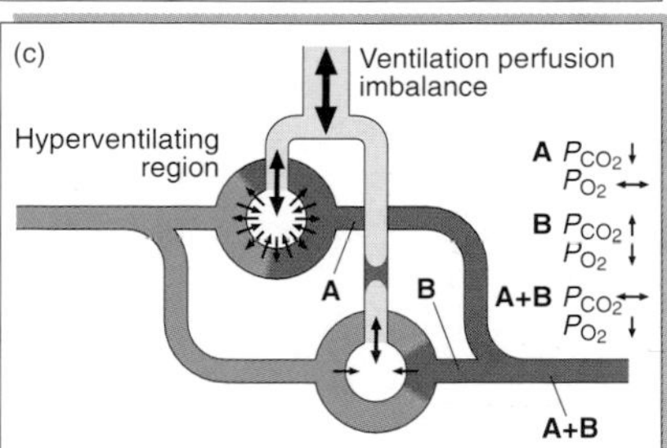

Fig. 4 **Blood gases in (a) normal circumstances, (b) hypoventilation and (c) where there is a ventilation/perfusion imbalance.**

OXYGEN THERAPY

In all respiratory diseases, oxygen therapy is a vital aspect of patient management but there is one caution. Some patients with chronic bronchitis become insensitive to respiratory stimulation by carbon dioxide. This insensitivity may develop over many years, and only the existing hypoxia keeps respiration going. Treating such patients with high concentrations of oxygen only serves to reduce respiration further. PCO_2 rises, acidosis worsens and the patient may become comatose.

Case history 16

A 58-year-old male was admitted with a history of chronic obstructive airways disease for many years. On examination he was cyanosed, breathless and there was marked systemic oedema. A blood sample gave the following results:

Arterial blood gases:

H^+	PCO_2	HCO_3^-	PO_2
nmol/l	*kPa*	*mmol/l*	*kPa*
44	9.3	40	4.0

- Describe the acid–base disorder.
- What type of respiratory problem is present?

Comment on page 153.

Oxygen transport

- Oxygen is carried in blood mostly bound to haemoglobin. Arterial blood PO_2 determines how much oxygen is bound to haemoglobin, although above a PO_2 of 10 kPa the haemoglobin is usually fully saturated.
- Measurements of haemoglobin and blood oxygen saturation are necessary to assess oxygen availability where the patient is anaemic, or if factors affecting the ability of the haemoglobin to bind oxygen, such as carbon monoxide, are present.
- Delivery of oxygen to the tissues also depends on cardiac output and peripheral perfusion.
- Respiratory failure is defined as an arterial PO_2 of less than 8 kPa in a patient breathing air.
- Hypoxia with CO_2 retention is seen where there is impaired ventilation.
- Hypoxia without CO_2 retention is seen commonly when there is ventilation/perfusion imbalance.

ACID–BASE DISORDERS: Diagnosis and Management

SPECIMENS FOR BLOOD GAS ANALYSIS

$[H^+]$ and PCO_2 are measured directly in an *arterial* blood sample. This is usually taken from the brachial or radial arteries into a syringe which contains a small volume of heparin as an anticoagulant. It is important to exclude air from the syringe before and after the blood is collected. Any air bubbles in the syringe when the sample has been taken should be expelled before the syringe is capped for immediate transport to the laboratory. Ideally, the syringe and its contents should be placed in ice during transit.

Acid–base problems may be discussed by referring to the three 'components' of the bicarbonate buffer system. In practice, blood gas analyzers measure the $[H^+]$ of the sample and its PCO_2. There is no need to measure the third parameter, the bicarbonate. By the law of mass action:

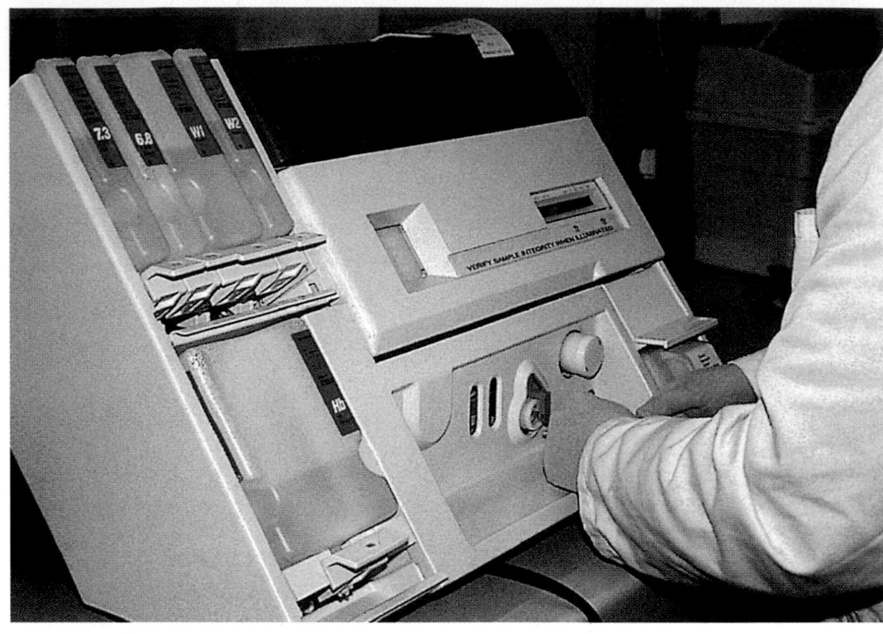

Fig. 1 **Blood gas analyzer.**

$$[H^+] \propto \frac{PCO_2}{[HCO_3^-]}$$

If any two of the variables are known, the third can always be calculated. Indeed, blood gas analyzers (Fig. 1) are programmed to provide this information which is printed out on the report form and usually includes the measured PO_2 as well. There are a multitude of other calculated values on some blood gas analyzer print outs, such as base excess and standard bicarbonate. These may be mostly disregarded in the routine assessment of a patient's acid–base balance.

Bicarbonate concentration is also determined directly as part of the electrolyte profile of tests on the laboratory's main analyzer, usually on a serum specimen obtained from a venous blood sample. These results are not identical to the print-out from the blood gas analyzer nor should this be expected since they include dissolved carbon dioxide, carbonic acid and other carbamino compounds. However, for practical purposes the results are similar and should not differ by more than 3 mmol/l. They may, therefore, be interpreted in the same way. A low bicarbonate in an electrolyte profile will usually indicate the presence of a metabolic acidosis.

INTERPRETING RESULTS

The predicted compensatory responses in $[HCO_3^-]$ or PCO_2 when $[H^+]$ changes as a result of primary acid–base disorders are shown in Table 1.

A practical approach to the interpretation of blood gas results is shown in Figure 2. The steps in classifying the acid–base disorder are:

- Look first at the $[H^+]$. Decide if an acidosis or an alkalosis is present.
- If the $[H^+]$ is elevated, decide what is the primary cause of the acidosis. Look at the PCO_2. If this is elevated, then there is a respiratory acidosis. Look at the bicarbonate. If this is decreased, there is a metabolic acidosis.
- If the $[H^+]$ is decreased, decide what is the primary cause of the alkalosis. Look at the PCO_2. If low, then there is a respiratory alkalosis. Look at the bicarbonate. If this is high, then there is a metabolic alkalosis.
- Having decided on the primary acid–base disorder, look to see if there is compensation. There will be a change in the other component (the one which was not used to determine the primary disorder), in the direction which 'compensates' for the primary disorder. If there is not, the acid–base disorder may be uncompensated. If the change is in the *opposite* direction then a second acid–base disorder may be present. Even if there is compensation consider the possibility that there is a second acid–base problem which mimics the compensatory response.
- If there is compensation, decide if the disorder is fully compensated or partially compensated. If fully compensated, the resulting $[H^+]$ will be within the reference limits.

Table 1 **Primary acid–base disorders and compensatory responses**

Primary disorder	Compensatory response
$\uparrow PCO_2$ (Respiratory acidosis)	$\uparrow HCO_3^-$
$\downarrow PCO_2$ (Respiratory alkalosis)	$\downarrow HCO_3^-$
$\downarrow HCO_3^-$ (Metabolic acidosis)	$\downarrow PCO_2$
$\uparrow HCO_3^-$ (Metabolic alkalosis)	$\uparrow PCO_2$

CLINICAL CASES

The above practical advice is best illustrated by four case examples.

- A patient with chronic bronchitis. Blood gas results are: $[H^+]$ = 44 nmol/l; PCO_2 = 9.5 kPa; $[HCO_3^-]$ = 39 mmol/l. *A compensated respiratory acidosis* is present.
- A patient who has had an acute asthmatic attack. Blood gas results are: $[H^+]$ = 24 nmol/l; PCO_2 = 2.5 kPa; $[HCO_3^-]$ = 20 mmol/l. An acute, and hence *uncompensated, respiratory alkalosis* is present.

- A young man with a history of dyspepsia and excessive alcohol intake who gives a 24-hour history of vomiting. Blood gas results are: $[H^+]$ = 28 nmol/l; PCO_2 = 7.2 kPa; $[HCO_3^-]$ = 48 mmol/l. This is a *partially compensated metabolic alkalosis*.
- A 50-year-old man with a two-week history of vomiting and diarrhoea. On examination he is dehydrated and his breathing is deep and noisy. Blood gas results are: $[H^+]$ = 64 nmol/l; PCO_2 = 2.8 kPa; $[HCO_3^-]$ = 8 mmol/l. These results show a *partially compensated metabolic acidosis*.

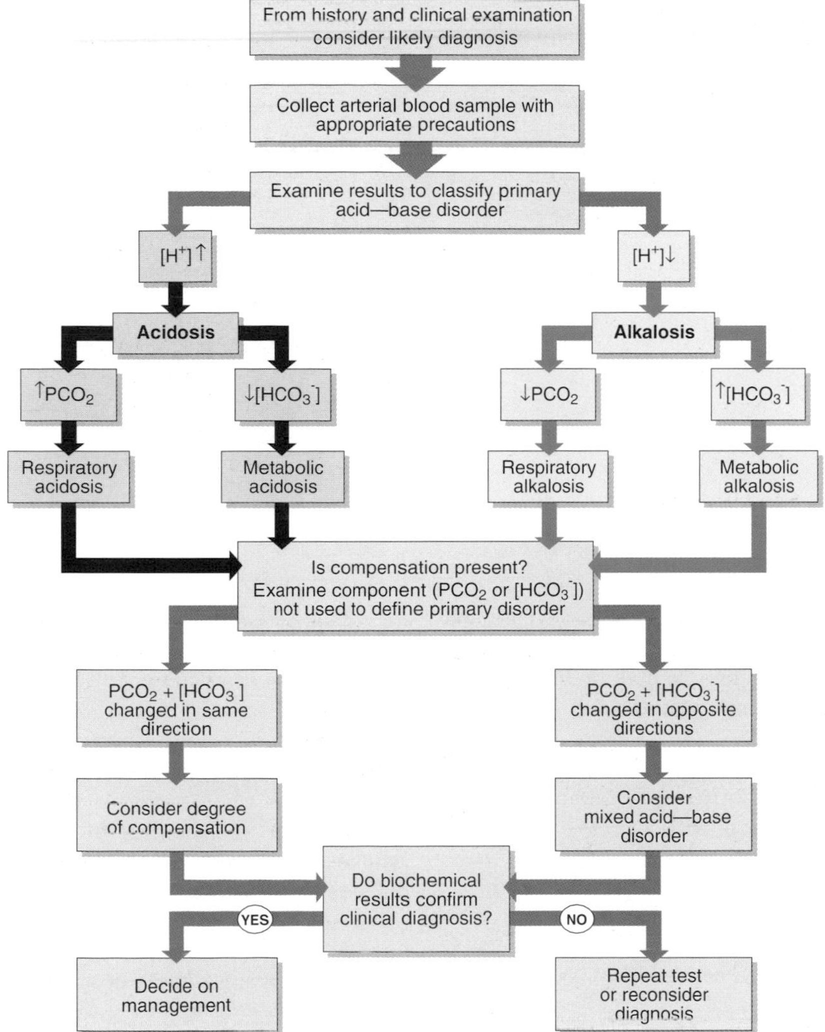

Fig. 2 **Acid–base disorders: diagnosis and management.**

MANAGEMENT OF ACID–BASE DISORDERS

Many acid–base disorders are secondary to some other disorder. In most cases the appropriate management of the acid–base disorder is to treat the underlying illness. This may involve:

- fluid therapy and insulin in diabetic ketoacidosis
- artificially ventilating by intermittent positive pressure ventilation (IPPV)
- improving GFR by restoring blood volume.

In cases where there is a life-threatening acidosis, the infusion of sodium bicarbonate may be considered. The circumstances when this might be appropriate include severe diabetic ketoacidosis. Sodium bicarbonate must always be used with caution. Careful monitoring of the patient by repeatedly measuring the blood gases may be necessary.

Clinical note

Overcompensation of an acid–base disorder does not occur physiologically but may be induced by the inappropriate use of artificial ventilation or intravenous bicarbonate solutions.

Case history 17

A 56-year-old woman was admitted seriously ill and confused. The patient had systemic oedema and was being treated with frusemide. On admission the following biochemical results were obtained:

Na^+	K^+	Cl^-	HCO_3^-	Urea	H^+	PCO_2	PO_2
		mmol/l			*nmol/l*	*kPa*	*kPa*
135	2.6	59	53	6.8	33	9.3	12

- What is the evidence that this patient has a mixed acid–base disorder? Identify the components.
- Explain the aetiology of the present blood gas and electrolyte results.
- How should the patient be treated?

Comment on page 153.

Acid–base disorders: diagnosis and management

- Care should be taken to exclude air from the arterial blood sample taken for blood gas analysis, and speedy transportation to the laboratory should be arranged.
- Blood gas analyzers measure $[H^+]$ and PCO_2 directly and calculate $[HCO_3^-]$. This calculated bicarbonate is similar but not identical to the bicarbonate concentration obtained from the electrolyte profile in a serum sample.
- Acid–base disorders can be classified as acidosis or alkalosis, compensated or uncompensated, fully or partially compensated.
- The clinical status of the patient and the blood gas results should always match up.
- Management of acid–base disorders should be directed towards the correction of the underlying illness.

PROTEINS AND ENZYMES

PLASMA PROTEINS

Plasma contains a variety of proteins with different functions. There are many characterized proteins whose function remains to be determined. The biochemistry laboratory routinely measures 'total protein' and 'albumin' concentrations, usually in a serum specimen, and reports the 'globulin' fraction as the difference between the first two results. Other proteins (e.g. immunoglobulins) are measured as classes, and immunochemical methods are available for measuring specific proteins and hormones. Enzymes are measured both by determining their activity and by immunochemical methods to assess their mass.

Simple electrophoresis of a serum sample separates its proteins into five bands, and is especially useful in demonstrating the presence of a paraprotein (pp. 46–47), derived from neoplastic cells.

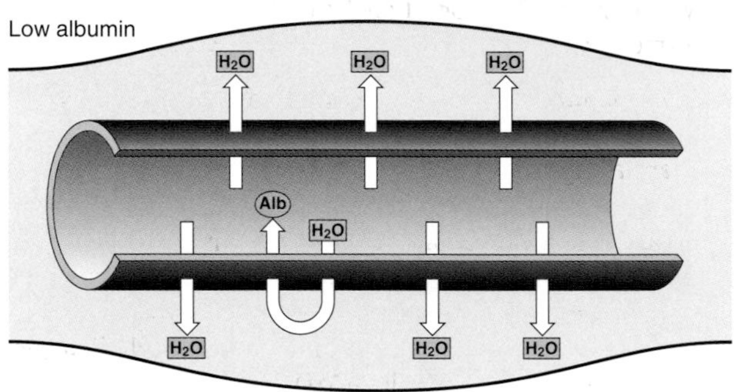

Fig. 1 **Pathogenesis of oedema in hypoalbuminaemia.**

TOTAL PROTEIN

Changes in total protein concentration are common. An elevated total protein concentration may mean the presence of a paraprotein. A decreased total protein usually means that the albumin concentration is low.

ALBUMIN

Albumin is the major plasma protein and is synthesized and secreted by the liver. It accounts for about 50% of the total hepatic protein production. Albumin has a biological half-life in plasma of about 20 days and a significant decrease in albumin concentration in plasma is slow to occur if there is reduced synthesis. Albumin makes the biggest contribution to the plasma oncotic pressure. If the albumin concentration falls very low, oedema is the result (Fig. 1). There are three main reasons for the occurrence of a low plasma albumin concentration:

- *Decreased synthesis.* This may be due to malnutrition or malabsorption. Decreased synthesis is also a feature of advanced chronic liver disease.
- *Abnormal distribution or dilution.* Hypoalbuminaemia can be induced by overhydration or if there is increased capillary permeability as occurs in septicaemia.
- *Abnormal excretion or degradation.* The causes include the nephrotic syndrome, protein-losing enteropathies, burns, haemorrhage and catabolic states.

Although serum albumin measurements have been used to monitor a patient's response to long-term nutritional support, they are unreliable and insensitive.

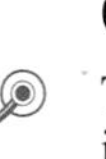

Clinical note

The only non-specific index of the presence of disease, comparable to C-reactive protein (CRP), is the erythrocyte sedimentation rate (ESR). This, in part, reflects the intensity of the acute phase response. The rate of change of ESR is much less than that of CRP and it reflects the clinical status of the patient less well. It is also affected by the number and morphology of the red cells. CRP can now be measured with relative ease and its determination is preferred over ESR in most pathological conditions. ESR as a non-specific indicator of disease may be helpful, for example, in the investigation of paraproteinaemias which do not necessarily provoke an acute phase response.

SPECIFIC PROTEINS

Measurement of a number of specific proteins gives useful information in the diagnosis and management of disease (Table 1). Characteristic changes in the concentration of certain plasma proteins are seen following surgery or trauma, or during infection or tumour growth. The proteins involved are called acute phase reactants (pp. 102–103). These acute phase proteins may be used to monitor progress of the condition or its treatment.

Table 1 **Specific proteins which are measured in serum**

Protein name	Function	Reason for assay
α_1-antitrypsin	Protease inhibitor	Reduced in α_1-antitrypsin deficiency
β_2-microglobulin	A subunit of the HLA antigen on all cell membranes	Raised in renal tubular dysfunction
Caeruloplasmin	Oxidizing enzyme	Reduced in Wilson's disease
C-reactive protein (CRP)	Involved in immune response	Increased in acute illness, especially infection
Ferritin	Binds iron in tissues	Gives an indication of body iron stores
Haptoglobin	Binds haemoglobin	Reduced in haemolytic conditions
Thyroid-binding globulin (TBG)	Thyroid hormone binding	Investigation of thyroid disease
Sex hormone binding globulin (SHBG)	Binds testosterone and oestradiol	Investigation of raised testosterone
Transferrin	Iron transport	Assessing response to nutritional support

ENZYMES

SERUM ENZYMES IN DISEASE

Enzymes may be classified in two groups. Some, such as the enzymes of the coagulation cascade, have a defined function in blood. Others were originally cell constituents, or were made within cells to be secreted into the gastrointestinal tract. They appear in the blood incidentally and their measurement is of value in diagnosis. Damage to the tissues of origin, or proliferation of the cells from which these enzymes arise, will lead to an increase in the activity of these enzymes in plasma (Fig. 2). It should be noted that increases in serum enzyme activity are only roughly proportional to the extent of tissue damage.

Enzymes that have been shown to have a diagnostic value are:

- *Acid phosphatase:* a tumour marker in prostatic carcinoma.
- *Alanine aminotransferase (ALT):* an indicator of hepatocellular damage.
- *Alkaline phosphatase:* increases in cholestatic liver disease and is a marker of osteoblast activity in bone disease.
- *Amylase:* an indicator of cell damage in acute pancreatitis.
- *Aspartate aminotransferase (AST):* an indicator of hepatocellular damage, or as as a marker of muscle damage, such as a myocardial infarction (MI).
- *Creatine kinase:* a marker of muscle damage and acute MI.
- *γ-glutamyl transpeptidase:* a sensitive marker of liver cell damage.
- *Lactate dehydrogenase:* a marker of muscle damage.

A further enzyme of practical interest is cholinesterase. Cholinesterase, normally involved in the process of neuromuscular conduction, incidentally hydrolyses succinylcholine, a muscle-relaxing drug used in anaesthesia. Patients with abnormal cholinesterase may fail to hydrolyze the drug normally and as a result suffer prolonged paralysis after anaesthesia. This is called scoline apnoea. Cholinesterase measurements are also useful in the diagnosis of poisoning with pesticides which are cholinesterase inhibitors.

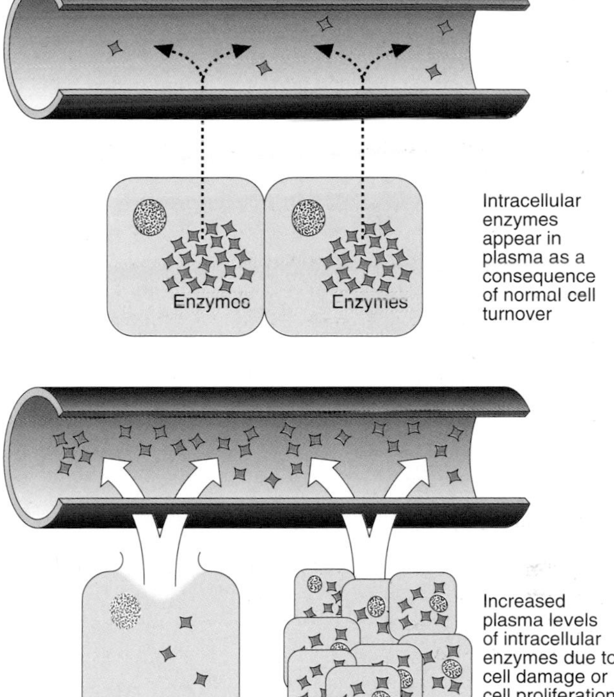

Fig. 2 **Plasma levels of intracellular enzymes.**

ISOENZYME DETERMINATION

Some enzymes are present in the plasma in two or more molecular forms. These variants are known as isoenzymes, and although they have different structures they perform the same catalytic function. Different isoenzymes may arise from different tissues and their specific detection may give clues to the site of pathology. Alkaline phosphatase isoenzymes may distinguish between bone and liver disease, especially in patients in whom metastases of bone or liver are suspected. A specific isoenzyme of creatine kinase (CK MB) is useful in the early detection of myocardial infarction. Heart muscle contains proportionally more of this isoenzyme than skeletal muscle, and raised levels of CK MB indicate that a myocardial infarction has occurred.

Case history 18

Eight months after an attack of acute glomerulonephritis, a 38-year-old housewife was hospitalized for investigation of progressive bilateral leg oedema. On examination, she was normotensive and exhibited pitting oedema of both ankles and dullness over her lung bases. Her face was pale and puffy and she admitted to frequent minor intercurrent infections.

- What is your tentative diagnosis?
- What biochemical analyses would you request, and in what order?
- What results would be consistent with your diagnosis?

Comment on page 154.

Proteins and enzymes

- An increase in total protein concentration in a serum specimen is usually due to an increase in the globulin fraction and may indicate the presence of a paraprotein.
- A decreased total protein concentration is usually due to hypoalbuminaemia.
- Albumin is the main determinant of plasma oncotic pressure. A very low albumin leads to oedema.
- Increased enzyme activities in serum indicate cell damage or increased cell proliferation.
- Isoenzymes are forms of an enzyme which are structurally different but have similar catalytic properties. Measurement of the isoenzymes of alkaline phosphatase and creatine kinase are of clinical value.

IMMUNOGLOBULINS

Immunoglobulins, or antibodies, are proteins produced by the plasma cells of the bone marrow as part of the immune response. The plasma cells are B lymphocytes transformed after exposure to a foreign (or occasionally an endogenous) antigen.

STRUCTURE

All immunoglobulins have the same basic structure and consist of two identical 'light' and two identical 'heavy' polypeptide chains, held together by disulphide bridges (Fig. 1). The 'light' chains may be either of two types: kappa or lambda. The heavy chains may be of five types: alpha, gamma, delta, epsilon and mu. The immunoglobulins are named after their heavy chain type, as IgA, IgG, IgD, IgE and IgM.

The molecules are characterized by two functional areas:

- The *Fab*, or *variable end* is the area which recognizes and binds to the antigen.
- The *Fc end*, is responsible for interaction with other components of the immune system, e.g. complement and T helper cells.

The various classes of immunoglobulins have different tertiary structure and functions (Table 1). The major antibodies in the plasma are IgG, IgA and IgM.

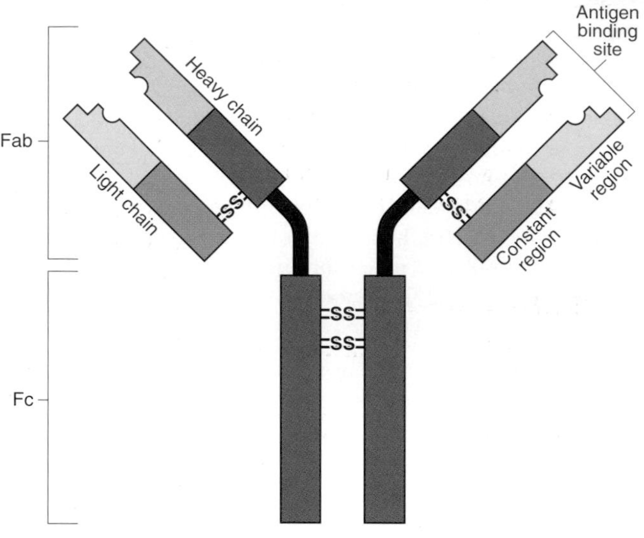

Fig. 1 **Structure of an immunoglobulin.**

ELECTROPHORESIS OF SERUM PROTEINS

Electrophoresis may be carried out to study a number of protein abnormalities. The normal pattern is shown in Figure 2(a). Immunoglobulins are detected primarily in the gamma globulin area on electrophoresis. Serum should be used for electrophoresis, as the fibrinogen of plasma gives a discrete band which can easily be mistaken for a paraprotein. Electrophoresis can show gross deficiency or excess of immunoglobulins and whether discrete bands (paraproteins) are present. (Figs 2b and c). A quantitative measure of each protein class may be obtained by scanning the electrophoresis strip (Fig. 3).

Table 1 **Classes of Immunoglobulin**

Immunoglobulin	Structure	Location	Action
IgG	Monomer	ECF	Neutralizes toxins, activates complement
IgA	Dimer	ECF+secretions	Antimicrobial
IgM	Pentamer	Mainly intravascular	First to be made in immune response
IgD	Monomer	ECF+cell membrane	Cell surface antigen receptors
IgE	Monomer	ECF	Antiallergenic, antiparasitic

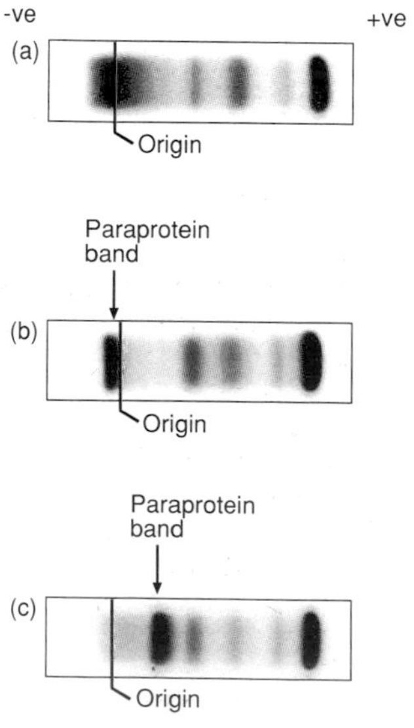

Fig. 2 **Electrophoresis of serum proteins. (a)** Normal pattern; **(b)** and **(c)** sera with paraprotein bands.

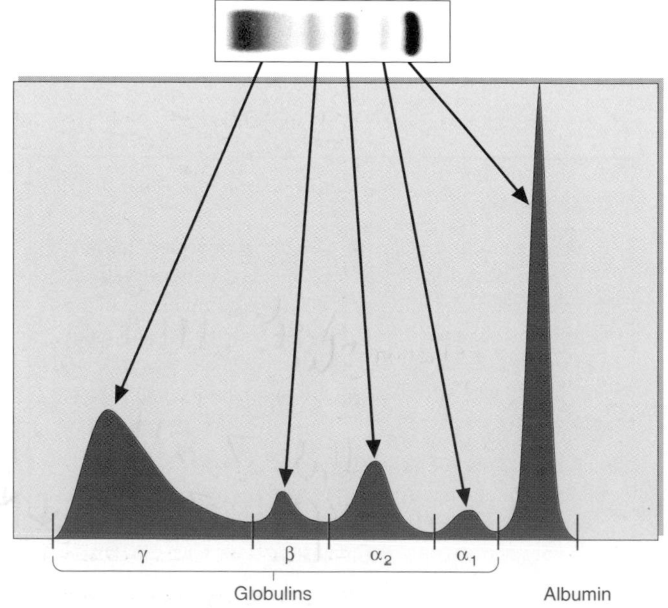

Fig. 3 **Scan of an electrophoresis strip.**

MEASUREMENT

Immunoglobulins may be measured in a number of ways, the necessity for the request often being triggered by an observed increase in the 'globulin' fraction (p. 44). If an abnormality is detected, then the particular type of immunoglobulin, or indeed of light or heavy chains where these are produced alone, may be confirmed by immunofixation or quantitatively by other means.

INCREASED IMMUNOGLOBULINS

Immunoglobulins may be increased non-specifically in a wide variety of infections and also in autoimmune disease. This increased synthesis comes from a number of cell lines, each producing its own specific immunoglobulin. The response is therefore said to be 'polyclonal' and results in a diffuse increase in protein mass throughout the gamma globulin region on electrophoresis. In contrast, cells from a single clone all make identical antibodies. As the cells multiply the immunoglobulin production becomes large enough to be observed on electrophoresis as a single discrete band. This may be an intact immunoglobulin or a fragment and is called a paraprotein.

Paraproteins

Paraproteins are found in myeloma, in Waldenström's macroglobulinaemia and in heavy chain diseases. These are malignant conditions. The paraproteins may arise from any of the immunoglobulin classes. Monoclonal light chains are produced in excess of heavy chains in 50% of cases of myeloma, and in 15% of cases only light chains are found. These light chains are small enough to spill into the urine where they are known as Bence–Jones protein. Serum electrophoresis may not show the presence of light chains, and urine electrophoresis after concentration may be required to demonstrate the paraprotein.

Myeloma is characterized by bony metastases, and bone pain is often the presenting symptom. In the face of increasing synthesis of abnormal immunoglobulins, other bone marrow function is reduced, and there is a decline in red and white cell and platelet formation and decreased production of normal immunoglobulins. Anaemia and susceptibility to infection are the consequences. Treatment of myeloma involves the use of bone marrow suppressive drugs. Plasmapheresis (replacement of the patient's plasma with normal plasma, with retention of his or her own cellular components) has been used in the treatment of myeloma and macroglobulinaemia.

Occasionally paraproteins are found in patients where there is no associated pathology. This is called benign paraproteinaemia, but such a diagnosis should be made only after the possibility of myeloma has been excluded by the failure of the disease to progress, as gauged by no increase in the concentration of the paraprotein in serum with time. Regular and careful follow-up of such patients is required.

Table 2 **Causes of hypogammaglobulinaemia**

Type	Specific causes
Physiological	Levels of IgA and IgM are low at birth
Genetic	Bruton's X-linked agammaglobulinopathy
Acquired	Malnutrition Malignancy Infections, e.g. HIV, measles Immunosuppressant drugs, e.g. azathioprine, cyclosporine

DEFICIENCIES OR ABSENCE OF IMMUNOGLOBULINS

Deficiencies or absence of immunoglobulins can occur as a result of infection, genetic abnormalities or the effects of therapy (Table 2). Where the situation is irreversible, replacement therapy has been used, either by addition of immunoglobulin-rich plasma or by the transplanting of bone marrow containing competent plasma cells.

Case history 19

A 45-year-old man presented with severe back pain and malaise. He had lost 3 kg weight in 3 months. His blood film showed many primitive RBCs and WBCs. His bone marrow biopsy showed an excess of plasma cells. He did not have a paraprotein band on serum electrophoresis. Analysis of concentrated urine revealed an excess of free monoclonal light chains.

- What is the diagnosis?

Comment on page 154.

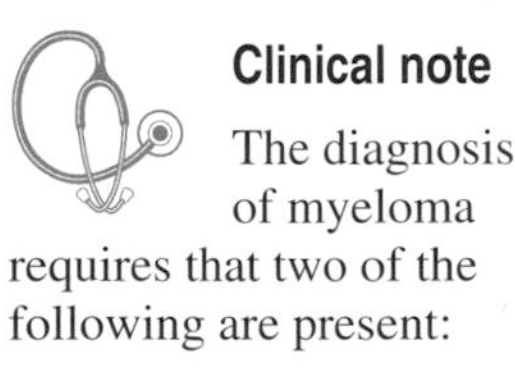

Clinical note

The diagnosis of myeloma requires that two of the following are present:

- a paraprotein in serum or urine
- plasma cell infiltration in bone marrow
- radiological evidence of bone lesions (Fig. 4).

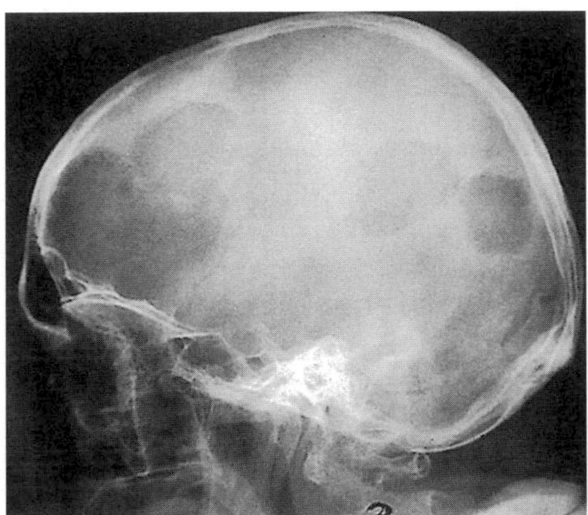

Fig. 4 **Skull X-ray showing myeloma.**

Immunoglobulins

- Electrophoresis of serum may confirm the presence of a paraprotein in a specimen from a patient with a raised globulin fraction.
- Some myelomas produce immunological light chains only. This is best demonstrated by urine electrophoresis.
- Immunoglobulin measurements can give information on:
  - immune deficiency
  - response to infection.
- Serial study of immunoglobulin levels can be of help in following the progression of disease or in monitoring of treatment.

MYOCARDIAL INFARCTION

Myocardial infarction (MI), also known as coronary thrombosis, is one of the commonest causes of mortality and morbidity in adults. MI is usually diagnosed by a history of crushing chest pain, characteristic ECG changes and cardiac muscle enzyme release.

PATHOLOGY

MI occurs when the supply of blood to the coronary muscle is reduced below a critical value, usually as a result of atheromatous plaque rupture and overlying thrombosis. This may be presaged by less catastrophic episodes of chest pain (angina pectoris) due to reduction of coronary perfusion caused by the narrowing of the arteries by atheromatous plaque (Fig. 1).

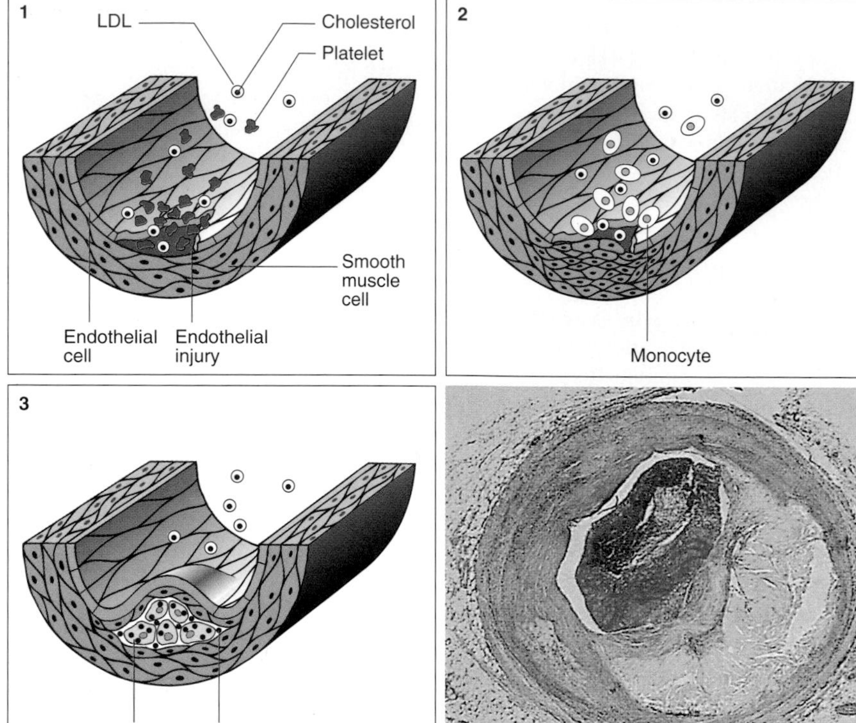

Fig. 1 **Development of atheroma in coronary arteries, with histopathological section (bottom right).**

DIAGNOSIS

Diagnosis is often well indicated by the history, although there are other sources of apparent cardiac pain. ECG changes characteristic of an MI are normally observed. However, the characteristic ECG pattern may not be present for up to 24 h after the infarction.The changes from a normal ECG to an uncomplicated infarction pattern vary somewhat with the site and degree of the area of damage. A typical change is shown in Figure 2. A new infarction in a previously damaged heart will give an ECG pattern which is more difficult to interpret.

Early diagnosis is important, since the earlier the treatment is begun, the better the prognosis. Treatment with streptokinase or other agents which reduce intravascular thrombosis should not be started unless a definite diagnosis has been made.

Biochemical tests complement the ECG findings. Three enzymes are commonly used in the diagnosis and follow-up of the MI. These are:

- creatine kinase (CK)
- aspartate aminotransferase (AST)
- lactate dehydrogenase (LDH).

The activity of these enzymes in serum following an MI is shown in Figure 3. Creatine kinase levels rise rapidly, peaking at 24 h, with slower rises being shown by AST and LDH. The more rapid fall in CK also allows for its use in the diagnosis of re-infarction, which sometimes occurs in patients while still in hospital. Note that in the first four hours after the infarction the enzymes may not be raised.

While there is a relationship between the size of the infarction and the amount of enzyme released into the plasma, the use of enzyme levels to predict the severity of the infarction has not proved very useful in practice. This is usually gauged by assessing cardiac function after the patient has stabilized. The development of cardiac arrhythmias, which is influenced by the site as well as the size

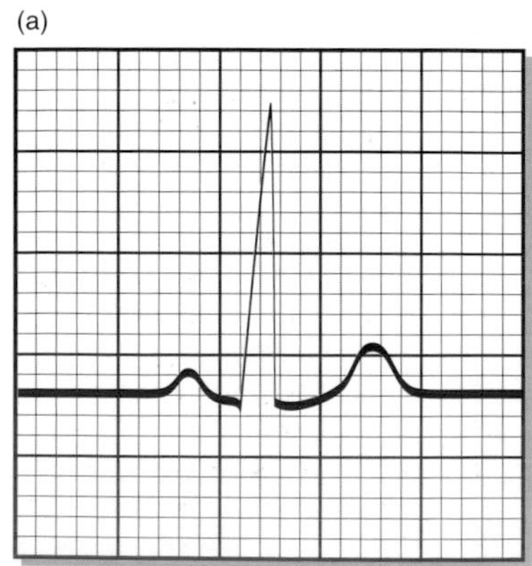

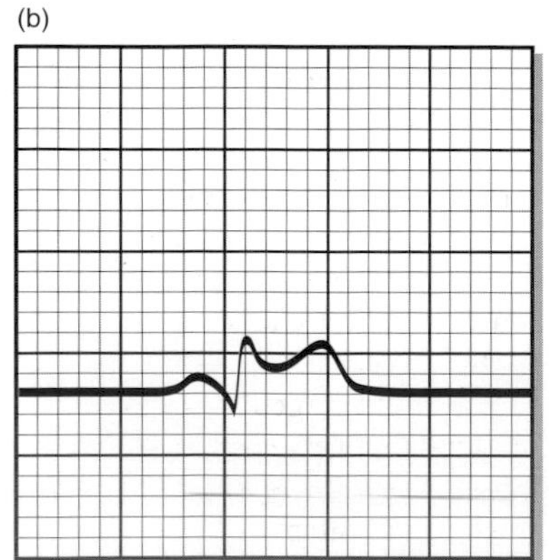

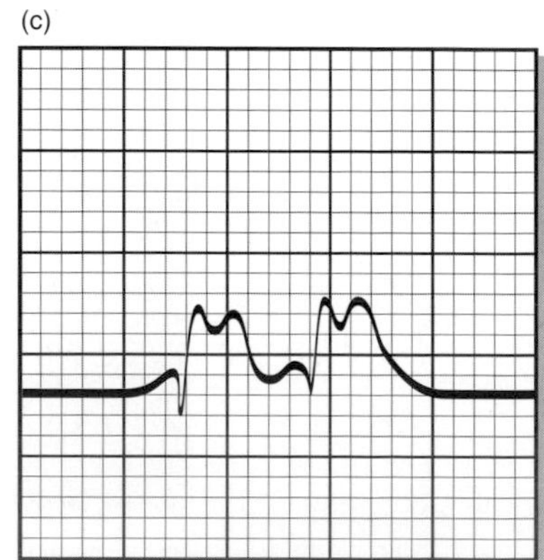

Fig. 2 **ECG changes following an MI. (a)** Normal ECG. **(b)** 2 hr after onset of chest pain. Note elevated ST segment. **(c)** 24 hr later the patient had a further episode of chest pain.

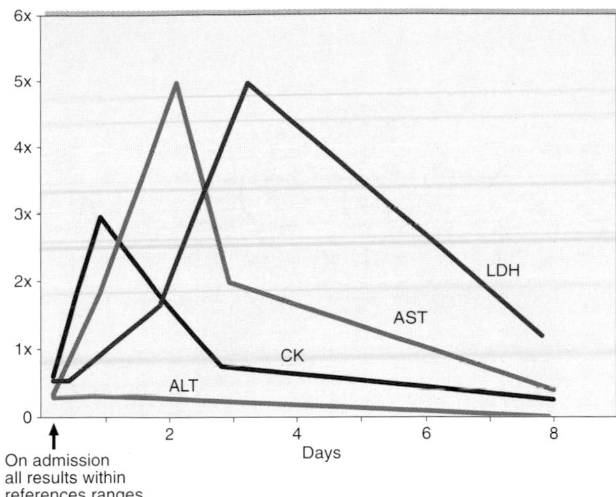

Fig. 3 **Enzymes in serum following an uncomplicated MI.**

of the infarction, is a major determinant of death in these patients.

Creatine kinase

CK is also released from damaged skeletal muscle. Although the predominant isoenzyme in cardiac muscle cells is the same as that in skeletal muscle (CK-MM), heart cells contain another CK isoenzyme, CK-MB. This isoenzyme is a more specific indicator of cardiac muscle damage, and is increasingly used (rather than total CK) in the investigation of MI.

Aspartate and alanine aminotransferases

AST release is not specific to MI, but is also found in many acute pathologies affecting the liver and skeletal muscle. The enzyme alanine aminotransferase (ALT) is sometimes measured as part of the 'cardiac enzyme' profile of tests (Fig. 3). ALT is found in high concentration in liver rather than muscle, and a normal ALT in the face of a raised AST confirms that liver pathology is not contributing to the raised enzyme levels. Approximately 25% of patients with pulmonary embolus, which features in the differential diagnosis of MI and which may or may not cause chest pain, show a raised AST concentration, and most also show an elevated LDH.

Lactate dehydrogenase

Like the other enzymes used in the diagnosis of MI, LDH is not specific to cardiac muscle, being found in liver and red cells. Although there is a measurable difference between the LDH_1 isoenzyme in heart and the LDH_5 isoenzyme in liver, the red cells can also release LDH_1. Blood for LDH measurement must therefore not be allowed to remain unseparated before analysis, or in vitro haemolysis will invalidate the LDH measurements.

Other biochemical indicators

Two other tests which are proving useful in MI are:

- *Myoglobin.* Detectable 1–3 hrs after infarction. It may be the earliest indicator of such an event and, as such, is useful for triage of chest pain patients who are seen in the emergency department.
- *Troponin I and T.* Cardiac troponins I and T are highly sensitive and specific markers for acute MI. Like CK-MB they are released from damaged cardiac muscle cells within 3–12 hrs of the infarction, but they remain elevated for much longer.
  Troponin T may take 2 weeks to return to normal levels, while increases in troponin I resolve within 5–10 days.
  The troponins have been used successfully in the diagnosis of MI and in the risk stratification of patients with unstable angina.

These molecular markers of myocardial necrosis are being increasingly used in clinical practice, but there is still debate about which is the preferred marker.

SUPPORT FOLLOWING MI

The progression of coronary heart disease can be significantly delayed and reversed in patients with established disease. In addition to treating any arrhythmias, heart failure or residual angina, patients may have modifiable risk factors such as hyperlipidaemia, diabetes mellitus, hypertension and smoking, which with appropriate treatment and counselling may be minimized.

Case history 20

A 52-year-old man presented at the Accident and Emergency department with severe chest pain which had been present for the past hour. He had previously attended the chest pain clinic and had a 2-year history of angina of effort.

- What specific tests would you request from the biochemistry laboratory?

Comment on page 154.

Clinical note

The classical feature of a myocardial infarction is crushing chest pain radiating down the left arm. Not all patients with an MI experience this. In addition to the many variants of angina-like pain, it is recognized that a sizeable proportion of MIs are 'silent', and are subsequently only detected by ECG.

In one European heart study, 2% of middle-aged men showed definite ECG evidence of a previously unrecognized myocardial infarction.

Myocardial infarction

- To make a diagnosis of myocardial infarction, two of the following must be present:
  - severe chest pain
  - ECG changes indicative of myocardial infarction
  - cardiac enzyme release.
- The cardiac enzymes are creatine kinase, aspartate aminotransferase and lactate dehydrogenase.
- A specific CK isoenzyme (CK-MB) is a more specific indicator of cardiac muscle damage than total CK, and can be detected in serum soon after an MI has occurred.
- Cardiac troponins are used as specific markers in MI and unstable angina.
- Early diagnosis of MI is important so that therapy can be started promptly.

LIVER FUNCTION TESTS

INTRODUCTION

The liver plays a major role in protein, carbohydrate and lipid homeostasis (Fig. 1). The metabolic pathways of glycolysis, the Krebs cycle, amino acid synthesis and degradation, and the processes of oxidative phosphorylation are all carried out in the hepatocytes which are well endowed with mitochondria. The liver contains an extensive reticulo-endothelial system for the synthesis and breakdown of blood cells. Liver cells metabolize, detoxify and excrete both endogenous and exogenous compounds. Excretion of water-soluble end products from the metabolism of both nutrients and toxins, and of digestive aids such as bile acids, occurs into the biliary tree.

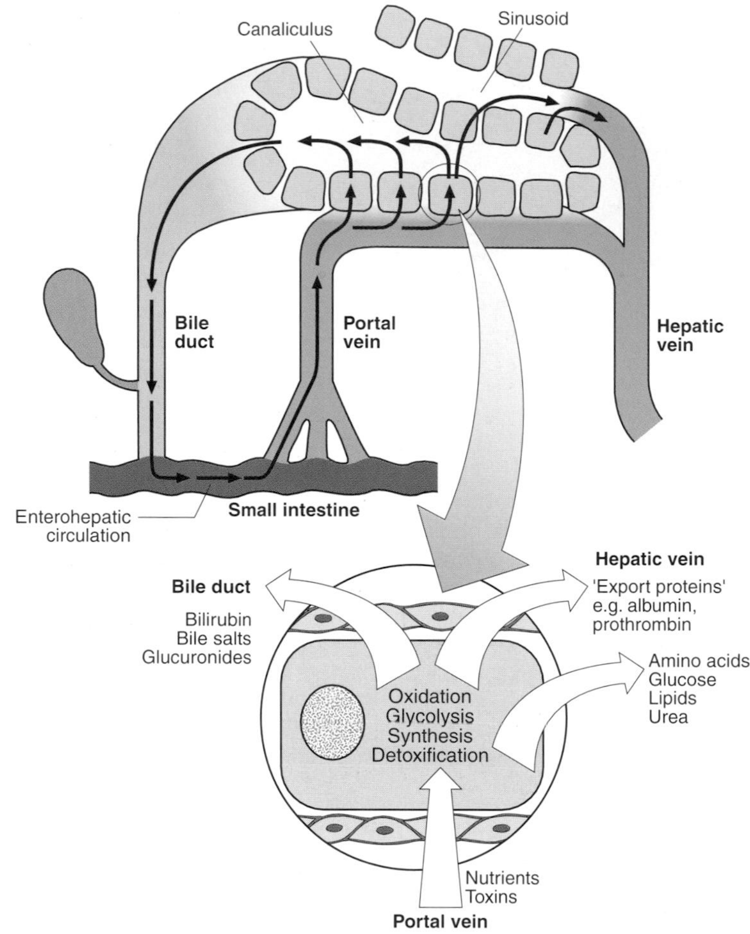

Fig. 1 **Liver function.**

LIVER FUNCTION TESTS

What are usually called liver function tests (LFTs) do not assess quantitatively the capacity of that tissue to carry out any of the functions which are described above. 'LFTs' are measurements of blood components which simply provide a lead to the existence, the extent and the type of liver damage. Usually, a request for LFTs will provide results for bilirubin, the aminotransferases and alkaline phosphatase in a serum specimen. Knowledge of the serum albumin concentration may also be of some value in the investigation of liver disease. These biochemical investigations can assist in differentiating the following:

- obstruction to the biliary tract
- acute hepatocellular damage
- chronic liver disease.

Serum total bilirubin concentration and serum alkaline phosphatase activity are indices of cholestasis, a blockage of bile flow. The serum aminotransferase activities are a measure of the integrity of liver cells. The serum albumin concentration is a crude measure of the liver's synthetic capacity, although it is affected by many other factors.

Bilirubin

Bilirubin is derived from haem, an iron-containing protoporphyrin mainly found in haemoglobin (Fig. 2). An adult normally produces about 450 μmol of bilirubin daily. It is insoluble in water and is transported in plasma almost totally bound to albumin. It is taken up by liver cells and conjugated to form mono- and di-glucuronides which are much more soluble in water than unconjugated bilirubin. The conjugated bilirubin is excreted into the bile. Normal bile contains bilirubin monoglucuronide as 25% and the diglucuronide as 75% of the total, accompanied by traces of unconjugated bilirubin. The main functional constituents of the bile are the bile salts which are involved in fat digestion and absorption from the small intestine. Serum bile acid concentrations are more sensitive indices of hepatic transport function than are total bilirubin measurements.

In the terminal ileum and colon the bilirubin conjugates are attacked by bacteria to form a group of compounds which are known collectively as *stercobilinogen*, most of which are excreted in faeces. Some are absorbed and eventually re-excreted from the body by way of bile. Small amounts of these tetrapyrroles are found in urine in which they are known as *urobilinogen*.

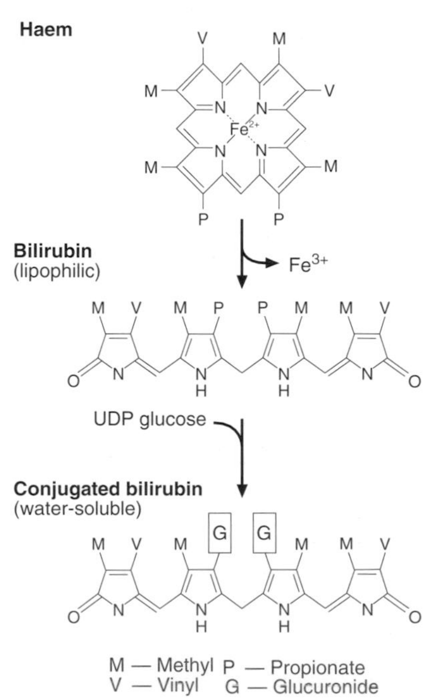

Fig. 2 **Structure of bilirubin and conjugated bilirubin.**

When the biliary tract becomes blocked, bilirubin is not excreted and serum concentrations rise. The patient becomes jaundiced. The jaundiced patient is described further on pages 52–53.

The aminotransferases (AST and ALT)

The activities of two aminotransferases, AST and ALT, are widely used in clinical practice as a sensitive, albeit non-specific index, of acute damage to hepatocytes irrespective of its aetiology. Causes of liver damage include hepatitis, no matter the causative agent, and toxic injury which may accompany any one of a large number of insults to the liver, including drug overdose. Acute liver damage due to shock, severe hypoxia and acute cardiac failure are also seen (see pp. 54–55).

Alkaline phosphatase (ALP)

Increases in alkaline phosphatase activity in liver disease are the result of increased synthesis of the enzyme by cells lining the bile canaliculi, usually in response to cholestasis, which may be either intra- or extra-hepatic. Cholestasis, even of short duration, results in an increased enzyme activity to at least twice the upper end of the reference interval. High alkaline phosphatase activity may also occur in infiltrative diseases of the liver, when space occupying lesions (e.g. tumours) are present. It also occurs in cirrhosis.

Liver is not the sole source of alkaline phosphatase activity. Substantial amounts are present in bone, small intestine, placenta and kidney. In normal blood, the alkaline phosphatase activity is derived mainly from bone and liver, with small amounts from intestine. Placental alkaline phosphatase appears in the maternal blood in the third trimester of pregnancy. Occasionally, the cause of a raised alkaline phosphatase will not be immediately apparent. The liver and bone isoenzymes can be separated by electrophoresis. However, an elevated γGT (see below) would suggest that the liver is the source of the increased alkaline phosphatase.

Case history 21

A 60-year-old female with a history of breast carcinoma treated by mastectomy three years previously is now complaining of general malaise and bone pain. Biochemistry showed that fluid and electrolytes, total protein, albumin and calcium values were all normal. LFTs were as follows:

Bilirubin	AST	ALT	Alkaline phosphatase	γGT
μmol/l	*U/l*			
7	33	38	890	32

- Evaluate these results and suggest a likely diagnosis.

Comment on page 154.

Gamma glutamyl transpeptidase (γGT)

γGT is a microsomal enzyme which is widely distributed in tissues including liver and renal tubules. The activity of γGT in plasma is raised whenever there is cholestasis, and it is a very sensitive index of liver pathology. It is also affected by ingestion of alcohol, even in the absence of recognizable liver disease. Drugs such as phenytoin induce enzyme activity. In acute hepatic damage, changes in γGT activity parallel those of the aminotransferases.

Plasma proteins

Albumin is the major protein product of the liver. It has a long biological half-life in plasma (15-19 days), and therefore significant falls in albumin concentration are slow to occur if synthesis is suddenly reduced. Hypoalbuminaemia is a feature of advanced chronic liver disease. It can also occur in *severe* acute liver damage.

The prothrombin time, which is a measure of the activities of certain coagulation factors made by the liver, is sometimes used as an indicator of hepatic synthetic function. Prothrombin has a very short half-life, and an increased prothrombin time may be the earliest indicator of hepatocellular damage.

The total serum globulin concentration is sometimes used as a crude measure of the severity of liver disease.

Alpha-fetoprotein (AFP) is synthesized by the fetal liver. In normal adults it is present in plasma at low concentrations (<20 μg/l). Measurement of AFP is of value in the investigation of hepatocellular carcinoma in which serum concentrations are increased in 80–90% of cases. AFP is also used as a marker for germ cell tumours (pp. 130–131).

Other proteins such as α_1-antitrypsin and caeruloplasmin are measured in the diagnosis of specific diseases affecting the liver (p. 55).

Clinical note

Imaging techniques play an important role in the investigation of liver disease. The arrow highlights an area of defective isotope uptake indicating the presence of a liver metastasis in a patient with disseminated malignant disease.

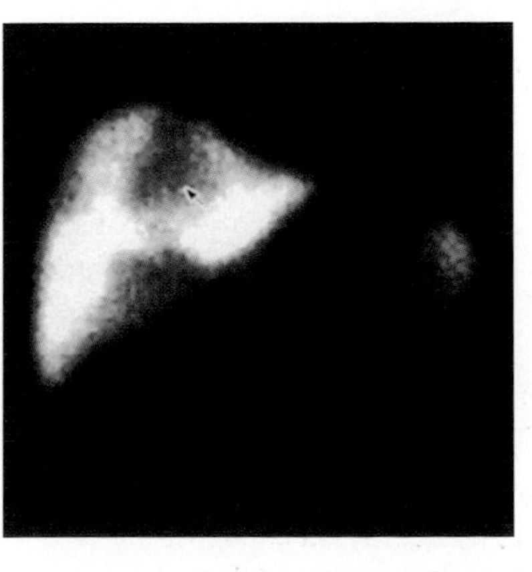
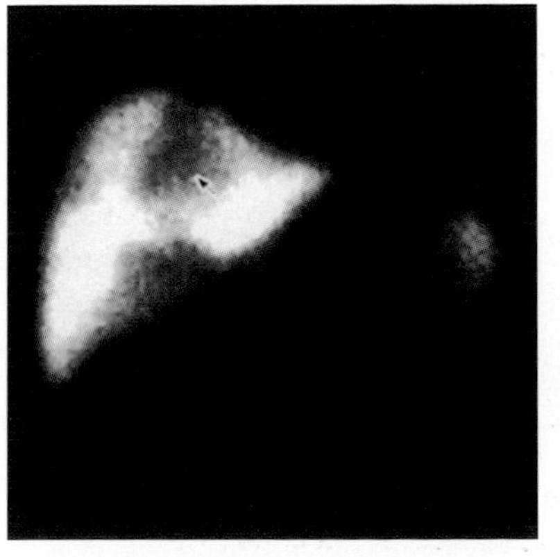

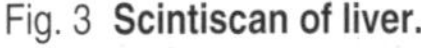
Fig. 3 **Scintiscan of liver.**

Liver function tests

- A request for LFTs will usually generate results for bilirubin, the aminotransferases and alkaline phosphatase.
- Raised activities of the aminotransferases (AST and ALT) indicate hepatocellular damage.
- Increased bilirubin concentration and increased alkaline phosphatase activity indicate the presence of cholestasis, a blockage in bile flow.
- Serial use of LFTs is of most value in following the progress or resolution of liver disease.
- Measurement of γ glutamyl transpeptidase can give an indication of hepatocellular enzyme induction due to drugs or alcohol.

JAUNDICE

Jaundice is a yellow discoloration of the skin or sclera (Fig.1). This is due to the presence of bilirubin in the plasma and is not usually detectable until the concentration is greater than about 40 μmol/l. Normally the bilirubin concentration in plasma is less than 22 μmol/l.

Bilirubin is derived from the tetrapyrrole prosthetic group found in haemoglobin and the cytochromes. It is normally conjugated with glucuronic acid to make it more soluble, and excreted in the bile (Fig. 2). There are three main reasons why bilirubin levels in the blood may rise (Fig. 3):

- *Haemolysis*. The increased haemoglobin breakdown produces bilirubin which overloads the conjugating mechanism.
- *Failure of the conjugating mechanism within the hepatocyte.*
- *Obstruction in the biliary system.*

Both conjugated bilirubin and unconjugated bilirubin may be present in plasma. Conjugated bilirubin is water soluble. Unconjugated bilirubin is not water soluble and binds to albumin from which it may be transferred to other proteins such as those in cell membranes. It is neurotoxic, and if levels rise too high in neonates, permanent brain damage can occur.

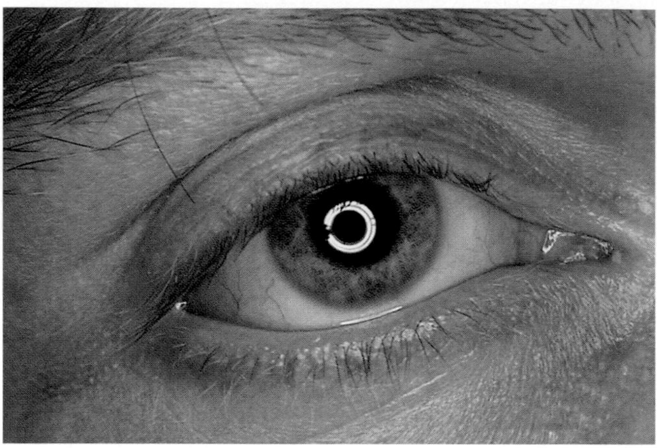

Fig. 1 **Jaundice in the sclera of an eye.**

Biochemical tests (LFTs) include measurement of serum AST and ALT as markers of hepatocellular damage, as well as bilirubin and alkaline phosphatase which are indicators of cholestasis.

BIOCHEMICAL TESTS

Bilirubin metabolites are responsible for the brown coloration of faeces. If bilirubin does not reach the gut, stools become pale in colour. Bilirubin in the gut is metabolized by bacteria to produce stercobilinogen. This is partly reabsorbed and re-excreted in the urine as urobilinogen, and may be detected by simple biochemical tests. When high levels of conjugated bilirubin are being excreted, urine may be a deep orange colour, particularly if allowed to stand.

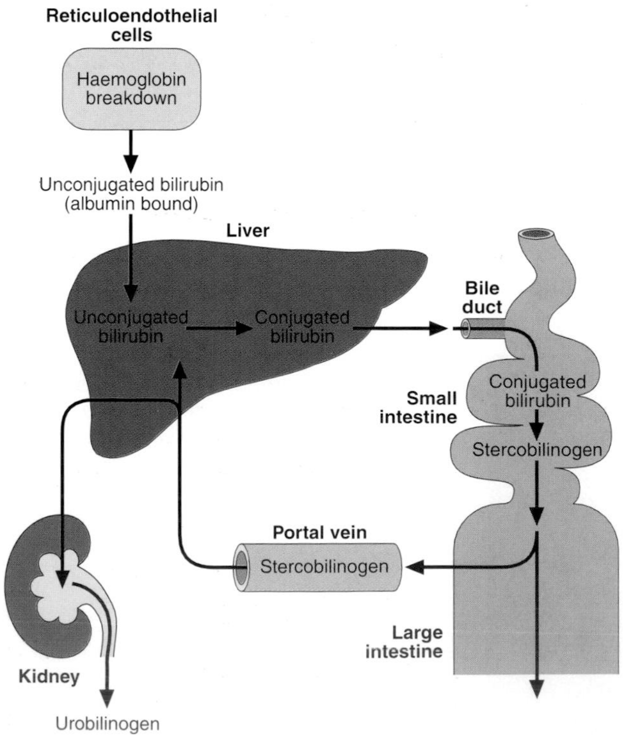

Fig. 2 **Bilirubin metabolism.**

DIFFERENTIAL DIAGNOSIS

Jaundice may be a consequence of haemolysis, cholestasis or hepatocellular damage. The causes and features of these are summarized in Figure 3 and Table 1. In addition there are inherited disorders of bilirubin metabolism. Gilbert's disease is the most common and causes a mild unconjugated hyperbilirubinaemia because of defective conjugation of bilirubin.

Table 1 **Laboratory differential diagnosis of jaundice**

	Haemolytic	Cholestatic	Hepatocellular
Features	• Bilirubin usually <75 μmol/l • No bilirubin in urine • Reticulocytosis • Haemoglobin ↓ • Haptoglobin ↓ • LDH may ↑	• Bilirubin may be ↑↑↑ • Bilirubin in urine • Alk. Phos. usually >3x upper limit of reference range • AST, ALT + LDH usually modestly ↑	• AST + ALT ↑↑ • Bilirubin ↑ later • Bilirubin in urine • Alk. Phos. ↑ later

Haemolysis

Increased bilirubin production caused by haemolysis gives a predominantly unconjugated hyperbilirubinaemia. This is commonly encountered in babies. A rapidly rising bilirubin in a neonate should be carefully monitored. If the concentration approaches 200 μmol/l, phototherapy should be used to break down the molecule and reduce the level. If the concentration rises above 300 μmol/l, exchange transfusion may be necessary.

Extrahepatic biliary obstruction

Gallstones can partially or fully block the bile duct. Such a blockage is known as extrahepatic obstruction. If the blockage is complete, both bilirubin and alkaline phosphatase are raised. There is little or no urobilinogen in urine. Stools will be pale in colour. When the obstruction is removed, the stools regain their colour and urine again becomes positive for urobilinogen. If the blockage is only partial, alkaline phosphatase may be high although serum bilirubin may well be within the reference

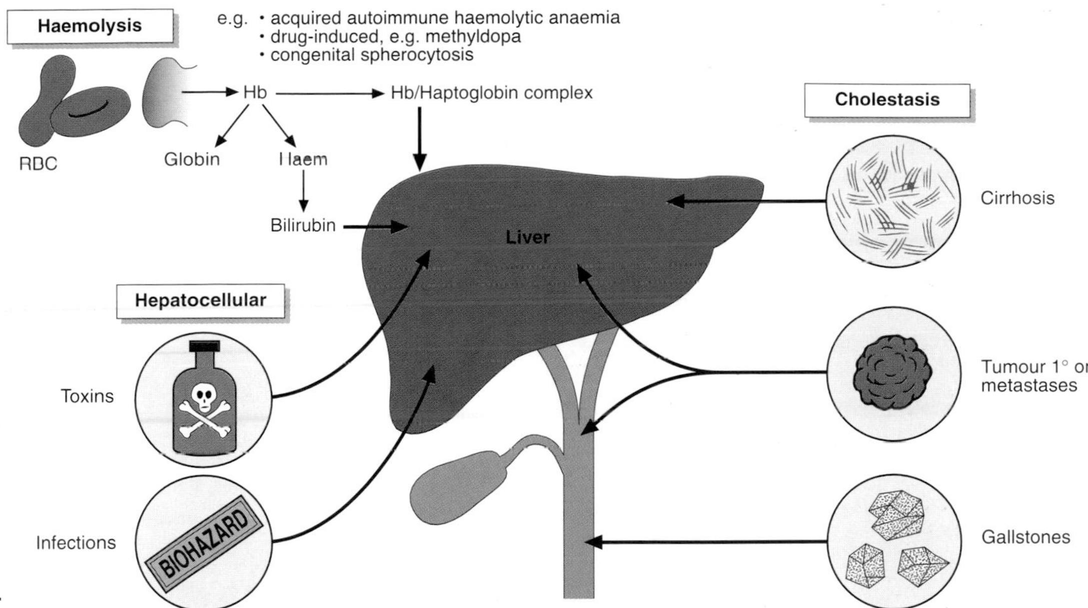

Fig. 3 **Causes of jaundice.**

range. This picture is classic of an isolated secondary neoplasm in the liver, partly disturbing the biliary tree. The normal functioning part of the liver is sufficient to process and excrete the bilirubin. The levels of alkaline phosphatase released into serum will mirror the degree of obstruction. Intrahepatic biliary obstruction is much more difficult to diagnose than extrahepatic obstruction. The bile canaliculi become blocked due to cirrhosis, liver cancer or infection. This leads to an increased concentration of conjugated bilirubin in serum.

Hepatocellular damage

Obstruction may be secondary to damage to the hepatocytes by infection or toxins, rather than damage to the biliary tract. The most common causes of acute jaundice seen in adults are viral hepatitis and paracetamol poisoning. In these cases, not only are the bilirubin and alkaline phosphatase levels raised, but AST and ALT are elevated indicating hepatocellular damage.

Clinical note

CT scanning is an invaluable tool in the investigation of the jaundiced patient. The dilated bile ducts are clearly visible in a CT scan of a patient with extrahepatic obstructive jaundice due to carcinoma of the head of the pancreas (Fig. 4).

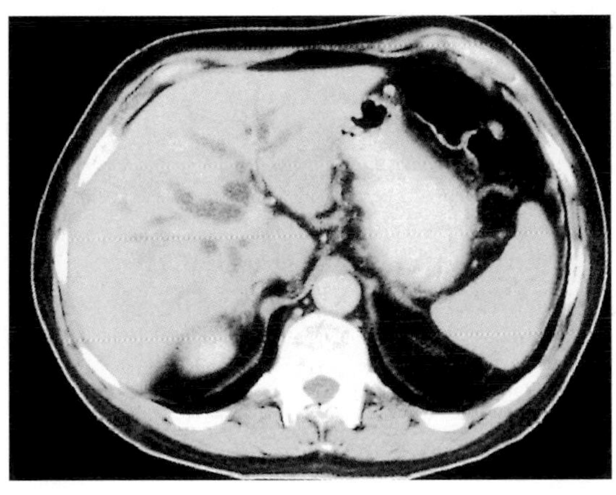

Fig. 4 **CT scan of liver and gall bladder.**

Case history 22

A 65-year-old man came to his GP's surgery with visible jaundice which he had noticed to be deepening in colour. He had no pain but had noticed some weight loss and that his stools were pale. He was a moderate drinker, and was not on any drug therapy. His LFTs were:

Bilirubin	AST	ALT	Alkaline phosphatase
μmol/l	*U/l*		
250	87	92	850

- What is the differential diagnosis?
- What other investigations would be helpful in making a diagnosis?

Comment on page 154.

Jaundice

- Jaundice indicates that there is an elevated concentration of bilirubin in serum.
- In neonates it is important to determine the concentration of unconjugated bilirubin in order to decide what treatment is required.
- In adults, the most common cause of jaundice is obstruction, and this is confirmed by the elevation of both bilirubin and alkaline phosphatase.

LIVER DISEASE

ACUTE LIVER DISEASE

Acute liver damage occurs for one of three reasons:

- poisoning
- infection
- inadequate perfusion.

INVESTIGATION

Biochemical markers of liver disease such as AST and ALT will indicate hepatocyte damage. Elevated serum bilirubin and alkaline phosphatase levels show the presence of cholestasis. Disease progression or recovery can be followed by serial measurements of LFTs.

Poisoning

The most well-documented poisons which affect the liver are paracetamol and carbon tetrachloride. These are metabolized by the intact liver in small amounts, but when present at high concentrations they give rise to toxic metabolites, leading to destruction of hepatocytes with massive release of enzymes. The capacity of the liver to withstand an insult is reduced if there is underlying liver damage due to alcohol, malnutrition or other chronic disease.

Some plant and fungal toxins can also cause catastrophic and fatal liver damage within 48 h (Fig. 1).

A third group of toxins are those which give rise to acute hepatocellular failure only in certain individuals who are susceptible. Important examples include sodium valproate, an anticonvulsant drug which gives rise to toxicity in some children, and halothane, an anaesthetic agent.

Liver infection

Both bacteria and viruses can give rise to infective hepatitis which causes many deaths worldwide. Hepatitis A, hepatitis B and hepatitis C are the most common.

OUTCOME

Acute liver damage can progress in three ways:

- It may resolve, as indeed it does in the majority of cases.
- It may progress to acute hepatic failure.
- It may lead to chronic hepatic damage.

Hepatic failure

Acute hepatic failure is a major medical emergency, since the failure of the complex metabolic functions of the liver cannot be compensated for by any other organ. In severe cases, much of the biochemical picture is disrupted. Electrolyte imbalance occurs, sodium and calcium concentrations may both fall. There may be severe metabolic acid–base disturbances and hypoglycaemia.

Hepatic failure may give rise to renal failure due to exposure of the glomeruli to toxins usually metabolized by the liver. There may be an increase in blood ammonia as a result of the failure to detoxify this to

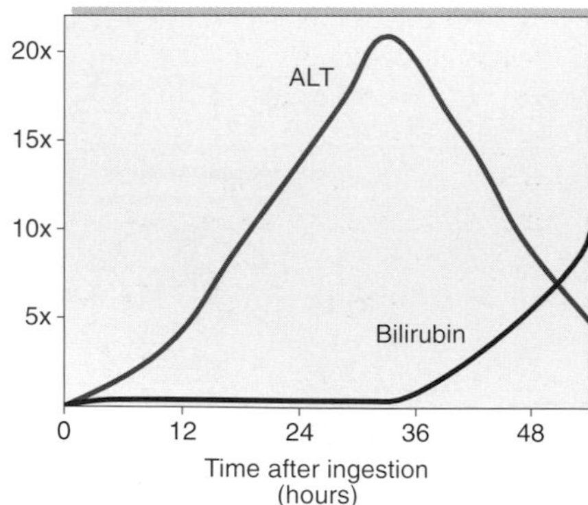

Fig. 1 **Pattern of LFTs following *Amanita phalloides* (a highly poisonous species of mushroom) toxicity.**

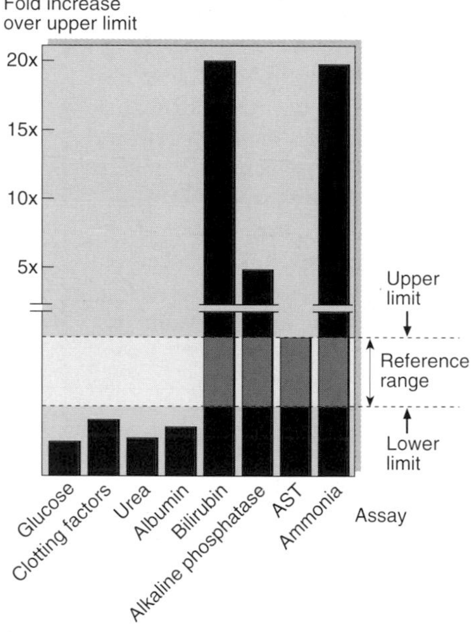

Fig. 2 **Biochemical findings in hepatic failure.**

Case history 23

A 49-year-old woman attended her GP with an 8-day history of anorexia, nausea and flu-like symptoms. She had noticed that her urine had been dark in colour over the past 2 days. Physical examination revealed tenderness in the right upper quadrant of the abdomen. LFTs were as follows:

Bilirubin	AST	ALT	Alkaline phosphatase	γGT	Total protein	Albumin
μmol/l			*U/l*		*g/l*	
63	936	2700	410	312	68	42

- Comment on these results.
- What is the differential diagnosis?

Comment on page 154.

urea. The pattern of abnormalities found in hepatic failure is shown in Figure 2.

In acute hepatocellular damage, albumin synthesis is reduced or ceases, leading to hypoalbuminaemia and the development of oedema and/or ascites. The failure of synthesis of clotting factors also leads to an increased tendency to haemorrhage or, in severe cases, to intravascular coagulation.

Recovery from acute hepatocellular damage may take some weeks, during which monitoring of LFTs is helpful in detecting relapse and assisting prognosis.

CHRONIC LIVER DISEASE

Three forms of chronic liver damage are:

- alcoholic fatty liver
- chronic active hepatitis
- primary biliary cirrhosis.

All of these conditions may progress to cirrhosis, a disease characterized by shrinking of the liver with disorganization of its architecture and the development of fibrosis in the remaining hepatocellular tissue (Fig. 3).

AETIOLOGY

Cirrhosis is the terminal stage of chronic liver damage and only occasionally follows an acute course. The most common causes of cirrhosis are:

- chronic excess alcohol ingestion
- viral hepatitis (particularly hepatitis B)
- autoimmune diseases.

Cirrhosis is not reversible, although in alcoholics the preceding stage, that of chronic fatty liver, does respond to abstention from alcohol. For reasons that are not clear, only about 30% of alcoholics progress to cirrhosis.

CLINICAL FEATURES

There are no good biochemical indicators of cirrhosis in the early and stable period which may last for many years. In the terminal stages the features include:

- developing jaundice
- encephalopathy, which may be related to toxins which are not removed from the plasma
- ascites due to reduced albumin synthesis
- bleeding tendencies
- terminal liver failure.

However, the cirrhotic liver has a reserve of function despite its macro- and microscopic appearance. The major complaints in cirrhosis may be difficulties in coping with food, especially fatty

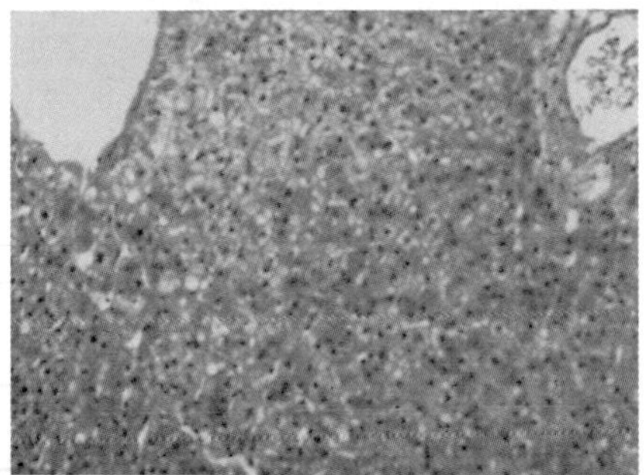

(a)

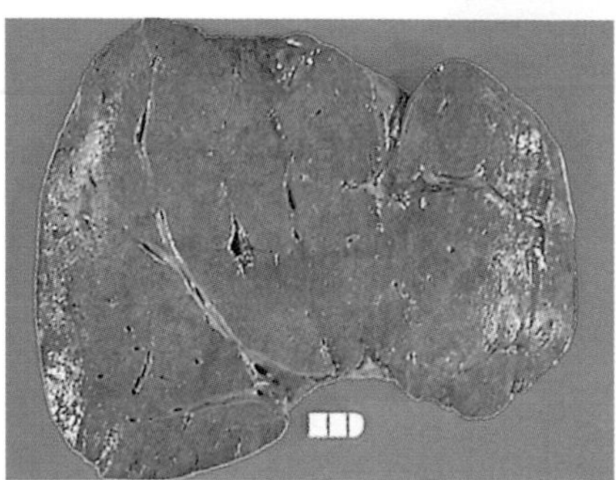

(b)

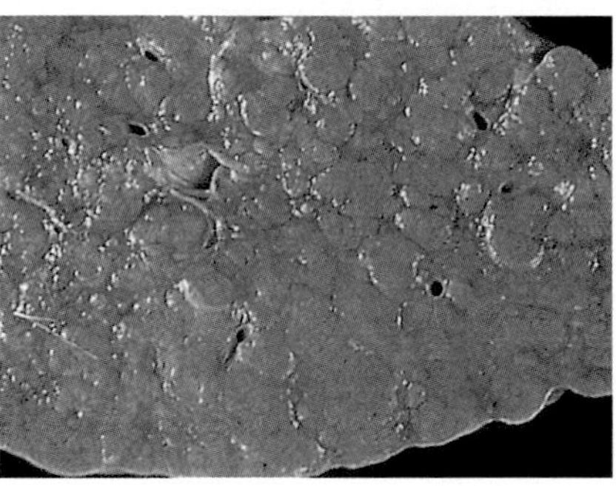

(c)

Fig. 3 **Appearance of normal and diseased liver.** **(a)** Normal liver histology. **(b)** Fatty liver. **(c)** Cirrhotic liver.

meals. Patients with cirrhosis have a reduced capacity to metabolize drugs. Some patients with cirrhosis suffer badly from itch, due to the disruption of the biliary architecture and subsequent failure to excrete bile acids, which accumulate in the skin. The immunological response of patients with cirrhosis may well be reduced, leading to increased susceptibility to infection.

UNUSUAL CAUSES OF CIRRHOSIS

Cirrhosis can develop in children as a result of α_1-antitrypsin deficiency or Wilson's disease, and in adults due to haemochromatosis. α_1-antitrypsin deficiency can be detected in newborn infants in whom there may be a prolonged period of jaundice for several weeks. In some cases this progresses to juvenile cirrhosis. Haemochromatosis is a disorder of iron absorption, associated with deposition of iron in the hepatocytes and other tissues which can lead to liver failure. The diagnosis is by measurement of serum iron, transferrin and ferritin (p. 107). Wilson's disease is an inherited disorder of copper metabolism which leads to failure in copper excretion, low concentrations of caeruloplasmin, and deposition of copper in the liver and other tissues (p. 108).

OTHER LIVER PROBLEMS

The liver is a common site of secondary metastases from a wide variety of primary tumours, and jaundice may be the first indication of the presence of cancer in some patients.

Primary hepatoma is associated with a number of conditions such as cirrhosis or hepatitis, although a number of causative carcinogens, such as aflatoxins generated by specific fungi infecting foodstuffs, have been identified. Alpha-fetoprotein is a useful marker of primary hepatic tumours (pp. 130–131).

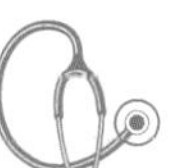

Clinical note

Liver biopsy is the most important way of making a specific diagnosis. Before attempting a needle biopsy it is essential that the patient's blood coagulation status is confirmed to be satisfactory.

Liver disease

- Acute liver damage is caused by shock, toxins or infection.
- Biochemical monitoring of liver disease is by sequential measurements of the aminotransferases, bilirubin and alkaline phosphatase.
- In acute liver damage there is usually intrahepatic obstruction as well as hepatocellular damage.
- Severe cases of acute liver damage may progress to hepatocellular failure.
- Cirrhosis is the end point of both acute and chronic liver damage, as well as being caused by a number of metabolic and autoimmune diseases.
- Biochemical tests may be of little value in making a specific diagnosis. A liver biopsy is frequently more helpful.

GLUCOSE METABOLISM AND DIABETES MELLITUS

Dietary carbohydrate is digested in the gastrointestinal tract to simple monosaccharides which are then absorbed. Starch provides glucose directly, while fructose (from dietary sucrose) and galactose (from dietary lactose) are absorbed and also converted into glucose in the liver. Glucose is the common carbohydrate currency of the body. Figure 1 shows the different metabolic processes which affect the blood glucose concentration. This level is, as always, the result of a balance between input and output, synthesis and catabolism.

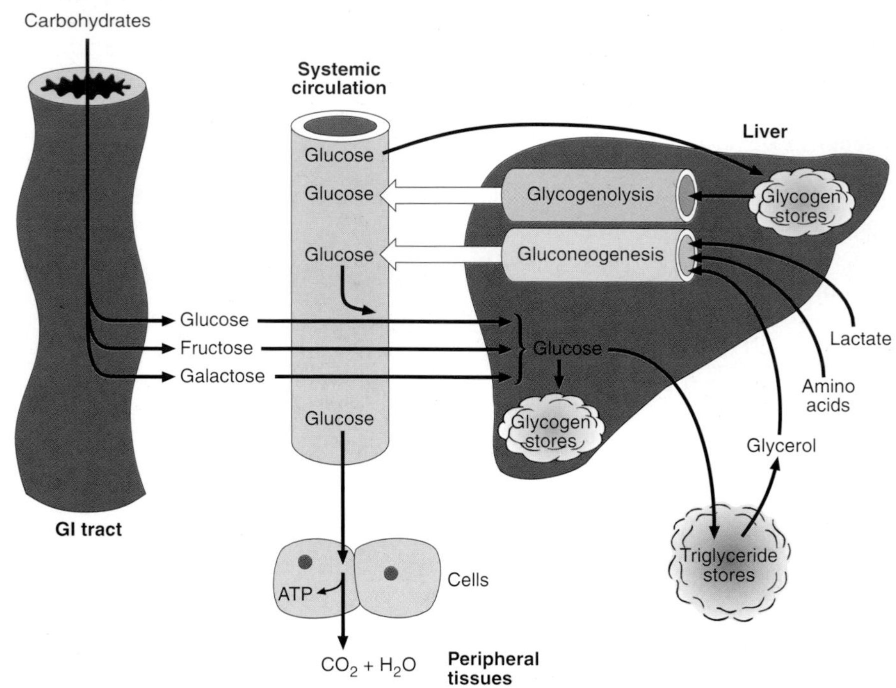

Fig. 1 **Glucose homeostasis.**

INSULIN

Insulin is the principal hormone affecting blood glucose levels, and an understanding of its actions is an important prerequisite to the study of diabetes mellitus. Insulin is a small protein synthesized in the beta cells of the islets of Langerhans of the pancreas. It acts through membrane receptors and its main target tissues are liver, muscle and adipose tissue.

The overall effect of insulin is to promote cellular uptake and storage of metabolic fuels and these actions are shown in Figure 2. It should be noted that glucose cannot enter the cells of most body tissues in the absence of insulin.

The effects of insulin are opposed by other hormones, glucagon, adrenaline, glucocorticoids and growth hormone. The blood glucose concentration is the result of a balance between these different endocrine forces.

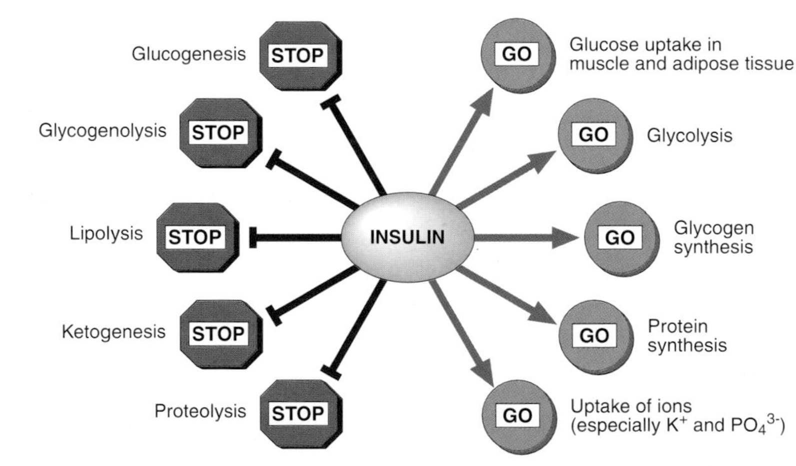

Fig. 2 **The actions of insulin.**

DIABETES MELLITUS

Diabetes mellitus is the commonest endocrine disorder encountered in clinical practice. It may be defined as a syndrome characterized by hyperglycaemia due to an absolute or relative lack of insulin and/or insulin resistance.

Primary diabetes mellitus is generally subclassified into insulin dependent diabetes mellitus (IDDM) or non-insulin dependent diabetes mellitus (NIDDM). These clinical entities differ in epidemiology, clinical features and pathophysiology. The contrasting features of IDDM and NIDDM are shown in Table 1.

Secondary diabetes mellitus may result from pancreatic disease, endocrine disease such as Cushing's syndrome, drug therapy, and, rarely, insulin receptor abnormalities.

Insulin dependent diabetes mellitus (IDDM)

IDDM accounts for approximately 15% of all diabetics. It can occur at any age but is most common in the young, with a peak incidence between 9 and 14 years of age. The absolute lack of insulin is a consequence of the autoimmune destruction of insulin-producing beta cells. There may be an environmental precipitating factor such as a viral infection. The presence of islet cell antibodies in serum predicts future development of diabetes.

Table 1 **Insulin dependent diabetes mellitus (IDDM) versus non-insulin dependent diabetes mellitus (NIDDM).**

Main Features	IDDM	NIDDM
Epidemiology		
Frequency in Northern Europe	0.02–0.4%	1–3%
Predominance	N. European Caucasians	Worldwide Lowest in rural areas of developing countries
Clinical Characteristics		
Age	<30yrs	>40yrs
Weight	Low	Normal or increased
Onset	Rapid	Slow
Ketosis	Common	Under stress
Endogenous insulin	Low/absent	Present
HLA associations	Yes	No
Islet cell antibodies	Yes	No
Pathophysiology		
Aetiology	Autoimmune destruction of pancreatic islet cells	Unclear. Impaired insulin secretion and insulin resistance
Genetic associations	Polygenic	Strong
Environmental factors	Viruses and toxins implicated	Obesity, physical inactivity

Non-insulin dependent diabetes mellitus (NIDDM)

NIDDM accounts for approximately 85% of all diabetics and can occur at any age. It is most common between 40 and 80 years. In this condition there is resistance of peripheral tissues to the actions of insulin, so that the insulin level may be normal or even high. Obesity is the most commonly associated clinical feature.

LATE COMPLICATIONS OF DIABETES MELLITUS

Diabetes mellitus is not only characterized by the presence of hyperglycaemia but also by the occurrence of late complications:

- *Microangiopathy* is defined as abnormalities in the walls of small blood vessels, the most prominent feature of which is thickening of the basement membrane.
- *Retinopathy* may lead to blindness because of vitreous haemorrhage from proliferating retinal vessels, and maculopathy as a result of exudates from vessels or oedema affecting the macula (Fig. 3).
- *Nephropathy* leads ultimately to renal failure. In the early stage there is kidney hyperfunction, associated with an increased GFR, increased glomerular size and microalbuminuria. In the late stage, there is increasing proteinuria and a marked decline in renal function, resulting in uraemia.
- *Neuropathy* may become evident as diarrhoea, postural hypotension, impotence, neurogenic bladder and neuropathic foot ulcers due to microangiopathy of nerve blood vessels and abnormal glucose metabolism in nerve cells.
- *Macroangiopathy (or accelerated atherosclerosis)* leads to premature coronary heart disease. The exact mechanisms for increased susceptibility to atherosclerosis in diabetics are unknown; however, hyperlipidaemia and increased protein glycation may play a role. The most common form of hyperlipidaemia observed in diabetics is hypertriglyceridaemia with increased plasma VLDL-cholesterol and decreased HDL-cholesterol.

Approximately 60% of diabetic patients die of vascular disease and 35% of coronary heart disease. Blindness is 25 times and chronic renal failure 17 times more common in the diabetic. There is increasing evidence that tight glycaemic control delays the onset of these sequelae.

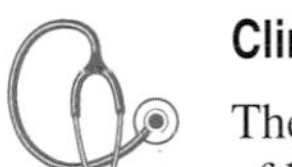

Clinical note

The clinical symptoms of hyperglycaemia include polyuria, polydipsia, lassitude, weight loss, pruritus vulvae and balanitis. These symptoms are common to both NIDDM and IDDM but are more pronounced in IDDM. It is important to remember that patients with NIDDM may be completely asymptomatic.

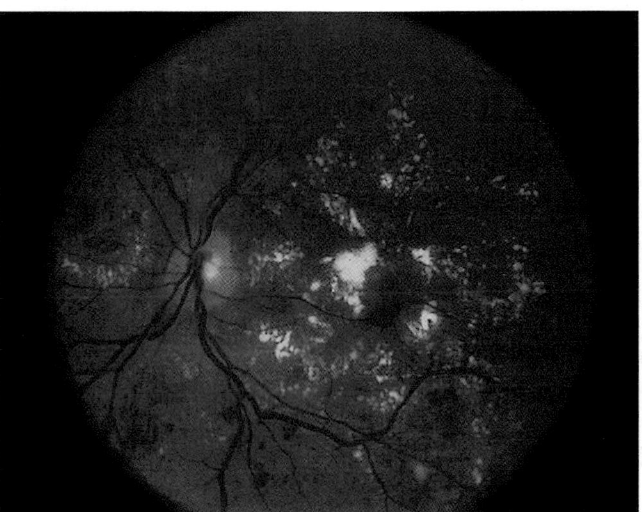

Fig. 3 **Diabetic retinopathy**

Glucose metabolism and diabetes mellitus

- Glucose is the carbohydrate currency of the body, all other carbohydrates being converted to glucose after digestion and absorption.
- Insulin controls blood glucose by promoting the storage of metabolic fuels.
- Diabetes mellitus is characterized by hyperglycaemia, absolute or relative insulin lack and late complications.
- Insulin dependent diabetes mellitus (IDDM) is caused by a complete lack of insulin and is most common in the young.
- Non-insulin dependent diabetes mellitus (NIDDM) accounts for 85% of all diabetics and can occur at any age.
- Late complications of diabetes mellitus are a result of micro- and macroangiopathies.

DIAGNOSIS AND MONITORING OF DIABETES MELLITUS

The diagnosis of diabetes mellitus must be made with care since it has far-reaching medical and social consequences. A number of biochemical tests are used in association with clinical assessment both for the initial diagnosis of this condition and the long-term monitoring of patients.

URINE TESTING

Glucose in urine

Glycosuria allows for a good first-line screening test for diabetes mellitus; most occupational health checks and hospital admissions will include a urinary glucose test. Normally glucose does not appear in the urine until the the plasma glucose rises above 10 mmol/l or thereabouts. However, in some healthy individuals, glucose may spill over into the urine at much lower plasma concentrations. These individuals are said to have a low renal threshold for glucose and have glycosuria without having diabetes mellitus. Conversely, the renal glucose threshold increases with age and as a result many diabetics will not have glycosuria. It is important when interpreting urinary glucose measurements to remember that the urine glucose level is a reflection of integrated glycaemia over the time of the formation of the urine and does not reflect the exact level of blood glucose at the time of testing.

A number of simple sideroom or home test kits are available for urine glucose measurement.

Ketones in urine/plasma

Ketone bodies (acetone, acetoacetate and ß-hydroxybutyrate) may accumulate in the plasma of a diabetic patient. Their presence is by no means diagnostic of ketoacidosis, a serious condition. Ketones may be present in a normal subject as a result of simple prolonged fasting. Dry reagent strips which detect acetoacetate but not ß-hydroxybutyrate might therefore provide an underestimate of ketonaemia / ketonuria.

BLOOD GLUCOSE

Glucose is routinely measured in the laboratory on blood specimens which have been collected into tubes containing fluoride, an inhibitor of glycolysis. Because of the need sometimes to obtain rapid blood glucose results and the widespread self-monitoring of diabetic patients, blood glucose is also assessed outside the laboratory using test strips.

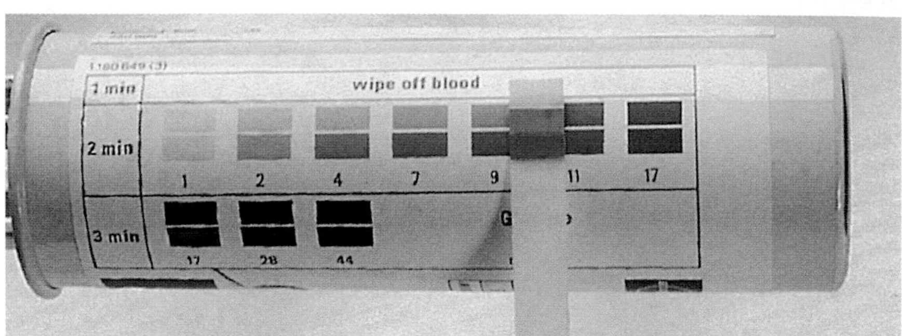

Fig. 1 **Blood glucose test container showing colour test results for comparison.**

The modern tests employ specific enzymatic reactions and provide a fairly accurate measurement over the broad range of blood glucose concentrations. The concentration of glucose can be read visually (Fig. 1) or with the aid of portable reflectance meters. It is important to follow the measuring procedure exactly. Improper storage of reagent strips can affect the results. Any grossly abnormal or unexpected results should be confirmed in the laboratory.

The World Health Organization has published guidelines for the diagnosis of diabetes mellitus on the basis of blood glucose results and the response to an oral glucose load. These are shown in Table 1 and are further discussed below.

Random blood glucose (RBG)

RBG is the only test required in an emergency. An RBG of less than 8 mmol/l should be expected in non-diabetics. RBG higher than 11 mmol/l usually indicates diabetes mellitus (Table 1).

Fasting blood glucose (FBG)

FBG is measured after an overnight fast (at least 10 hours). An FBG is better than RBG for diagnostic purposes. In non-diabetics it is usually lower than 6 mmol/l. Fasting values of 6–8 mmol/l should be interpreted as borderline. FBG equal to or above 8 mmol/l on two occasions is diagnostic for diabetes mellitus. It is important in each case to recognize the differences between measurements performed on whole blood, plasma or capillary samples (Table 1).

Oral glucose tolerance test (OGTT)

Classically, the diagnosis of diabetes is made on the basis of a patient's response to an oral glucose load. A baseline blood sample is first taken after an overnight fast. The patient is then given 75 g of glucose orally, in about 300 ml of water, to be drunk within 5 minutes. Plasma glucose levels are measured every 30 minutes for 2 hours. Urine may also be tested for glucose at time 0 and after 2 hours. The patient should be sitting comfortably throughout the test, should not smoke or exercise and should have been on a normal diet for at least 3 days prior to the test. Normal and diabetic responses to an oral glucose load are shown in Figure 2.

Table 1 **WHO criteria for the diagnosis of diabetes mellitus and impaired glucose tolerance (IGT).**

Random glucose sample (mmol/l)	Diabetes likely	Diabetes uncertain	Diabetes unlikely
Venous plasma	≥11.1	5.5–<11.1	<5.5
Venous blood	≥10.0	4.4–<10.0	<4.4
Capillary plasma	≥12.2	5.5–<12.2	<5.5
Capillary blood	≥11.1	4.4–<11.1	<4.4

Standardized OGTT (mmol/l)		Diabetes	IGT
Venous plasma	Fasting	≥7.8	<7.8
	2h	≥11.1	7.8–<11.1
Venous blood	Fasting	≥6.7	<6.7
	2h	≥10.0	6.7–<10.0
Capillary plasma	Fasting	≥7.8	<7.8
	2h	≥12.2	8.9–<12.2
Capillary blood	Fasting	≥6.7	<6.7
	2h	≥11.1	7.8–<11.1

Indications

Many OGTTs are performed unnecessarily. There are relatively few indications for the test. These include:

- borderline fasting or post-prandial blood glucose
- persistent glycosuria
- glycosuria in pregnant women
- pregnant women with a family history of diabetes mellitus and those who previously had large babies or unexplained fetal loss.

It is important to note that the OGTT is of little value in hospitalized patients or in patients immediately after a severe illness.

Interpretation of an OGTT

The interpretation of an OGTT is summarized in Table 1. In asymptomatic patients, OGTT should be interpreted as diagnostic of diabetes mellitus only when there is an increased 2 h glucose level, and the blood glucose is also equal to or greater than 11 mmol/l at some other point during the test. If the patient has a normal fasting plasma glucose and only the 2 h value in the diabetic range, the test should be repeated after approximately 6 weeks. Impaired glucose tolerance (IGT) should not be regarded as a disease. It signals that the patient is at an intermediate stage between normality and diabetes mellitus and is at an increased risk of developing diabetes. Such patients should be followed up yearly, and dietary treatment may be used.

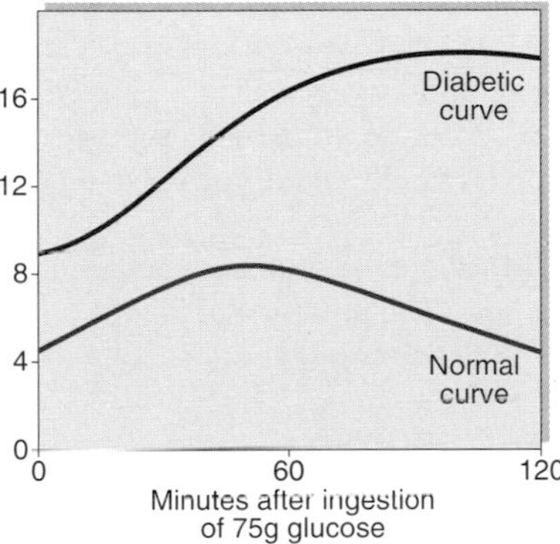

Fig. 2 **Plasma glucose levels following an oral glucose load in normal and diabetic subjects.**

LONG-TERM INDICES OF DIABETIC CONTROL

A high concentration of glucose in the ECF leads to its non-enzymatic attachment to the lysine residues of a variety of proteins. This is called glycation. The extent of this process depends on the ambient glucose level. It is virtually irreversible at physiological hydrogen ion concentration and therefore the glucose molecule will remain attached until the protein molecule is degraded. The concentration of glycated protein is therefore a reflection of a mean blood glucose level prevailing in the extracellular fluid during the life of that protein.

Haemoglobin A_{1c} or glycated haemoglobin

Glycated haemoglobin reflects the mean glycaemia over 2 months prior to its measurement, the half-life of haemoglobin. This test is accepted as a good index of diabetic control and is used routinely in most diabetic clinics to complement the information from single blood glucose levels, or indeed a patient's log of his or her own blood glucose measurements.

Fructosamine

Many other proteins in addition to haemoglobin are glycated when exposed to glucose in the blood. An indication of the extent of this glycation can be obtained by measuring fructosamine, the ketoamine product of non-enzymatic glycation. As albumin is the most abundant plasma protein, glycated albumin is the major contributor to serum fructosamine measurements. As this protein has a shorter half-life than haemoglobin, fructosamine measurements are complementary to Hb A_{1c} providing an index of glucose control over the 3 weeks prior to its measurement.

Microalbuminuria

Microalbuminuria may be defined as an albumin excretion rate intermediate between normality (2.5–25 mg/day) and macroalbuminuria (>250 mg/day). The small increase in urinary albumin excretion is not detected by simple albumin stick tests and requires confirmation by careful quantitation in a 24h urine specimen. The importance of microalbuminuria in the diabetic patient is that it is a signal of early, reversible renal damage.

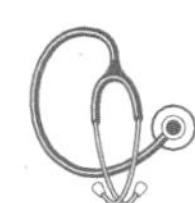

Clinical note

The glucose result log book kept by insulin-dependent diabetics who perform home monitoring may at first sight appear to show good and consistent glucose control. This may not always represent the truth. The clinician should determine the true level of control by close questioning and objective assessments such as Hb A_{1c} or fructosamine.

Case history 24

Interpret these results from the four oral glucose tolerance tests below.

75 g glucose was given at time 0.

Case number	Clinical details on request form	Minutes post glucose load — venous plasma glucose mmol/l — 0	30	60	90	120
(i)	Male, 65 yrs, obese ?NIDDM	8.8	13.8	17.5	16.8	16.7
(ii)	Female, 62 yrs, presented to dental hospital with 'burning mouth'	6.0	11.7	15.2	16.4	17.0
(iii)	Male, 41 yrs, glycosuria at works medical	7.4	9.5	10.8	10.1	9.5
(iv)	Female, 75 yrs, high RBG result	5.0	8.6	10.7	11.0	10.2

Comments on page 154.

Diagnosis and monitoring of diabetes mellitus

- The diagnosis of diabetes mellitus is made on the basis of blood glucose concentrations either alone or in response to an oral glucose load.
- In asymptomatic patients the results of an oral glucose tolerance test should be interpreted as diagnostic of diabetes mellitus only when there is an increased 2 h glucose concentration, and the blood glucose is also equal to or greater than 11 mmol/l at some other point during the test.
- Hb A_{1c} and fructosamine are measures of protein glycation and serve as indices of long-term glucose control.
- Microalbuminuria is a measure of early, reversible, diabetic nephropathy.

DIABETIC KETOACIDOSIS

HOW DIABETIC KETOACIDOSIS DEVELOPS

The most common precipitating factors in the development of diabetic ketoacidosis (DKA) are infection, myocardial infarction, trauma or omission of insulin. All metabolic disturbances seen in DKA are the indirect or direct consequences of the lack of insulin (Fig. 1). Decreased glucose transport into tissues leads to hyperglycaemia which gives rise to glycosuria. Increased lipolysis causes over-production of fatty acids, some of which are converted into ketones, giving ketonaemia, metabolic acidosis and ketonuria. Glycosuria causes an osmotic diuresis, which leads to the loss of water and electrolytes — sodium, potassium, calcium, magnesium, phosphate and chloride. Dehydration, if severe, produces pre-renal uraemia and may lead to hypovolaemic shock. The severe metabolic acidosis is partially compensated by an increased ventilation rate (Kussmaul breathing). Frequent vomiting is also usually present and accentuates the loss of water and electrolytes. Thus the development of DKA is a series of interlocking vicious circles all of which must be broken to aid the restoration of normal carbohydrate and lipid metabolism.

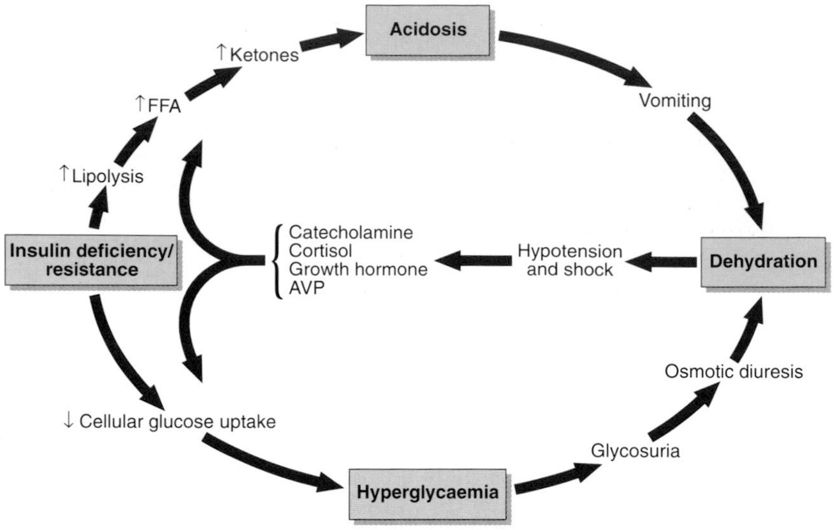

Fig. 1 **The development of diabetic ketoacidosis.**

TREATMENT

The management of DKA requires the administration of three agents:

- *Fluids.* Patients with DKA are usually severely fluid depleted and it is essential to expand their ECF with saline to restore their circulation.
- *Insulin.* Intravenous insulin is most commonly used. Intramuscular insulin is an alternative when an infusion pump is not available or where venous access is difficult, e.g. in small children.
- *Potassium.* Despite apparently normal serum potassium levels, all patients with DKA have whole body potassium depletion which may be severe.

In most cases, rehydration and insulin therapy will correct the metabolic acidosis, and no further therapy is indicated. However, in the most severe cases when the hydrogen ion concentration is greater than 100 nmol/l, i.v. sodium bicarbonate may be indicated.

The detailed management of diabetic ketoacidosis is shown in Figure 2. The importance of good fluid charts, as in any serious fluid and electrolyte disorder, cannot be over-emphasized. The initial high input of physiological (0.9%) saline is cut back as the patient's fluid and electrolyte deficit improves. Intravenous insulin is given by continuous infusion using an automated pump, and potassium supplements are added to the fluid regimen. The hallmark of good management of a patient with DKA is close clinical and biochemical monitoring.

LABORATORY INVESTIGATIONS

Initially, urine (if available) should be tested for glucose and ketones, and blood checked for glucose using a test strip. Venous blood should be sent to the laboratory for plasma glucose and serum sodium, potassium, chloride, bicarbonate, urea and creatinine. An arterial blood sample should also be sent for measurement of blood gases.

It is important to highlight a clinically important consequence of laboratory methodology here. The presence of ketone bodies

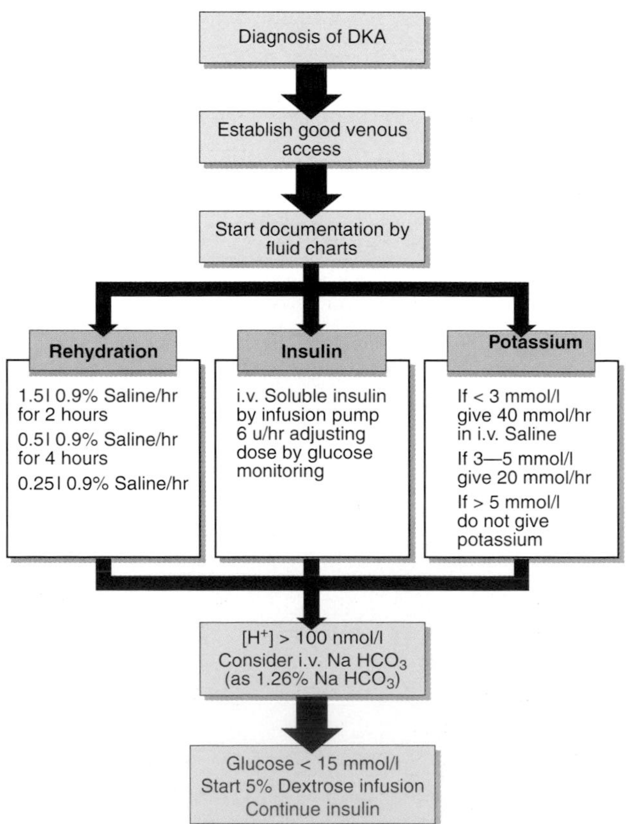

Fig. 2 **The management of diabetic ketoacidosis.**

in serum interferes with creatinine measurement; therefore serum creatinine can be falsely elevated in the acute stage. Reliable creatinine values are obtained only after ketonaemia subsides.

Amylase activity in serum is also increased in diabetic ketoacidosis. Pancreatitis should be considered as a precipitating factor only if there is persistent abdominal pain.

Blood glucose should be monitored hourly at the bedside until less than 15 mmol/l. Thereafter checks may continue 2-hourly. The plasma glucose should be confirmed in the laboratory every 2–4 hours. The frequency of monitoring of blood gases depends on the severity of DKA. In severe cases it should be performed 2-hourly at least for the first 4 hours. The serum potassium level should be checked every 2 hours for the first 6 hours, while urea and electrolytes should be measured at 4-hourly intervals (Fig. 3).

Two other forms of severe metabolic decompensation may occur in diabetics. These are hyperosmolar non-ketotic (HONK) coma and lactic acidosis. Table 1 shows the principal features of these conditions in comparison with DKA.

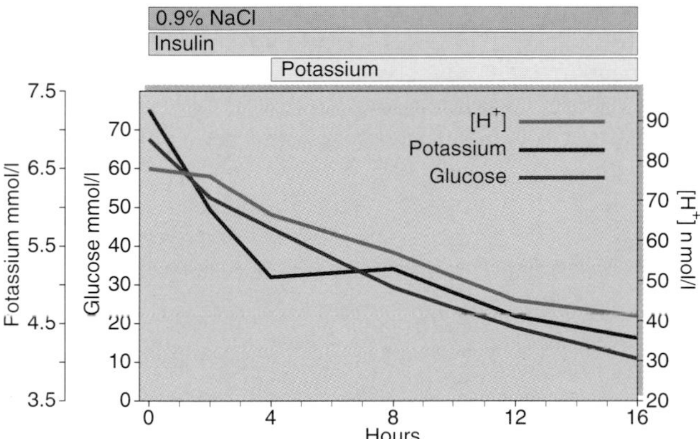

Fig. 3 **Effective treatment of a severe case of diabetic ketoacidosis.**

Table 1 **Principal features of three forms of metabolic decompensation in diabetes**

Features	Diabetic keto-acidosis (DKA)	Hyperosmolar non-ketotic coma (HONK)	Lactic acidosis
Plasma glucose	High	Very high	Variable
Ketones	Present	None	Variable
Acidosis	Moderate/Severe	None	Severe
Dehydration	Prominent	Prominent	Variable
Hyperventilation	Present	None	Present

Case history 25

A 22-year-old diabetic comes to the Accident and Emergency department. She gives a 2-day history of vomiting and abdominal pain. She is drowsy and her breathing is deep and rapid. There is a distinctive smell from her breath.

- What is the most likely diagnosis?
- Which bedside tests could you do to help you to confirm this diagnosis?
- Which laboratory tests would you request?

Comment on page 154.

HYPEROSMOLAR NON-KETOTIC (HONK) COMA

Diagnosis

HONK coma occurs mostly in elderly, non-insulin dependent diabetics, and develops relatively slowly over days or weeks. The level of insulin is sufficient to prevent ketosis but does not prevent hyperglycaemia and osmotic diuresis. Precipitating factors include severe illness, dehydration, glucocorticoids, diuretics, parenteral nutrition, dialysis and surgery. Extremely high blood glucose levels (above 35 mmol/l, and usually above 50 mmol/l) accompany severe dehydration resulting in impaired consciousness.

Treatment

Treatment is similar to that of DKA, with the following modifications. Rehydration should be slower to avoid neurological damage. Dilute (0.45%) saline has been used where the serum sodium level is above 160 mmol/l. However, recent data indicate that in most cases the use of physiological (0.9%) saline is sufficient. The insulin dose requirements are usually lower than in DKA.

LACTIC ACIDOSIS

Diagnosis

Type I lactic acidosis occurs in hypoxic subjects and is due to an excessive production of lactate by peripheral tissues. Hypoxia is not a feature of type II lactic acidosis which is probably caused by the impaired metabolism of lactate in the liver. Both are characterized by an extreme metabolic acidosis ([H⁺] above 100 nmol/l). There is a high anion gap with low or absent ketones, and high blood lactate concentrations.

Treatment

Large amounts of intravenous sodium bicarbonate may be required to correct the acidosis. Alternatively the patient may be dialysed against a bicarbonate-containing solution.

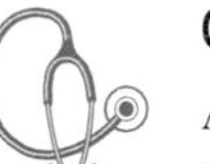

Clinical note

Always screen for infections in the diabetic patient presenting with DKA, as this is a common precipitating factor. Blood, urine, sputum and any wound fluids should be sent for culture at the earliest opportunity and certainly before antibiotics are introduced.

Diabetic ketoacidosis

- Diabetic ketoacidosis arises from a number of metabolic problems caused by insulin lack.
- Treatment is by intravenous fluids, insulin and potassium.
- Only in the most severe cases of DKA should sodium bicarbonate be used.
- Close clinical and biochemical monitoring are required to tailor the management protocol to the individual patient.
- Other, much less common, severe metabolic disturbances of carbohydrate metabolism are hyperosmolar non-ketotic coma and lactic acidosis.

HYPOGLYCAEMIA

Hypoglycaemia is a laboratory 'diagnosis' which is usually taken to mean a blood glucose level below 2.5 mmol/l. Hypoglycaemia may be due to a number of underlying conditions including endocrine disorders, liver disease, inborn errors of metabolism and gastrointestinal surgery. The cause is an imbalance between glucose intake, endogenous glucose production and glucose utilization. A low blood glucose level normally leads to the stimulation of catecholamine secretion and correction of hypoglycaemia through suppression of insulin secretion and stimulation of glucagon, cortisol and growth hormone. The catecholamine surge accounts for the signs and symptoms most commonly seen in hypoglycaemia, i.e. sweating, shaking, tachycardia, nausea and weakness. Hypoglycaemia decreases the glucose fuel supply to the brain and may lead to brain damage particularly in infants.

CLINICAL EFFECTS

The clinical effects of hypoglycaemia depend upon the concentration of blood glucose and the speed with which the level has fallen. These effects are summarized in Figure 1.

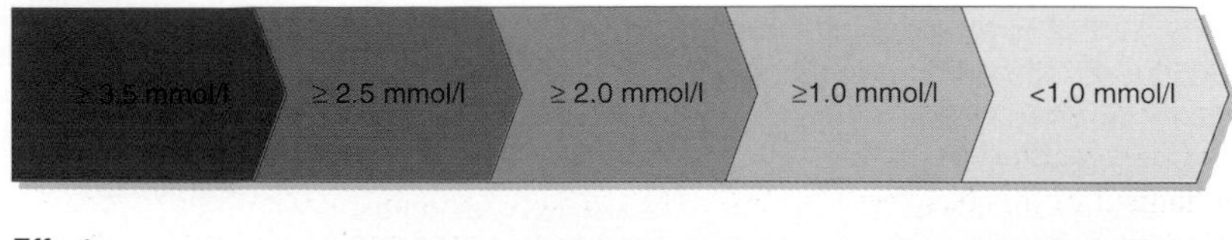

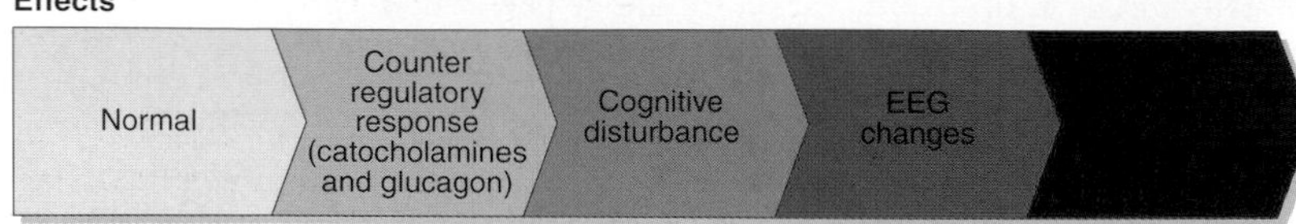

Fig. 1 **The clinical effects of hypoglycaemia.**

LABORATORY INVESTIGATION

The biochemistry laboratory can confirm hypoglycaemia and may also provide some useful clues to the underlying cause.

- *Blood glucose.* The detection of hypoglycaemia is by blood glucose testing. Urine testing cannot detect hypoglycaemia.
- *Plasma insulin.* Insulin measurements can lead to the diagnosis or exclusion of insulinoma. They play no part in the diagnosis of diabetes mellitus.
- *Insulin/glucose ratio.* In order to make better diagnostic use of insulin measurements, the ratio of insulin and glucose concentrations, measured on the same sample, is reported.
- *Plasma C-peptide.* Insulin secretion in insulin-treated diabetics cannot be assessed by the measurement of plasma insulin since the insulin given therapeutically will also be measured in the assay. However, insulin and its associated connecting-peptide (or C-peptide) are secreted by the islet cells in equimolar amounts (Fig. 2) and thus measurement of C-peptide levels together with insulin can differentiate between hypoglycaemia due to insulinoma (high C-peptide) and that due to exogenous insulin (low C-peptide).

TREATMENT

Suspected hypoglycaemic patients require immediate treatment irrespective of the underlying cause. Blood glucose should be measured with a test strip and another blood sample sent to the laboratory. The clinician, however, should act on the basis of the test strip results. The aim in comatose or confused patients should be to correct the hypoglycaemia rapidly with either intravenous dextrose or intramuscular glucagon. Possible treatments for hypoglycaemia are summarized in Figure 3.

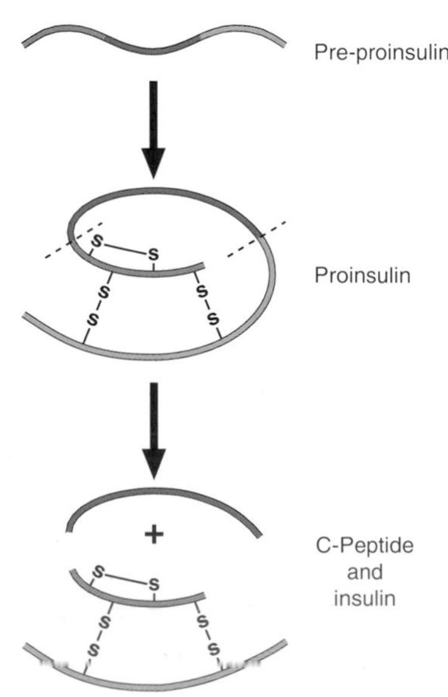

Fig. 2 **Insulin and C-peptide.**

SPECIFIC CAUSES OF HYPOGLYCAEMIA

Over 99% of all episodes of hypoglycaemia occur in insulin-dependent diabetic patients. It is essential that suspected hypoglycaemia be promptly treated in diabetic patients. Confirmation by measuring blood glucose is not usually necessary. Reasons for hypoglycaemia in the diabetic include:

- insufficient carbohydrate intake
- excess of insulin or sulphonylurea
- strenuous exercise
- excessive alcohol intake.

Other causes of hypoglycaemia may be conveniently discussed in two groups: those which produce hypoglycaemia in the *fasting* patient, and those in which the low glucose concentration is a response to a stimulus (*reactive* hypoglycaemia). The recognition and investigation of hypoglycaemia in the neonate is also important.

Fasting hypoglycaemia

Causes of fasting hypoglycaemia include:

- *Insulinoma.* β-cell islet tumours of the pancreas may produce insulin both inappropriately and in excess. These tumours are usually single and benign and may be part of the wider multiple endocrine neoplasia syndrome (MEN type 1, see p. 133) where there are associated tumours in two or more endocrine organs. Insulinomas produce hypoglycaemia classically in the fasting state and their diagnosis depends upon the demonstration of hypoglycaemia in the presence of inappropriately high serum insulin levels. The management of such tumours is by surgical excision.
- *Cancer.* Hypoglycaemia is associated with advanced malignancy.
- *Hepatic disease.* Although the liver

has large functional reserves, severe damage may result in hypoglycaemia.

- *Addison's disease.* Cortisol action is to maintain blood glucose concentration; glucocorticoid deficiency is a rare cause of hypoglycaemia.
- *Sepsis.* Severe infections may result in hypoglycaemia although the mechanism of this has not been fully explained.

Reactive hypoglycaemia

In reactive hypoglycaemia, patients may become hypoglycaemic in response to:

- *Drugs.* Factitious hypoglycaemia due to surreptitious insulin administration may be as common a cause as insulinoma. It is essential that both insulin and C-peptide are measured in all suspected cases.
- *Food: post-prandial hypoglycaemia.* A number of patients complain of hypoglycaemic-like symptoms after eating. In order to differentiate those individuals in whom a low blood glucose is causative it is best to obtain a blood glucose measurement when the patient has symptoms. Accelerated gastric emptying after gastric surgery ('dumping syndrome') may give rise to this condition, which may also be a feature of early diabetes mellitus. In some patients mild hypoglycaemia following a large meal or even an oral glucose tolerance test is thought to be due to an exaggerated insulin response (idiopathic post-prandial hypoglycaemia).
- *Alcohol.* Patients who ingest large amounts of alcohol after fasting or if they are malnourished may become hypoglycaemic. Hypoglycaemia should always be excluded in alcoholics who are admitted in a drowsy state.

Neonatal hypoglycaemia

The diagnosis and treatment of hypoglycaemia in the neonate is particularly important because of the high risk of hypoglycaemic brain damage (p. 149). There are a number of important causes:

- *Babies of diabetic mothers.* A fetus that is exposed to maternal hyperglycaemia will have pancreatic islet cell hyperplasia and elevated insulin levels. After delivery the neonate is unable to suppress its inappropriately high insulin levels and will develop hypoglycaemia.
- *Intra-uterine growth retardation.* Small-for-dates babies may have inadequate liver glycogen stores. This situation is further compromized by prematurity because glycogen is laid down mainly in the last four weeks of pregnancy.
- *Inborn errors of metabolism.* There are a large number of potential causes of hypoglycaemia in this category. Galactosaemia and glycogen storage disease are examples (pp. 146–147).

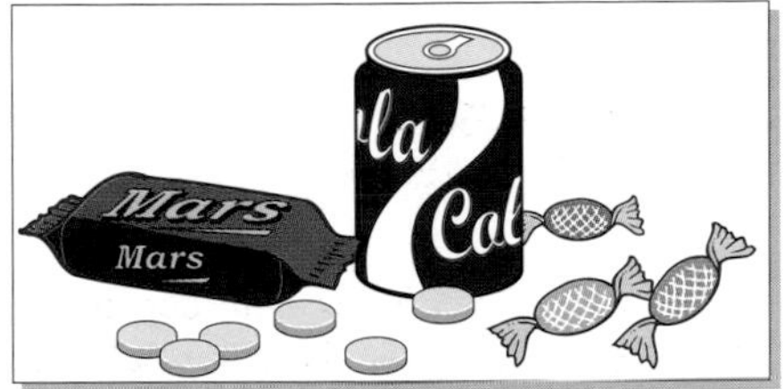

Oral glucose in conscious patient
If patient can swallow, give sweet drinks, sweets or glucose tablets

Oral glucose in comatose patient
If patient is unable to swallow, *as a first aid measure only*, jam, or commercially available glucose gels, may be smeared on inside of cheeks. This carries a risk of aspiration but may be useful especially in children

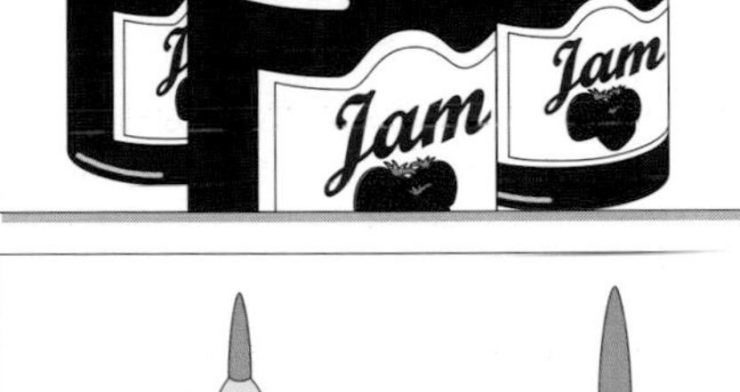

i.m. Glucagon
May be given to comatose patient. Many diabetics will have this available

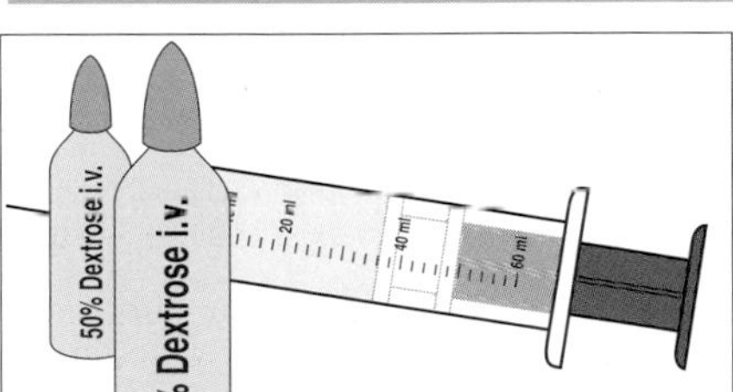

i.v. Glucose
Treatment of choice in comatose patient, but only available in patient care setting, while above treatments may be administered at home or at work

Fig. 3 **Treatment of hypoglycaemia.**

Clinical note

The use of 50% dextrose as an intravenous bolus has remarkable effects in reversing the signs and symptoms of hypoglycaemia. This solution is like syrup and may cause thrombophlebitis. Care must also be taken not to cause extravasation.

Case history 26

A 25-year-old woman with IDDM complained of repeated episodes of sleep disturbances, nightsweats and vivid, unpleasant dreams.

- What is the most likely cause of this woman's symptoms and how might the diagnosis be confirmed?

Comment on page 154.

Hypoglycaemia

- Hypoglycaemia is not a diagnosis but is a biochemical sign associated with a diverse group of diseases.
- Management is by glucose therapy irrespective of the underlying cause.
- Excess insulin, excess alcohol or low calorie intake in a diabetic patient are the most common causes of hypoglycaemia.
- Insulinoma is characterized by hypoglycaemia in the face of inappropriately high plasma insulin.
- Hypoglycaemia in the neonate may result in brain damage.

CALCIUM REGULATION AND HYPOCALCAEMIA

CALCIUM HOMEOSTASIS

The amount of calcium present in the extracellular fluid is very small in comparison to that stored in bone. Even in the adult, calcium in bone is not static; some bone is resorbed each day and the calcium returned to the ECF. To maintain calcium balance, an equal amount of bone formation must take place. Figure 1 shows how much calcium is exchanged between one compartment and another daily. Calcium is both absorbed from and secreted into the gut, but net absorption must equal urinary loss every day if balance is to be maintained.

Calcium homeostasis is modulated by hormones (Fig. 2). Parathyroid hormone (PTH) is the most important calcium regulator. It is a hormone of 84 amino acids, and is secreted from the parathyroid glands in response to a low unbound plasma calcium. PTH causes bone resorption and promotes calcium reabsorption in the renal tubules, preventing loss in the urine. 1,25-dihydroxycholecalciferol (1,25 DHCC) maintains intestinal calcium absorption. This sterol hormone is formed from vitamin D (cholecalciferol), following hydroxylation in the liver (at carbon-25) and kidney (at carbon–1). However, hydroxylation in the kidney is PTH dependent, and so even the absorption of calcium from the gut relies (albeit indirectly) on PTH.

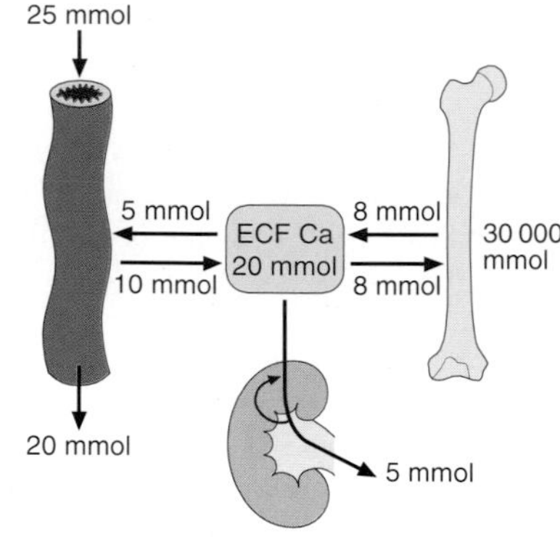

Fig. 1 **Normal calcium balance.** Calcium is exchanged each day, in the amounts shown, between the extracellular fluid and the gut, bone and kidney.

SERUM CALCIUM

A healthy person has a total serum calcium of around 2.4 mmol/l. About half is bound to protein, mostly to albumin. Binding is pH dependent and is decreased in acidosis, because the amino acid side chains on albumin become more positively charged. Conversely, binding is increased if an alkalosis is present. Hence, the percentage unbound calcium increases in acidosis and decreases if there is an alkalosis.

Unbound calcium is the biologically active fraction of the total calcium in plasma and maintenance of its concentration within tight limits is required for nerve function, membrane permeability, muscle contraction and glandular secretion. It is the unbound calcium concentration which is recognized by the parathyroid glands, and PTH acts to keep this concentration constant.

Although it is possible to measure the unbound calcium fraction (often erroneously called 'ionized' calcium), special equipment and collection techniques are required. So, laboratories routinely measure *total* calcium concentration (that is both the bound and unbound fractions) in a serum sample. Unfortunately, this gives rise to a problem in the interpretation of results. Changes in serum albumin concentration in patients cause changes in total calcium concentration. If albumin concentration falls, total serum calcium is low because the bound fraction is decreased. Unbound calcium is normal — maintained by PTH (Fig. 3). Remember that the homeostatic mechanisms for regulating plasma calcium respond to the unbound fraction, not to the total calcium. Patients with a low albumin (and that includes many in any hospital) have total serum calcium lower than the reference values, yet have normal unbound calcium. *These patients should not be thought of as hypocalcaemic.*

In order to circumvent this problem and to ensure that patients with a low albumin are not mistakenly labelled as hypocalcaemic, clinical biochemists use the convention of the 'adjusted calcium'. More importantly this also ensures that patients with an apparently normal total calcium and a low albumin are not overlooked when they are, in fact, hyper-calcaemic. Most laboratories measure both total calcium and albumin, and, if the albumin is abnormal, calculate what the total calcium would have been if the albumin had been normal. One such calculation is:

Adjusted calcium (mmol/l) = Total measured calcium + 0.02(47–albumin)

The measured calcium is 'adjusted' by 0.1 mmol/l for every 5 g/l that the albumin is less than 47.

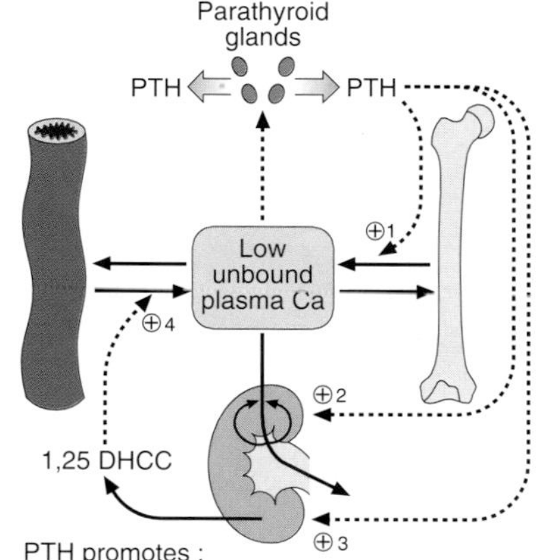

Fig. 2 **The effects of PTH in restoring a low plasma calcium to normal.**

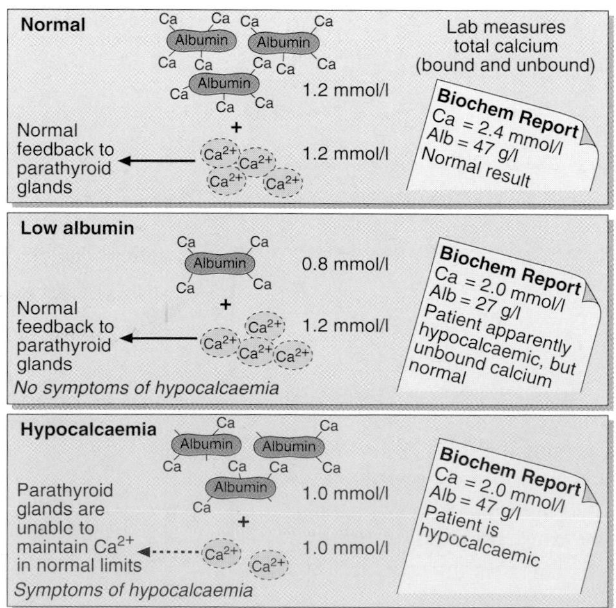

Fig. 3 **The binding of calcium to albumin.**

HYPOCALCAEMIA

Aetiology

The causes of hypocalcaemia include:

- *Hypoparathyroidism:* idiopathic, after neck surgery, or occasionally due to magnesium deficiency.
- *Vitamin D deficiency.* This may be due to malabsorption, or an inadequate diet with little exposure to sunlight. It may lead to the bone disorders, osteomalacia in adults and rickets in children (see pp. 70–71).
- *Renal disease.* The diseased kidneys fail to synthesize 1,25 DHCC (see pp. 26–27). Increased PTH secretion in response to the hypocalcaemia may lead to bone disease if untreated.
- *Pseudohypoparathyroidism.* PTH is secreted but there is failure of target tissue receptors to respond to the hormone.
- *Rarer causes* such as malignancy, acute rhabdomyolysis, acute pancreatitis, or bone marrow transplantation.

Clinical features

The clinical features of hypocalcaemia include:

- neurologic features such as tingling, tetany, and mental changes
- cardiovascular signs such as an abnormal ECG
- cataracts.

A strategy for the investigation and differential diagnosis of hypocalcaemia is shown in Figure 4.

Treatment

The management calls for the treatment of the cause of the hypocalcaemia, if this is possible. Oral calcium supplements are commonly prescribed in mild disorders. 1,25 DHCC, or the synthetic vitamin D metabolite 1α-hydroxycholecalciferol, can be given.

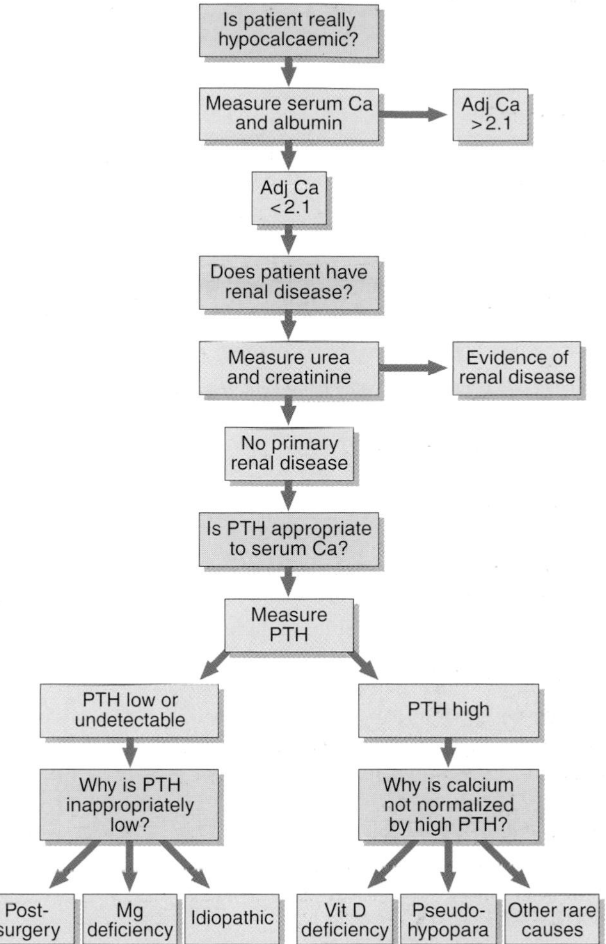

Fig. 4 **The investigation of hypocalcaemia.**

Clinical note

Trousseau's sign is the most reliable indication of latent tetany. A sphygmomanometer cuff is inflated to above systolic pressure for at least 2 minutes while observing the hand. A positive response will be the appearance of a typical carpal spasm, which relaxes some 5 seconds or so after the cuff is released.

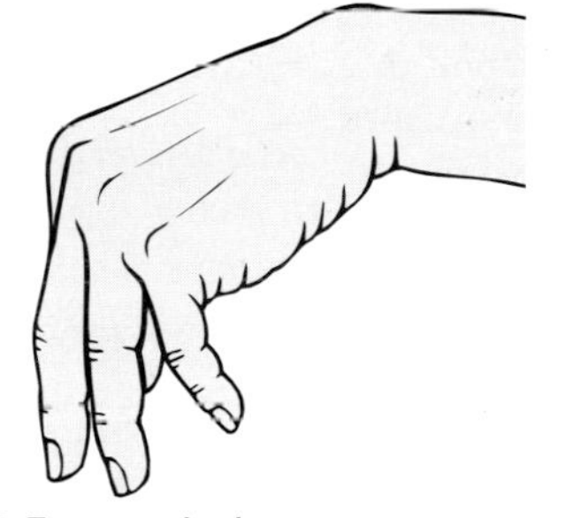

Fig. 5 **Trousseau's sign.**

Case history 27

A 70-year-old woman attended her GP complaining of generalized bone pain. Biochemistry results on a serum specimen taken at the surgery showed the following:

Calcium	Phosphate	Albumin	Ca (adj)
mmol/l	*mmol/l*	*g/l*	*mmol/l*
1.80	1.1	39	1.96

- What further investigations would be appropriate?

Comment on page 154.

Calcium regulation and hypocalcaemia

- 'Adjusted calcium' should be used to avoid the problems of interpreting the total calcium concentration in patients who have abnormal serum albumin concentrations.
- If a hypocalcaemic patient has low or undetectable PTH in serum, he/she is hypoparathyroid.
- If PTH concentrations are appropriately elevated to the low calcium, then the reason for the hypocalcaemia is most likely to be vitamin D deficiency.
- Patients with chronic renal failure often have hypocalcaemia due to the inability of renal cells to make 1,25 dihydroxycholecalciferol. Secondary hyperparathyroidism and bone disease may result.

HYPERCALCAEMIA

The commonest causes of hypercalcaemia are primary hyperparathyroidism and hypercalcaemia of malignancy.

Patients today are unlikely to present with gross bone disease or severe renal calculi as a consequence of untreated primary hyperparathyroidism. General practitioners who are aware of the telltale signs and symptoms of hypercalcaemia can identify this disorder before gross bone abnormalities or renal problems have had time to develop. The widespread use of multichannel analyzers in screening mode in clinical biochemistry laboratories can detect unsuspected hypercalcaemia even before symptoms become apparent. A high serum calcium concentration may be an unexpected finding in a patient in any clinic or hospital ward, as the symptoms of hypercalcaemia are nonspecific. All such findings should be followed up.

CLINICAL FEATURES

Symptoms of hypercalcaemia include:

- neurological and psychiatric features such as lethargy, confusion, irritability and depression
- gastrointestinal problems such as anorexia, abdominal pain, nausea and vomiting, and constipation
- renal features such as thirst and polyuria, and renal calculi
- cardiac arrhythmias.

DIAGNOSIS

A diagnostic decision chart is shown in Figure 1. *Primary hyperparathyroidism* is most often due to a single parathyroid adenoma which secretes PTH independently of feedback control by plasma calcium. *Hypercalcaemia associated with malignancy* is the commonest cause of a high calcium in a hospital population. Some tumours secrete a protein called PTHrP (parathyroid hormone-related protein) which has PTH-like properties.

Rarer causes of hypercalcaemia include:

- *Inappropriate dosage of vitamin D or metabolites,* e.g. in the treatment of hypoparathyroidism or renal disease.
- *Granulomatous diseases* (such as sarcoidosis or tuberculosis) or certain tumours (such as lymphomas) synthesize 1,25 dihydroxycholecalciferol.
- *Thyrotoxicosis* very occasionally leads to increased bone turnover and hypercalcaemia.
- *Diuretic therapy:* the hypercalcaemia is usually mild.
- *Immobilization:* especially in young people and patients with Paget's disease.
- *Renal disease.* Long-standing secondary hyperparathyoidism may lead to PTH secretion becoming independent of calcium feedback. This is termed tertiary hyperparathyroidism.
- *Calcium therapy.* Patients are routinely given calcium-containing solutions during cardiac surgery, and may have transient hypercalcaemia afterwards.
- *Diuretic phase of acute renal failure or in the recovery from severe rhabdomyolysis.*
- *Milk alkali syndrome:* the combination of an increased calcium intake together with bicarbonate, as in a patient self medicating with proprietary antacid, may cause severe hypercalcaemia, but the condition is very rare.

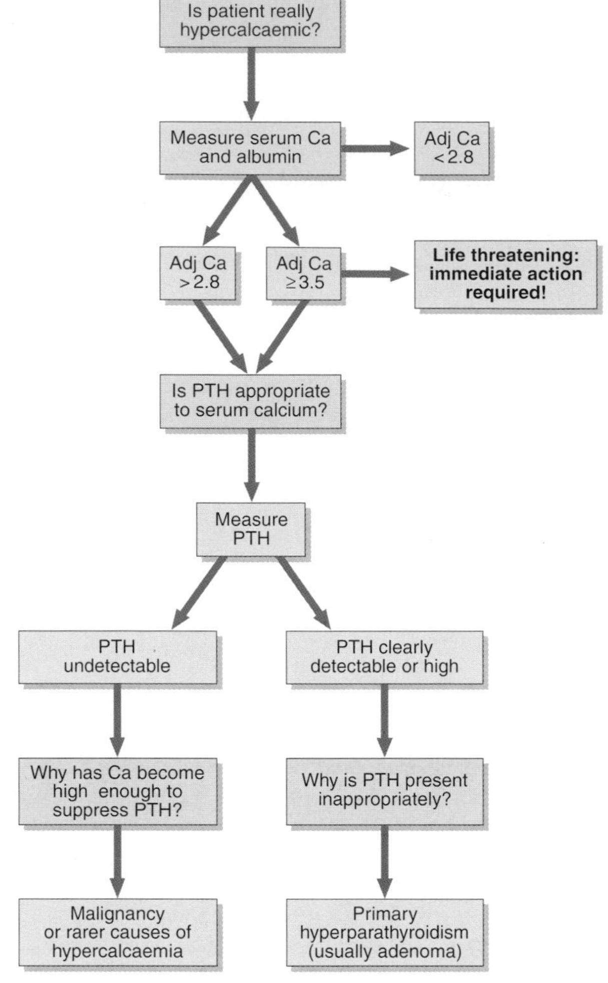

Fig. 1 **Investigation of hypercalcaemia.**

TREATMENT

Treatment is ***urgent*** if the adjusted serum calcium is greater than 3.5 mmol/l; the priority is to reduce it to a safe level. Intravenous saline is administered first to restore the glomerular filtration rate and promote a diuresis. Although steroids, mithramycin, calcitonin and intravenous phosphate have been used, compounds known as the bisphosphonates have been found to have the best calcium-lowering effects. Aminohydroxypropylidene diphosphonate (APD) has become the treatment of choice in patients with hypercalcaemia of malignancy (Fig. 2). It acts by inhibiting bone resorption.

The cause of the hypercalcaemia should be treated if possible. Surgical removal of a parathyroid adenoma usually provides a complete cure for a patient with primary hyperparathyoidism. Immediately after successful surgery, transient hypocalcaemia may have to be treated with vitamin D metabolites, until the remaining parathyroids begin to operate normally.

FAMILIAL HYPOCALCIURIC HYPERCALCAEMIA

Although a definitive differential diagnosis of hypercalcaemia can often be made, there is one rare condition where a wrong

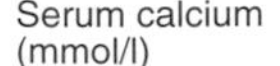

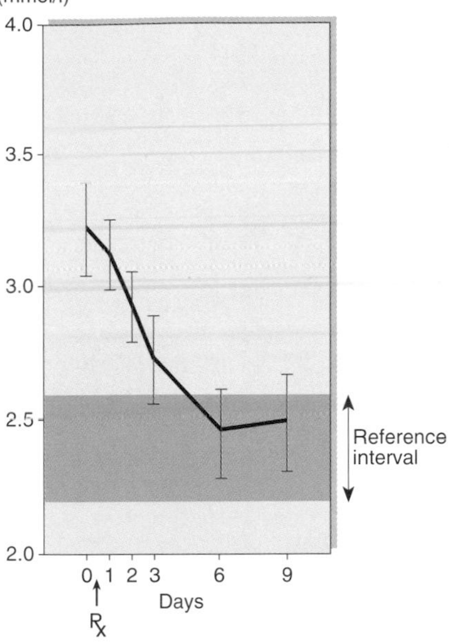

Fig. 2 **Treatment of hypercalcaemia of malignancy with APD.**
The graph shows the response of serum calcium in 12 patients treated with a single dose of the bisphosphonate 'Pamidronate' (APD), 30 mg in 500 ml 0.9% saline infused over 6 hours, after initial rehydration.

Case history 28

A 48-year-old woman came to her GP with a 12-month history of increasing tiredness and muscle fatigue. In recent weeks she had been increasingly thirsty and had polyuria. Her GP tested a urine sample for glucose, which he found to be negative, and then arranged that her urea and electrolytes be measured. He decided to request a calcium profile on the serum sample as well.

Biochemistry results in a serum specimen were:

Na^+	K^+	Cl^-	HCO_3^-	Urea	Creatinine
		mmol/l			*µmol/l*
149	3.5	109	20	7.5	160

Calcium	Phosphate	Albumin	Ca (adj)
mmol/l	*mmol/l*	*g/l*	*mmol/l*
3.30	0.51	35	3.54

- What are the most likely diagnoses in this patient?
- What other investigations would be appropriate?

Comment on page 155.

diagnosis can lead to unnecessary surgery. In familial hypocalciuric hypercalcaemia (FHH), a high plasma calcium is sensed by the parathyroids as normal; the patient has normal, detectable, levels of PTH, despite having hypercalcaemia. There are usually no symptoms of hypercalcaemia, but the patient may be labelled as primary hyperparathyroid, because of the detectable PTH in the face of a high serum calcium. On neck exploration, no parathyroid adenoma is found and it may be discovered subsequently that family members also have asymptomatic hypercalcaemia. Patients with the condition require no treatment; indeed, many would be better off remaining undiagnosed, such is the likelihood of unnecessary surgery.

The hypercalcaemia in FHH may be mild and without symptoms. It is sometimes possible to distinguish this condition from primary hyperparathyroidism on the basis of a urinary calcium excretion, which is inappropriately low for the serum calcium concentration in the patient with FHH. However, in practice, the urinary calcium excretion reference values in both conditions overlap. The possibility of FHH must always be considered when investigating the cause of asymptomatic hypercalcaemia in a relatively young patient.

Clinical note

If hypercalcaemia is not detected early, the high circulating PTH causes a characteristic pattern of bone resorption, known as osteitis fibrosa cystica shown in Figure 3. As awareness of hypercalcaemia has grown and detection methods have improved, such severe bone abnormalities are seen much less frequently.

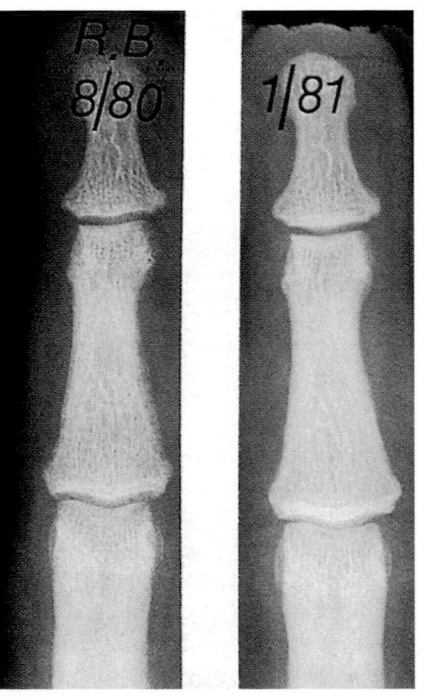

Fig. 3 **Classic subperiosteal resorption in a patient with severe primary hyperparathyroidism.**
(a) Radiograph shows resorption in the phalanges.
(b) Same finger 5 months after removal of parathyroid adenoma.

Hypercalcaemia

- Consideration of both serum calcium and albumin concentrations, as an 'adjusted' calcium, will give a correct assessment of the severity of the hypercalcaemia.
- Hypercalcaemia will most likely be due to the presence of a parathyroid adenoma, or will be associated with a malignancy. In the former, serum PTH will be high or inappropriately detectable, whereas in hypercalcaemia of malignancy the high calcium suppresses parathyroid function and serum PTH is undetectable.
- Serum calcium in excess of 3.5 mmol/l is life-threatening.
- Bisphosphonates such as APD have the ability to reduce serum calcium rapidly by inhibiting bone resorption.

PHOSPHATE AND MAGNESIUM

PHOSPHATE

Phosphate is abundant in the body and is an important intracellular and extracellular anion. Much of the phosphate inside cells is covalently attached to lipids and proteins. Phosphorylation and dephosphorylation of enzymes are important mechanisms in the regulation of metabolic activity. Most of the body's phosphate is in bone (Fig. 1). Phosphate changes accompany calcium deposition or resorption of bone. Control of ECF phosphate concentration is achieved by the kidney, where tubular reabsorption is reduced by PTH. The phosphate which is not reabsorbed in the renal tubule acts as an important urinary buffer.

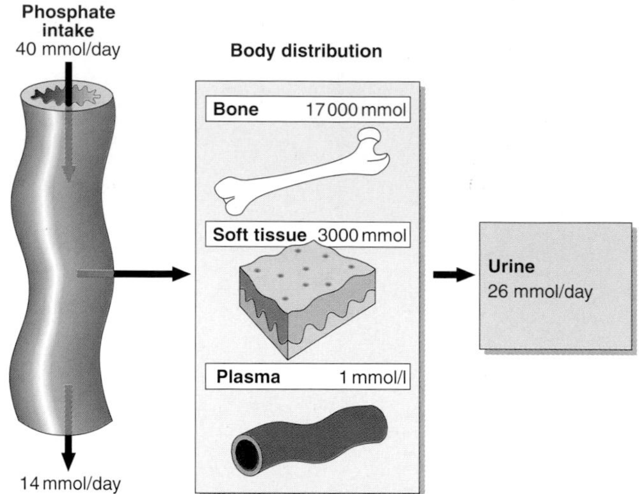

Fig. 1 **Normal phosphate balance.**

Plasma inorganic phosphate

At physiological hydrogen ion concentrations, phosphate exists in the ECF both as monohydrogen phosphate and as dihydrogen phosphate. Both forms are together termed 'phosphate', and the total is normally maintained within the limits of 0.80–1.40 mmol/l. Sometimes the term 'inorganic phosphate' is used to distinguish these forms from organically bound phosphate such as in ATP. Approximately 20% of plasma phosphate is attached to protein, although in contrast to the binding of calcium, this is of little significance.

In plasma, calcium and phosphate often have a reciprocal relationship. In particular, if phosphate rises, calcium falls.

HYPERPHOSPHATAEMIA

Persistent hyperphosphataemia may result in calcium phosphate deposition in soft tissues. Causes of a high serum phosphate concentration include:

- *Renal failure.* Phosphate excretion is impaired. This is the commonest cause of hyperphosphataemia.
- *Hypoparathyroidism.* The effect of a low circulating PTH decreases phosphate excretion by the kidneys, and this contributes to a high serum concentration.
- *Haemolysis.* This may occur intravascularly in the patient, or may be a consequence of an improper sampling procedure.
- *Pseudohypoparathyroidism.* There is tissue resistance to PTH.

HYPOPHOSPHATAEMIA

Severe hypophosphataemia (<0.3 mmol/l) is rare and causes muscle weakness which may lead to respiratory impairment. The symptomatic disorder requires immediate intravenous infusion of phosphate. Modest hypophosphataemia is much more common.

Causes of a low serum phosphate include:

- *Hyperparathyroidism.* The effect of a high PTH is to increase phosphate excretion by the kidneys and this contributes to a low serum concentration.
- *Congenital defects of tubular phosphate reabsorption.* In these conditions phosphate is lost from the body.
- *Ingestion of non-absorbable antacids, such as aluminium hydroxide.* These prevent phosphate absorption.
- *Treatment of diabetic ketoacidosis.* The effect of insulin in causing the shift of glucose into cells may cause similar shifts of phosphate which may result in hypophosphataemia.
- *Severe dietary deficiency.* Hypophosphataemia is frequently encountered when starved patients are first fed.
- *Oncogenic hypophosphataemia.* This is a rare cause of severe hypophosphataemia, and the causative factor produced by the tumour remains to be identified.

MAGNESIUM

Although the biological and biochemical importance of magnesium ions (Mg^{2+}) are well understood, the role of this cation in clinical medicine is sometimes overlooked. Magnesium ions are the second most abundant intracellular cations, after potassium. Some 300 enzyme systems are magnesium activated, and most aspects of intracellular biochemistry are magnesium dependent, including glycolysis, oxidative metabolism and transmembrane transport of potassium and calcium.

As well as these intracellular functions, the electrical properties of cell membranes are affected by any reduction in the *extracellular* magnesium concentration. Any detailed consideration of magnesium biochemistry has to take into account the interactions between Mg^{2+}, K^+ and Ca^{2+} ions.

Magnesium influences the secretion of PTH by the parathyroid glands, and severe hypomagnesaemia may cause hypoparathyroidism.

Magnesium homeostasis

Since magnesium is an integral part of chlorophyll, green vegetables are an important dietary source, as are cereals and animal meats. An average dietary intake is around 15 mmol per day which generally meets the recommended dietary intake. Children and pregnant or lactating women have higher requirements. About 30% of the dietary magnesium is absorbed from the small intestine and widely distributed to all metabolically active tissue (Fig. 2).

Serum magnesium

Hypermagnesaemia is uncommon but is occasionally seen in renal failure. Hypomagnesaemia is usually associated with magnesium deficiency. The symptoms of hypomagnesaemia are very similar to those of hypocalcaemia: impaired neuromuscular function such as tetany, hyperirritability, tremor, convulsions and muscle weakness.

MAGNESIUM DEFICIENCY

Since magnesium is present in most common foodstuffs, low dietary intakes of magnesium are associated with general nutritional insufficiency. Symptomatic magnesium deficiency can be expected as a result of:

- dietary insufficiency accompanied by intestinal malabsorption, severe vomiting, diarrhoea or other causes of intestinal loss
- osmotic diuresis such as occurs in diabetes mellitus
- prolonged use of diuretic therapy especially when dietary intake has been marginal
- prolonged nasogastric suction
- cytotoxic drug therapy such as cisplatinum which impairs renal tubular reabsorption of magnesium
- treatment with the immunosuppressant drug, cyclosporin.

Laboratory diagnosis

The repeated demonstration of a magnesium concentration of less than 0.7 mmol/l in a serum specimen is evidence of marked intracellular depletion and of a clinical condition which may benefit from magnesium therapy. However, intracellular magnesium depletion may exist where the serum magnesium concentration is within the reference range. Research procedures are required to detect these marginal states. These include the use of NMR spectroscopy to detect 'free' Mg^{2+} inside cells, and direct determination of Mg^{2+} in peripheral blood white cells, or in muscle biopsy samples.

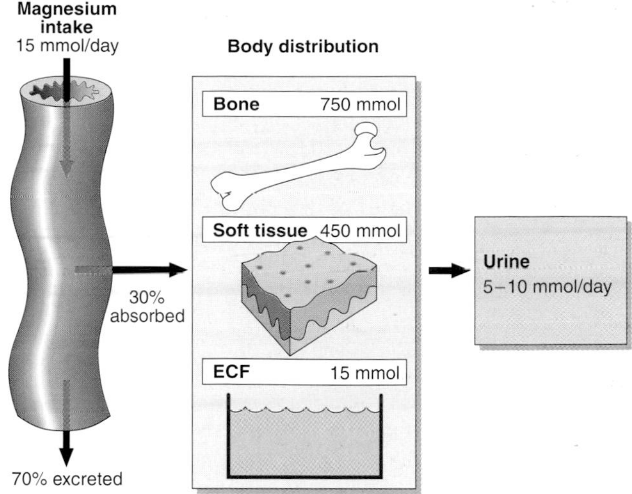

Fig. 2 **Normal magnesium balance.**

Management

The provision of magnesium supplements in oral diets is complicated by the fact that they often cause diarrhoea. A variety of oral, intramuscular and intravenous regimens have been proposed. Administration of magnesium salts, by whatever route, is contraindicated when there is a significant degree of renal impairment. In these circumstances any supplementation must be monitored carefully to avoid toxic effects associated with hypermagnesaemia.

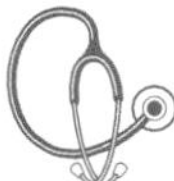

Clinical note

Magnesium supplements are increasingly being given after cardiac surgery and myocardial infarction to prevent cardiac arrhythmias.

Case history 29

A 46-year-old woman, known to have radiation enteritis with chronic diarrhoea and associated malabsorption syndrome, presented to the outpatient department complaining of severe tingling of recent onset in her hands and feet. The patient had a past history of hypocalcaemic tetany 18 months previously, but serum calcium had since remained normal on therapy with 1α-hydroxycholecalciferol, 0.75 μg daily, plus oral calcium supplements.

Calcium	Phosphate	Albumin	Calcium (adj)	Alk phos	Magnesium
mmol/l		*g/l*	*mmol/l*	*U/l*	*mmol/l*
1.30	1.1	39	1.46	110	0.25

The patient did not respond to treatment with increased calcium supplements and continued 1α–hydroxycholecalciferol.

- What would you predict the patient's PTH status to be?
- What treatment is appropriate and why?

Comment on page 155.

Phosphate and magnesium

- Hyperphosphataemia is commonly a consequence of renal impairment.
- Hypophosphataemia may be due to the effects of a high circulating parathyroid hormone concentration, or to congenital disorders of renal phosphate reabsorption.
- Magnesium deficiency results from a combination of poor dietary intake and increased urinary or intestinal losses.
- Magnesium deficiency may occur as a complication of intestinal disease or surgery, renal damage by nephrotoxins, diuretics or in diabetes.
- The demonstration of a low serum magnesium suggests severe deficiency, whereas marginal magnesium deficiency states may be present even when magnesium is within reference limits.

BONE DISEASE

The finding that a patient has hypercalcaemia or hypocalcaemia does not imply that there will be marked bone changes. Conversely, severe bone disease can occur whilst serum calcium levels appear quite normal. The main bone diseases are:

- osteoporosis
- osteomalacia and rickets
- Paget's disease.

BONE METABOLISM

Bone is constantly being broken down and reformed in the process of bone remodelling (Fig. 1). The clinician looking after patients with bone disease will certainly need to know to what extent bone is being broken down, and, indeed, if new bone is being made. Biochemical markers of bone resorption and bone formation can be useful in assessing the extent of disease, as well as monitoring treatment.

Hydroxyproline, from the breakdown of collagen, can be used to monitor bone resorption. However, urinary hydroxyproline is markedly influenced by dietary gelatin. Better markers of resorption are required. One candidate would seem to be another collagen degradation product: the fragments of the molecule containing the pyridinium cross links. Deoxypyridinoline is one such crosslink which is specific for bone, and not metabolized or influenced by diet.

The activity of the enzyme alkaline phosphatase has traditionally been used as an indicator of bone turnover. The osteoblasts which lay down the collagen framework and the mineral matrix of bone have high activity of this enzyme. Increased osteoblastic activity is seen as an elevated alkaline phosphatase activity in a serum specimen. Indeed, children who have active bone growth compared with adults have higher 'normal' alkaline phosphatase activity in serum. However alkaline phosphatase is also produced by the cells lining the bile canaliculi and is a marker for cholestasis. The bone isoenzyme of alkaline phosphatase may be measured, but there is need for a more specific and more sensitive marker.

Osteocalcin meets some of these requirements. It is made by osteoblasts and is an important noncollagenous constituent of bone. Not all of the osteocalcin which an osteoblast makes is incorporated into the bone matrix. Some is released into plasma, and provides a sensitive indicator of osteoblast activity. The test is available in specialized laboratories.

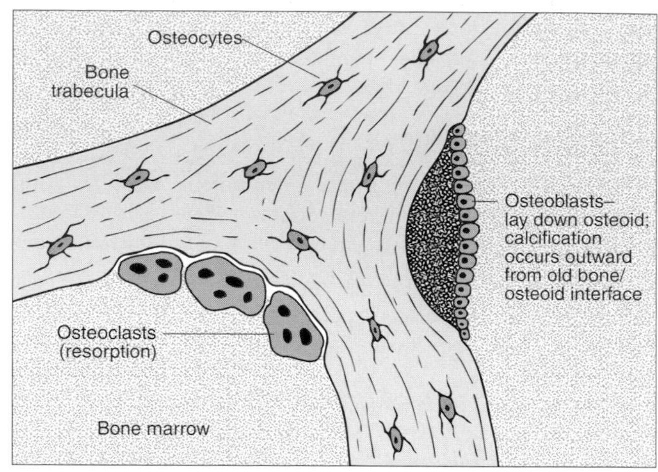

Fig. 1 **Bone remodelling.**

COMMON BONE DISORDERS

Osteoporosis

Osteoporosis is the commonest of bone disorders and is discussed separately on page 72.

Osteomalacia and rickets

Osteomalacia is the name given to defective bone mineralization in adults (Fig. 2). Rickets is characterized by defects of bone and cartilage mineralization in children. Vitamin D deficiency was once the most common reason for rickets and osteomalacia, but the addition of vitamin D to foodstuffs has almost eliminated the condition except in the elderly or housebound, the institutionalized, and in certain ethnic groups. Elderly Asian women with a predominantly vegetarian diet are particularly at risk. Vitamin D status can be assessed by measurement of the main circulating metabolite, 25-hydroxycholecalciferol, in a serum specimen. The metabolism of vitamin D is shown in Figure 3.

In severe osteomalacia due to vitamin D deficiency, serum calcium will fall, and there will be an appropriate increase in PTH secretion. Serum alkaline phosphatase activity will also be elevated.

The bony features of osteomalacia and rickets are also shared by other bone diseases (see later).

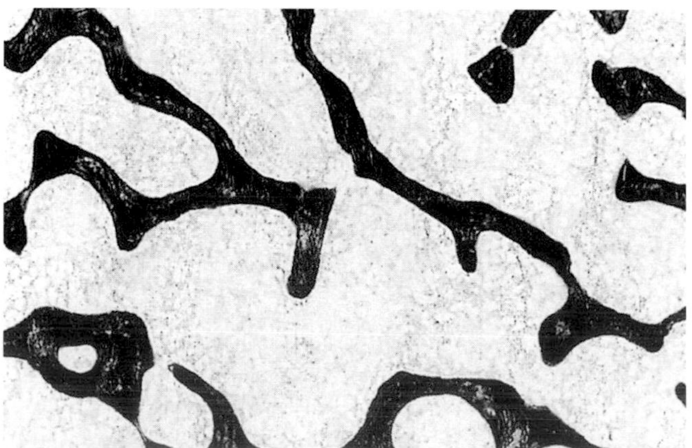

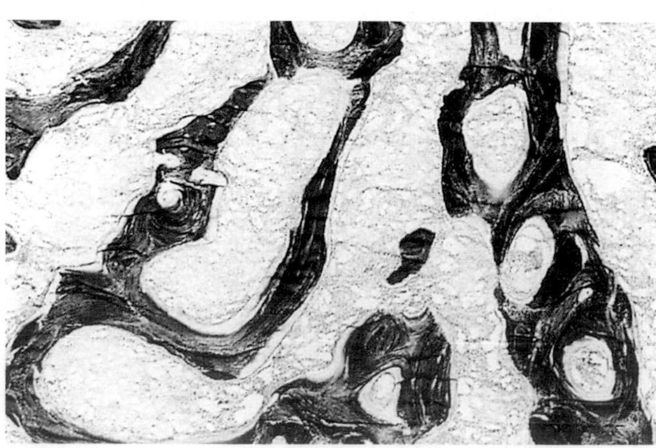

Fig. 2 **Bone biopsy showing normal (left) and osteomalacic (right) bone.**

Paget's Disease

Paget's disease is common and characterized by increased osteoclastic activity which leads to increased bone resorption. Increased osteoblastic activity repairs resorbed bone, but the new bone is laid down in a disorganized way. The clinical presentation is almost always bone pain which can be particularly severe. Serum alkaline phosphatase is high, and urinary hydroxyproline excretion is elevated. These provide a way of monitoring the progress of the disease. Although a viral cause for Paget's disease has been proposed, the aetiology remains obscure.

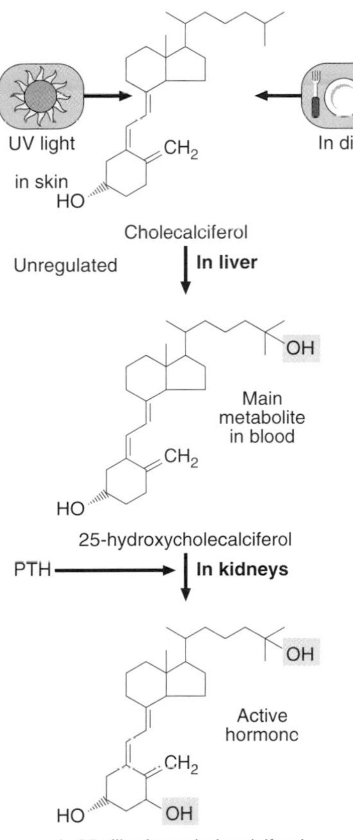

Fig. 3 **The main steps in the metabolism of vitamin D.**

Case history 30

A 66-year-old male presented to the bone clinic with severe pains in his right leg and pelvis. Radiological examination revealed Pagetic lesions in his legs, pelvis and also his skull. Biochemical results in a serum sample were unremarkable except for alkaline phosphatase which was grossly elevated at 2700 U/l. It was decided to treat him with a bisphosphonate drug.

- How would you monitor this patient's response?

Comment on page 155.

OTHER BONE DISEASES

Examples include:

- *Vitamin D dependent rickets, Types 1 and 2.* These are rare bone diseases resulting from genetic disorders leading to the inability to make the active vitamin D metabolite, or from receptor defects which do not allow the hormone to act.
- *Tumoral calcinosis.* This is characterized by ectopic calcification around the joints.
- *Hypophosphatasia.* This is a form of rickets or osteomalacia which results from a deficiency of alkaline phosphatase.
- *Hypophosphataemic rickets.* This is believed to be a consequence of a renal tubular defect in phosphate handling.
- *Osteopetrosis.* This condition is characterized by defective bone resorption.
- *Osteogenesis imperfecta.* Brittle bone syndrome, is an inherited disorder which occurs around once in every 20 000 births.

Diagnosis of these and other rare conditions may require help from specialized laboratories.

BIOCHEMISTRY TESTING IN CALCIUM DISORDERS OR BONE DISEASE

The role of the routine biochemistry laboratory in diagnosis and treatment of patients with calcium disorders and bone disease is to provide measurements of calcium, albumin, phosphate and alkaline phosphatase in a serum specimen as first line tests. Follow-up tests which may be requested include:

- PTH
- magnesium
- urine calcium excretion
- 25-hydroxycholecalciferol
- urine hydroxyproline excretion
- osteocalcin.

Characteristic biochemistry profiles in some common bone diseases are shown in Table 1.

Table 1 **Biochemical profiles in bone diseases**

Disease	Profile
Bone metastases	Calcium may be high, low or normal Phosphate may be high, low or normal PTH is usually low Alkaline phosphatase may be elevated or normal
Osteomalacia/Rickets	Calcium will tend to be low, or may be clearly decreased PTH will be elevated 25-hydroxycholecalciferol will be decreased if the disease is due to vitamin D deficiency
Paget's disease	Calcium is normal Alkaline phosphatase is grossly elevated
Osteoporosis	Biochemistry is unremarkable
Renal osteodystrophy	Calcium is decreased PTH is very high
Osteitis fibrosa cystica (primary hyperparathyroidism)	Calcium is elevated Phosphate is low or normal PTH is increased, or clearly detectable and thus 'inappropriate' to the hypercalcaemia

Bone disease

- Alkaline phosphatase is a marker for bone formation. Urinary hydroxyproline is a marker for bone resorption. Better markers for bone turnover are being evaluated.
- Osteomalacia due to vitamin D deficiency can be confirmed by finding a low 25-hydroxycholecalciferol concentration. In severe disease, alkaline phosphatase will be increased. Calcium may well fall and there will be an appropriate rise in PTH.
- The characteristic biochemical marker of Paget's disease is a grossly increased alkaline phosphatase activity, as a consequence of increased bone turnover.

OSTEOPOROSIS

OSTEOPOROSIS

Osteoporosis is a large public health problem. One in four women and one in twenty men over the age of 60 in Britain will have an osteoporosis related fracture. It is a major cause of morbidity and mortality in the elderly. Almost one third of orthopaedic beds are occupied by patients with this disease which was once dismissed as a normal part of ageing.

Osteoporosis is characterized by a reduction in bone mass per unit volume. The composition of the matrix is essentially normal, but there is just less of it. The cortical areas of bones are thinner than normal and the trabeculae are smaller and less extensive (Fig.1). Both sexes show a gradual bone loss throughout life but women lose bone rapidly in the post-menopausal years. This is called primary osteoporosis and is of unknown aetiology.

Accelerated bone loss leading to secondary osteoporosis may be caused by:

- certain drugs, especially long-term use of corticosteroids or heparin
- immobilization
- smoking
- alcohol
- Cushing's syndrome
- gonadal failure
- hyperthyroidism
- gastrointestinal disease.

Diagnosis

Serial measurements of bone density are required to demonstrate bone loss but frequently on presentation the diagnosis can be made from a single measurement. It may take months or years to quantitate the rate of bone loss with confidence.

For many patients the first indication of the disease is when they suffer a vertebral compression fracture, a fracture of the distal radius or a fractured neck of femur. Crush fractures of vertebrae may occur slowly and relatively painlessly over a period of time (Figs. 2 and 3).

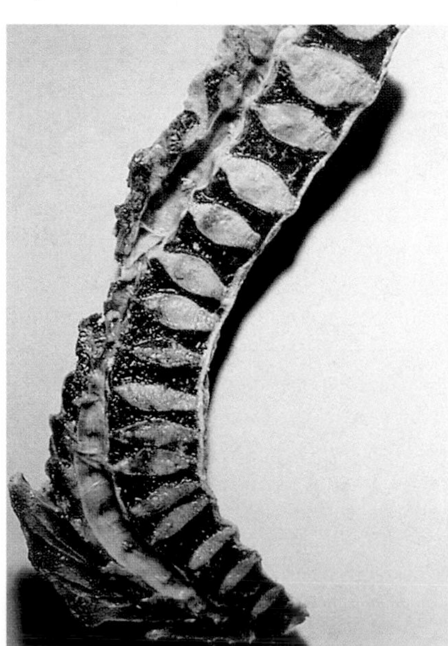

Fig. 2 **Crush fractures of vertebral bodies from patient with osteoporosis.** Reproduced by kind permission of Dr W. Kumthornthip.

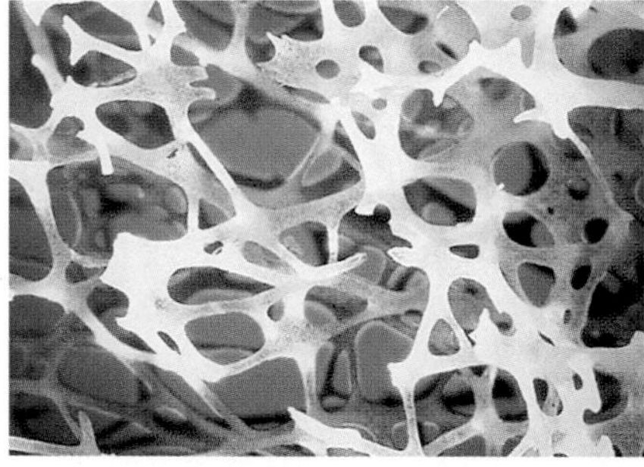

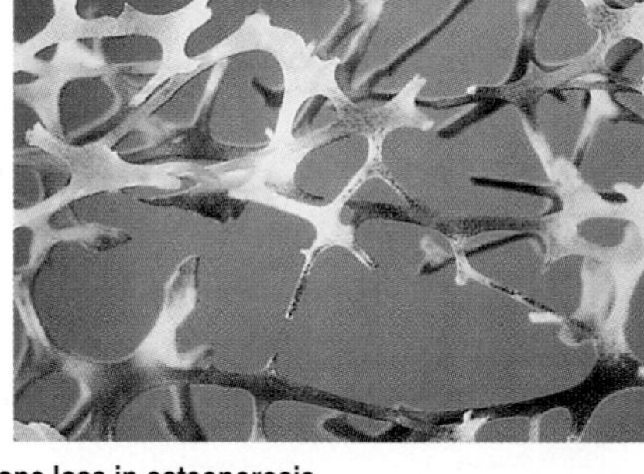

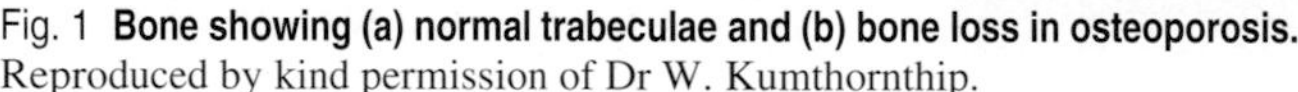

Fig. 1 **Bone showing (a) normal trabeculae and (b) bone loss in osteoporosis.** Reproduced by kind permission of Dr W. Kumthornthip.

The role of the clinical biochemistry laboratory

Biochemical tests cannot be used to diagnose primary osteoporosis or monitor accelerated bone loss because the results of the common biochemical analyses overlap in healthy subjects and patients with the disorder. Biochemical tests are of value in the diagnosis of hyperthyroidism, gonadal failure or Cushing's syndrome which cause secondary osteoporosis.

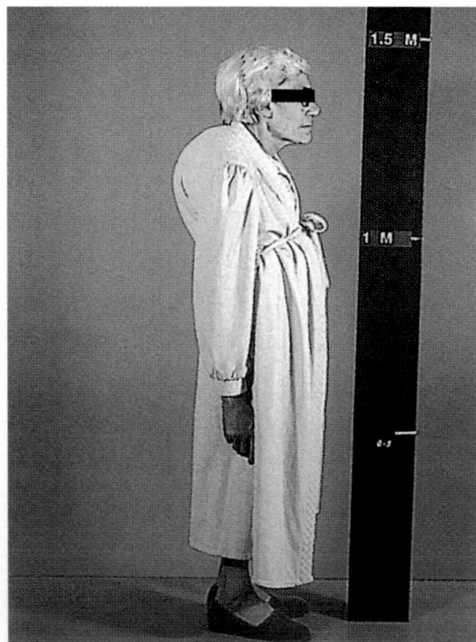

Fig. 3 **Elderly woman with so called 'Dowager's hump' from collapsed vertebrae due to osteoporosis.**

Osteoporosis may be present alongside osteomalacia (pages 70–71) in which case biochemical monitoring is helpful.

Treatment

Prevention, rather than cure, is the current goal. This should start in childhood with a good diet and exercise. The most powerful predictor of osteoporosis is the skeletal mass at 16 years of age.

Once skeletal maturity has been attained, it is the magnitude of the subsequent bone loss which may lead to osteoporosis. The use of corticosteroid drugs should be minimized. Stopping smoking is important. At the menopause, hormone replacement therapy is of benefit, not only for the relief of menopausal symptoms but also to prevent rapid bone loss. Indeed, cardiovascular protection also follows as an incidental benefit of such therapy.

When osteoporosis is established the treatment options are as yet unsatisfactory. Oral calcium supplements, oestrogens and fluoride have all been advocated. Bisphosphonates may be beneficial.

Osteoporosis

- Osteoporosis is a major cause of morbidity and mortality in the elderly.
- It is characterized by a reduction in bone mass per unit volume.
- Although both sexes show a gradual bone loss throughout life, women lose bone rapidly in the post-menopausal years. This 'primary osteoporosis' is of unknown aetiology.
- Bone loss causing secondary osteoporosis may be accelerated by a number of factors such as the use of corticosteroids, smoking and immobilization.

ENDOCRINOLOGY

ENDOCRINE CONTROL

BIOCHEMICAL REGULATORS

Endocrinology is the study of hormones, chemical agents which are secreted from specialized glands into the blood to influence the activity of cells at distant sites in the body. Hormones are just one type of biochemical regulator. Endocrinology has been recently expanded by the discovery of whole families of paracrine factors, which are not secreted into the circulation but act on adjacent cells. Some of these paracrine factors, which act to stimulate growth or to regulate the immune system, are identical to classical hormones and to neurotransmitters. In addition, some of these regulators of cellular activity appear to act in an autocrine fashion: they stimulate the very cell responsible for their synthesis (Fig. 1).

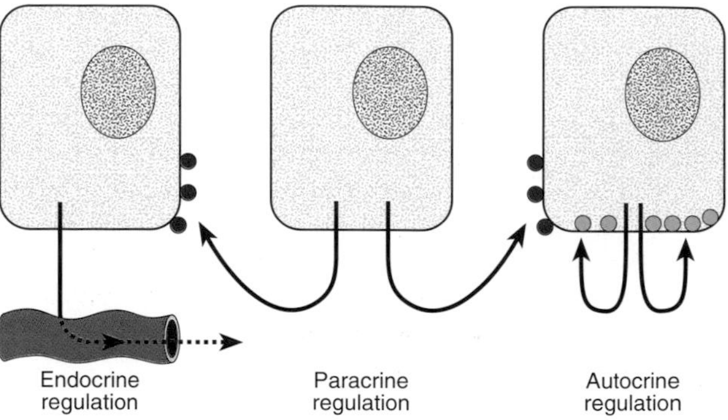

Fig. 1 **Biochemical regulation of cell function.**

All these regulators act via receptor proteins, which may be on the cell surface or within the target cells. The intracellular mechanisms whereby the hormone-receptor complex triggers a sequence of events culminating in a biological response are the subject of much current research.

TYPES OF HORMONE

Hormones fall into one of three broad classes on the basis of their structure:

- *Peptides or proteins.* Most hormones fall into this class. These may be small (the hypothalamic factor, thyrotrophin releasing hormone, has just three amino acids) or large (the pituitary gonadotrophins are glycoproteins with subunits).
- *Amino acid derivatives.* A few hormones fall into this class, e.g. adrenaline and the thyroid hormones.
- *Steroid hormones.* These are all derivatives of cholesterol.

Many hormones are members of families of related structure and reflect the process of molecular evolution. The steroid and thyroid hormones, which have diverse biological effects, are known now to act similarly, through one large superfamily of receptors which share structural and functional features.

Many hormones are commonly known just by their initials (Table 1).

Table 1 **Acronyms for some hormones**

Hormone	Acronym
Adrenocorticotrophic hormone	ACTH
Arginine vasopressin	AVP
Corticotrophin releasing hormone	CRH
Follicle stimulating hormone	FSH
Gonadotrophin releasing hormone	GnRH
Growth hormone	GH (or HGH)
Growth hormone releasing hormone	GHRH
Luteinizing hormone	LH
Parathyroid hormone	PTH
Thyroid stimulating hormone	TSH
Thyrotrophin releasing hormone	TRH
Thyroxine	T_4
Triiodothyronine	T_3

MEASUREMENT OF HORMONES

At one time it was the biological response to the hormone which formed the basis of bioassays for measuring hormone activity. The development of radioimmunoassays revolutionized the study of endocrinology, although measurement of structurally related hormones continues to be a problem for the clinical biochemistry laboratory. The use of monoclonal antibodies has allowed the development of more sensitive and more specific methods for measuring hormones. Sensitivity is paramount. Hormone concentrations in blood are sometimes very low. It is important for the laboratory to be able to measure subnormal concentrations of hormones and to be able to distinguish these from the lower limit of the reference range.

HORMONE BINDING IN PLASMA

Steroid and thyroid hormones bind to specific hormone binding glycoproteins in plasma. It is the unbound or 'free' fraction of the hormone in plasma which is biologically active; so measurement of free hormone status or binding protein levels may be important in the diagnosis of patients with thyroid or gonadal disorders.

FACTORS CONTROLLING HORMONE SECRETION

Hormone secretion is under a variety of influences:

- Stimulatory and inhibitory agents, such as hypothalamic peptides or neurotransmitters, may influence hormone synthesis or release.
- Many hormones, such as GnRH, are released in a pulsatile fashion.
- Some hormones exhibit a circadian rhythm. ACTH, and consequently cortisol, is a well known example, but prolactin, TSH, GH and even parathyroid hormone have peak secretion at different times during the day or night.
- Stress can increase hormone synthesis and release. Examples are ACTH, GH and prolactin.
- Hormones synthesized by target organ cells may feed back to the endocrine glands (Fig. 2).
- Changes in metabolic products as a result of hormone action may likewise exert feedback control.
- Other hormones or drugs may modulate normal endocrine responses.

As a result of the above, plasma hormone concentrations are normally variable (Fig. 3). Thus a single measurement of a hormone in peripheral plasma may suggest, incorrectly, that there is abnormal endocrine function. Dynamic tests have been developed to give clearer information about endocrine activity in the patient, especially those with suspected pituitary or adrenocortical disorders.

ENDOCRINE DISEASE

At its simplest, endocrine disease may be described as over- or under-secretion of hormone. In fact, there are other considerations (Table 2). For example, a patient may become hypocalcaemic because the parathyroid glands are

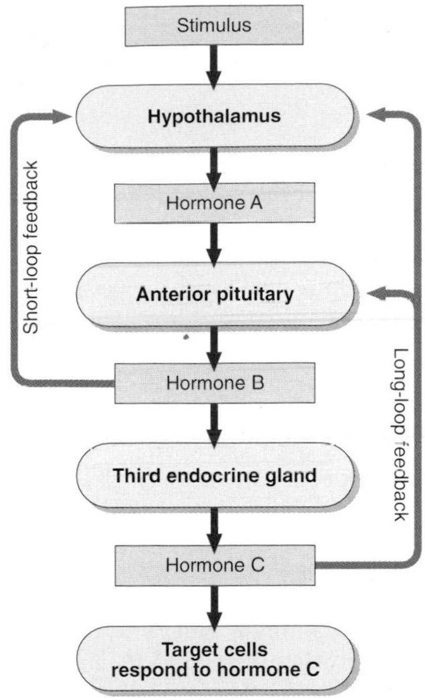

Fig. 2 **Feedback interactions in a hypothalamic-pituitary-endocrine gland system.**

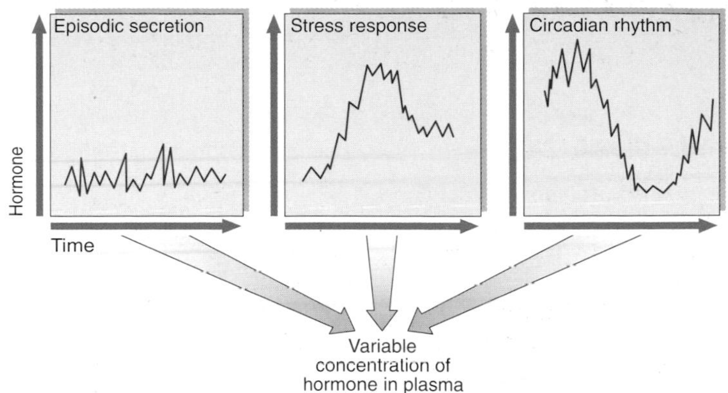

Fig. 3 **Reasons why a single blood hormone measurement may have little clinical value.**

unable to make sufficient hormone (hypoparathyroidism), or if there is a malfunctioning receptor mechanism in the target cells (pseudohypoparathyroidism). In practice, many endocrine diseases are managed without direct knowledge of the hormone concentration itself. Diagnosis and monitoring of diabetes mellitus, the commonest endocrine disorder, is carried out by measuring plasma glucose rather than insulin.

COMMONLY USED DYNAMIC TESTS IN THE INVESTIGATION OF ENDOCRINE DISEASE

Oral glucose tolerance test

The oral glucose tolerance test (see p. 58) is commonly used in the diagnosis of diabetes mellitus but is also used to investigate growth hormone response in acromegaly.

TRH test

TRH is given as an intravenous bolus, and in normal subjects, elicits a brisk release of both TSH and prolactin. Subnormal TSH responses are seen in thyrotoxicosis (excess feedback) and in cases of damage to the pituitary thyrotroph cells. The lack of prolactin response to TRH stimulation may be of value in the diagnosis of a prolactinoma.

GnRH test

In normal adults, GnRH elicits a marked release of LH and a smaller release of FSH. This test is frequently used to investigate possible damage to pituitary gonadotrophin secreting cells.

Synacthen test

Administration of a synthetic ACTH preparation (Synacthen) stimulates the adrenal cortex. An impaired cortisol response to Synacthen is seen in Addison's disease (primary adrenal failure).

Insulin-induced hypoglycaemia test (ITT)

Insulin is administered intravenously to make the patient hypoglycaemic. The response to this deliberately induced stress confirms or excludes the diagnosis of Cushing's syndrome. The test is also used in the investigation of growth hormone deficiency, and hypopituitarism. With the increased availability of the hypothalamic hormone CRH, it is likely that the CRH test will become more accepted as a means of investigating the hypothalamic–pituitary–adrenocortical axis.

Dexamethasone suppression tests

Dexamethasone is a synthetic cortisol analogue which is used to suppress pituitary production of ACTH and, hence, cortisol in the diagnosis and differential diagnosis of Cushing's syndrome.

Combined anterior pituitary function test (CAPFT)

The investigation of any pituitary disorder usually includes a CAPFT which comprises the simultaneous administration of insulin (stimulates ACTH, GH and prolactin), TRH (stimulates TSH and prolactin) and GnRH (stimulates FSH and LH). This complex test is discussed in detail on pages 76–77.

Table 2 **Examples of Endocrine Disease**

Oversecretion Cushing's disease where a pituitary adenoma secretes ACTH
Undersecretion Primary hypothyroidism where the thyroid gland is unable to make sufficient thyroid hormone despite continued stimulation by TSH
Failure of hormone responsiveness Pseudohypoparathyroidism where patients become hypocalcaemic despite elevated plasma PTH concentration because target organs lack a functioning receptor signalling mechanism

Clinical note

The overriding influence of stress on the endocrine system makes the diagnosis of endocrine disorders in the critically ill patient very difficult. Ill patients may have hyperglycaemia, high serum cortisol or abnormal thyroid hormone results. These could be misinterpreted as diabetes mellitus, Cushing's syndrome or thyroid disease.

Endocrine control

- Endocrinology is the study of hormones, a class of biochemical regulators which are secreted into blood to act at distant sites in the body.
- Hormone concentrations in plasma are very variable.
- For the clear demonstration of abnormalities of hormone secretion or regulation, dynamic tests are often necessary.

PITUITARY FUNCTION

THE PITUITARY GLAND

The pituitary gland is a complex structure of secretory cells, blood vessels and nervous tissue lying in a bony cavity at the base of the skull. Considering its importance in regulating so many bodily functions, the pituitary gland is really a very small organ, weighing only about 0.5 g. Most (75%) of the gland comprises the anterior pituitary or adenohypophysis; the remainder is the posterior pituitary, the neurohypophysis. Pituitary function is regulated by the hypothalamus, to which it is connected via the pituitary stalk which comprises portal blood capillaries and nerve fibres. The anterior pituitary is influenced by a variety of stimulatory and inhibitory hormones through these capillaries. The posterior pituitary is a collection of specialized nerve endings that derive from the hypothalamus.

Anterior pituitary hormones

The anterior pituitary hormones are:

- *TSH (thyroid stimulating hormone)* which acts specifically on the thyroid gland to elicit secretion of thyroid hormones. Disorders of the hypothalamic–pituitary–thyroid axis are described in detail on pages 80–85.
- *ACTH (adrenocorticotrophic hormone)* acts specifically on the adrenal cortex to elicit secretion of cortisol. Disorders of the hypothalamic–pituitary–adrenal axis are described in detail on pages 86–91.
- *LH (luteinizing hormone) and FSH (follicle stimulating hormone)*, known jointly as the gonadotrophins, act cooperatively on the ovaries in women and the testes in men to stimulate sex hormone secretion and reproductive processes (pp. 92–94).
- *GH (growth hormone)* acts directly on many tissues to modulate metabolism. Metabolic fuels (e.g. glucose, free fatty acids) in turn modify GH secretion. Growth hormone over- and under-secretion is described in more detail on pages 78–79.
- *Prolactin* acts directly on the mammary glands to control lactation. Gonadal function is impaired by elevated circulating prolactin concentrations.

The hypothalamic factors which control anterior pituitary hormone secretion are shown in Figure 1. Tumours secreting each of the anterior pituitary hormones have been identified. TSH and gonadotrophin secreting tumours are rare. GH and ACTH secreting tumours are more common. Prolactin secreting adenomas (prolactinomas) are the most common.

Hyperprolactinaemia

Hyperprolactinaemia is common and can cause infertility in both sexes. An early indication in women is amenorrhoea and galactorrhoea, whereas in men there may be no early signs and the first indication of the presence of a prolactinoma may be when a large growing tumour begins to interfere with the optic nerves. Causes of hyperprolactinaemia include:

- stress (venepuncture is sufficient to raise plasma prolactin in some patients)
- drugs (e.g. oestrogens, phenothiazines, metoclopramide, α-methyl dopa)
- primary hypothyroidism (prolactin is stimulated by the raised TRH)
- other pituitary disease.

If these causes are excluded, the differential diagnosis is between:

- a prolactinoma (a prolactin-secreting pituitary tumour, commonly a microadenoma)
- idiopathic hypersecretion which may be due to impaired secretion of dopamine, the hypothalamic factor which inhibits prolactin release.

Differentiating between these, after exclusion of stress, drugs and other disease, is by detailed pituitary radiology together with dynamic tests of prolactin secretion. A rise in serum prolactin following administration of TRH or metoclopramide, is observed in idiopathic hyperprolactinaemia but not in the presence of a pituitary tumour.

Posterior pituitary hormones

Hypothalamic neurones synthesize arginine vasopressin (AVP) and oxytocin which pass along axonal nerve fibres in the pituitary stalk to the posterior pituitary where they are stored in granules in the terminal bulbs of nerves in close proximity to systemic veins.

Secretion of AVP, also known as antidiuretic hormone (ADH), is stimulated by:

- increased plasma osmolality via hypothalamic osmoreceptors
- severe blood volume depletion via cardiac baroreceptors
- stress and nausea.

The role of AVP in fluid and electrolyte regulation is discussed on pages 14–15. A pituitary tumour arising in the anterior gland may cause impaired secretion of this posterior pituitary hormone, with consequent diabetes insipidus.

Oxytocin is released in response to suckling of the breast and uterine contraction at the onset of labour.

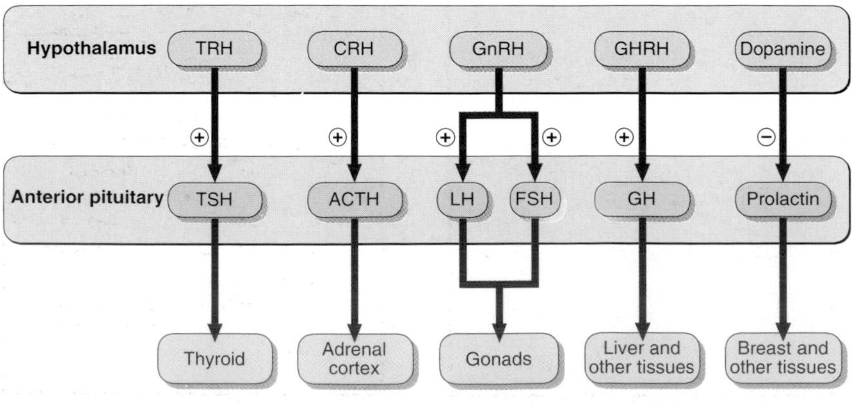

PITUITARY TUMOUR

Diagnosis

Pituitary tumours may be either functional (that is they secrete hormones) or non-functional. The incidence of different tumour types is shown in Figure 2. Local effects such as headaches, papilloedema and visual field defects caused by large tumours extending upwards to interfere with the optic nerves may be evident on clinical examination. There may be specific signs of hormone excess particularly in acromegaly, Cushing's syndrome and prolactinoma. There may be signs of hypopituitarism in skin, hair and musculature.

Fig. 1 **Hypothalamic factors which regulate anterior pituitary function.**

Radiological investigations seek evidence of an enlarged pituitary fossa. Plain skull X-ray, CT scans and magnetic resonance imaging (MRI) may be used.

The clinical biochemistry laboratory is commonly called upon to establish if there is excessive hormone secretion. Simple screening tests to eliminate other diagnoses are followed by more complicated dynamic tests. If a pituitary tumour is suspected, it is important to establish the extent of damage to other pituitary functions. The combined anterior pituitary function test (Fig. 3) is used here. TRH, GnRH and insulin are given from separate syringes. All hormones are measured at 0, 30 and 60 min, and cortisol and GH additionally at 45, 90 and 120 min. It is usual to assess basal thyroid function (thyroxine) and basal gonadal function (testosterone or oestradiol) at the same time.

A clinician must be on hand throughout the test, glucose and hydrocortisone should be available for intravenous administration if needed, and a carbohydrate meal should be given at the end of the test. The test is contraindicated in epilepsy or heart disease.

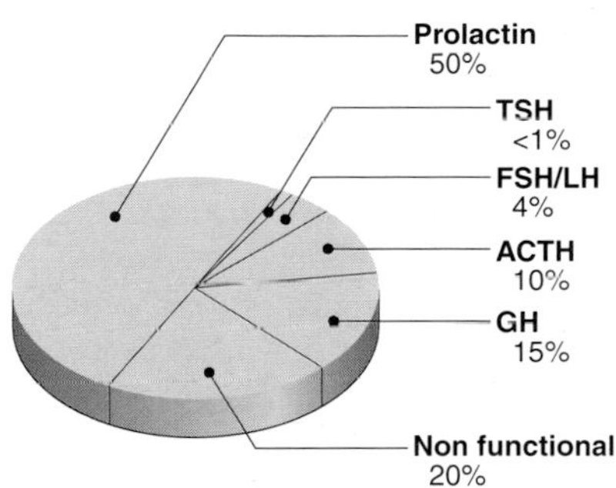

Fig. 2 **Incidence of different types of pituitary tumours.**

Because of its associated dangers, insulin-induced hypoglycaemia is being replaced by administration of GHRH and CRH to investigate GH and cortisol secretion. Thus, to investigate pituitary function, a combined TRH/GnRH/GHRH/CRH test may be carried out.

Treatment

The treatment of functional pituitary tumours varies. Microadenomas secreting prolactin are the most common and may be managed medically or surgically. Large suprasellar prolactinomas may be shrunk with dopamine agonist drugs before surgery. Other options for treatment include external irradiation or radioactive implants.

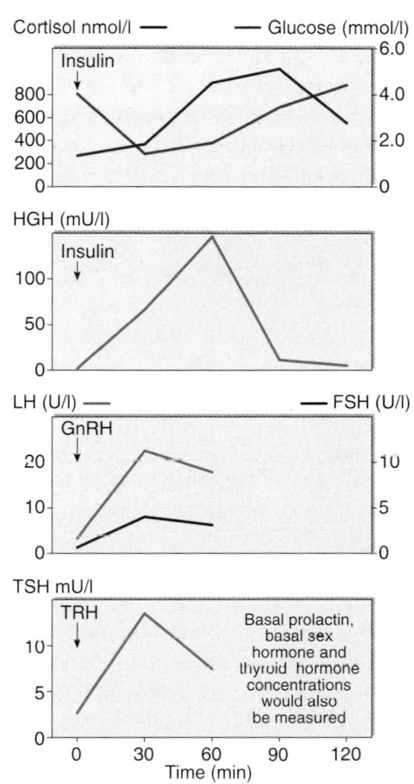

Fig. 3 **Normal responses in a combined anterior pituitary function test.**

HYPOPITUITARISM

There are many causes of hypopituitarism, a relatively uncommon condition in which there is failure of one or more pituitary functions. These causes include:

- tumour
- infarction
- trauma
- congenital malformation
- infection
- hypothalamic disorder.

The clinical presentation of hypopituitarism depends on the age of the patient. In infancy, short stature or impaired development may point to the condition. In the reproductive years, women may present with amenorrhoea or infertility. Men may present with decreased libido or a lack of male secondary sex characteristics. Elderly patients may complain of symptoms relating to ACTH or TSH deficiency such as hypoglycaemia or hypothermia.

Clinical note

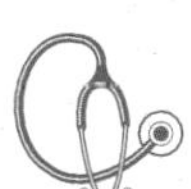

Imaging techniques are very important in the diagnosis of pituitary tumours in conjunction with the biochemical findings.

Case history 31

A 36-year-old man complained of impaired vision while driving, particularly at night. After clinical and initial biochemical assessment, a combined anterior pituitary stimulation test was performed (i.v. insulin 0.1 U/kg, TRH 200 μg, GnRH 100 μg).

Time (min)	Glucose mmol/l	Cortisol nmol/l	GH mU/l	PRL mU/l	FSH U/l	LH U/l	TSH mU/l	T_4 nmol/l	Testosterone nmol/l
0	3.6	320	1.5	17 000	<0.7	<1.0	<1.0	32	6.1
30	0.9	310	1.7	16 400	0.8	3.7	2.7		
60	1.8	380	1.6	18 000	1.2	3.7	4.1		
90	2.7	370	1.4						
120	3.3	230	1.4						

- A lower than normal dose of insulin was used. Why?
- What is the most likely diagnosis?
- What precautions should be taken before surgery?

Comment on page 155.

Pituitary function

- Adenomas secreting each of the anterior pituitary hormones have been identified.
- Around 20% of pituitary tumours appear not to secrete hormone.
- It is important to establish if a pituitary tumour, whether hormone secreting or not, has interfered with the other hypothalamic–pituitary connections.
- Hyperprolactinaemia is common. Once stress, drugs or other disease have been eliminated as possible causes, dynamic tests and detailed radiology are used to differentiate between prolactinoma and idiopathic hypersecretion.
- Hypopituitarism is uncommon; the clinical presentation depends on the age of the patient.

GROWTH DISORDERS AND ACROMEGALY

NORMAL GROWTH

Growth in children can be divided into three stages (Fig. 1). Rapid growth occurs during the first 2 years of life; the rate is influenced by conditions in utero, as well as the adequacy of nutrition in the postnatal period. The next stage is relatively steady growth for around 9 years and is controlled mainly by growth hormone (GH). If the pituitary does not produce sufficient growth hormone, the yearly growth rate during this period may be halved and the child will be of short stature. The growth spurt at puberty is caused by the effect of the sex hormones in addition to continuing GH secretion. The regulation of GH secretion is outlined in Figure 2.

GH is only one of many hormones involved in growth. Others are thyroxine, cortisol, the sex steroids, insulin, and a number of paracrine 'growth factors', particularly the somatomedins or insulin-like growth factors (IGFs) which mediate the growth promoting effects of growth hormone.

GROWTH HORMONE INSUFFICIENCY

Growth hormone insufficiency is a rare cause of impaired physical growth. It is important to differentiate between children whose slow growth or growth failure is due to illness or disease and those whose short stature is a normal variant of the population. It is usual to classify children with short stature into two groups: those with normal features and those who have an abnormal appearance. Causes of short stature are:

- having parents who are both short
- inherited diseases such as achondroplasia, the commonest cause of severe dwarfism
- poor nutrition
- systemic chronic illness, such as renal disease, gastrointestinal disorders or respiratory disease
- psychological factors such as emotional deprivation
- hormonal disorders.

Growth hormone deficiency is only one possible endocrine cause. Others include hypothyroidism and Cushing's syndrome.

Standard graphs relating age and height are available for the normal population. Accurate measurements of height should be made to establish whether a child is small for chronological age. These measurements are repeated after 6 and 12 months to assess the growth rate. The height of the parents should also be assessed. The bone age is important for the prognosis of a child with short stature; this is determined by radiological examination of hand and wrist. In most growth disorders bone age is delayed and by itself is of little diagnostic value, but taken together with height and chronological age, a prediction of final height may be obtained.

Any child whose height for age falls below the 3rd centile on a standard chart, or who exhibits a slow growth rate, requires further investigation. If GH deficiency is diagnosed, and treatment is required, then the earlier it is given the better the chance that the child will eventually reach normal size.

Tests of growth hormone insufficiency

Growth hormone deficiency may be present from birth or due to later pituitary failure. A variety of stimulation tests have been used to evaluate GH deficiency. Serum GH concentrations rise in response to exercise, and this may be used as a preliminary screening test. They also rise during sleep, and high concentrations in a nocturnal sample may exclude GH deficiency. The lack of GH response to clonidine, a potent stimulant of GH secretion, is diagnostic. Some centres have now abandoned the use of insulin-induced hypoglycaemia as a diagnostic test in children because of its hazards.

The GH response to stimulation may be blunted before puberty, and priming with the appropriate sex steroid is necessary before investigating GH reserve.

Increasingly, urinary growth hormone measurements are being used to assess possible GH lack in children. Random

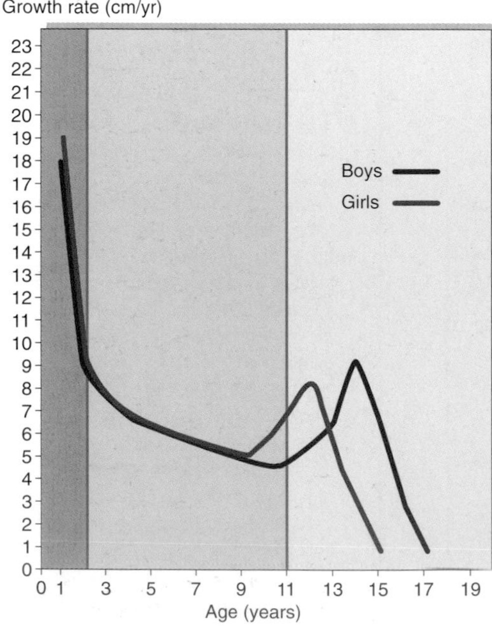

Fig. 1 **Median height velocity curve for boys and girls showing the three growth stages.**

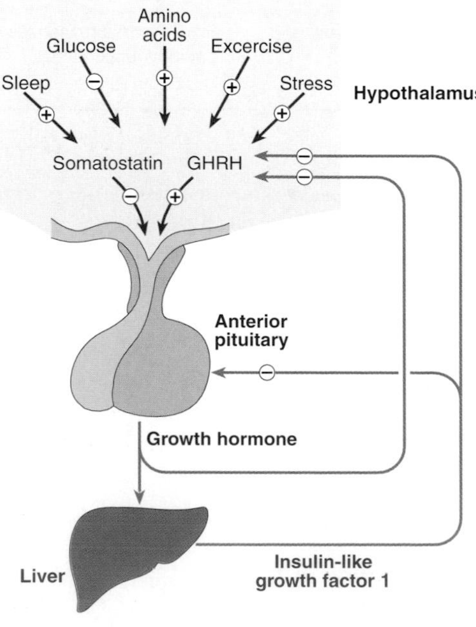

Fig. 2 **The normal regulation of GH secretion.**

serum IGF 1 determinations may be of value. Levels within reference limits exclude GH deficiency.

Treatment

Genetically engineered GH is available and is used in the treatment of that small group of children with proven GH deficiency.

EXCESSIVE GROWTH

Growth hormone excess in children is characterized by extremely rapid linear growth (gigantism). The condition is rare and is most often due to a pituitary tumour. Other causes of tall stature in children include:

- *Congenital adrenal hyperplasia.*
- *Hyperthyroidism.* An increased growth rate, with advanced bone age, is a feature of hyperthyroidism in children, or hypothyroid children over-replaced with thyroxine.
- *Inherited disorders* such as Klinefelter's syndrome (a 47 XXY karyotype).

ACROMEGALY

Increased GH secretion later in life, after fusion of bony epiphyses, causes acromegaly (Fig. 3). The most likely cause is a pituitary adenoma. Clinical features include:

- coarse facial features
- soft tissue thickening, e.g the lips
- characteristic 'spade-like' hands
- protruding jaw (prognathism)
- sweating
- impaired glucose tolerance or diabetes mellitus.

Diagnosis

Basal serum GH concentrations are elevated but since growth hormone secretion is both episodic and responsive to stress, a single sample may give unreliable results. The oral glucose tolerance test, commonly used in the investigation of diabetes mellitus, is used in the diagnosis of acromegaly. A normal person will suppress GH in plasma in response to a glucose load, this being the expected metabolic response of a hormone which primarily regulates catabolic pathways of metabolism. The acromegalic patient's GH levels do not suppress in response to the elevated glucose concentrations (Fig. 4), there being at best only a slight fall in GH concentration, and in some patients a paradoxical rise in GH may even be observed.

Elevated concentrations of IGF 1 in serum confirm the diagnosis of acromegaly. Single IGF 1 measurements may in future replace the need for multiple GH determinations during suppression tests.

When investigating any pituitary tumour it is important to assess if there is disruption of other pituitary hormone secretion by means of a combined anterior pituitary function test (p. 77).

Treatment

GH secreting tumours may be treated in three ways:

- by surgery
- with radiotherapy
- with drugs such as octreotide (a somatostatin analogue) and bromocriptine.

Occasionally patients will require all three modes of treatment. Clinically it is difficult to be sure of the success of treatment. Biochemical evidence of recurrence can be monitored by measuring IGF 1 concentrations and by assessing GH response to the oral glucose tolerance test at intervals.

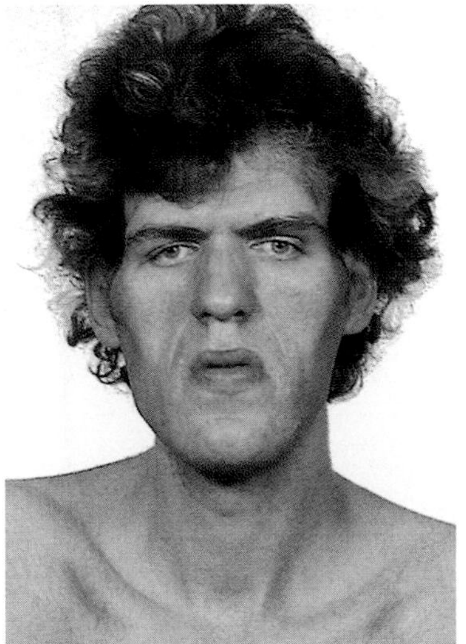

Fig. 3 **Clinical picture of an acromegalic patient.**

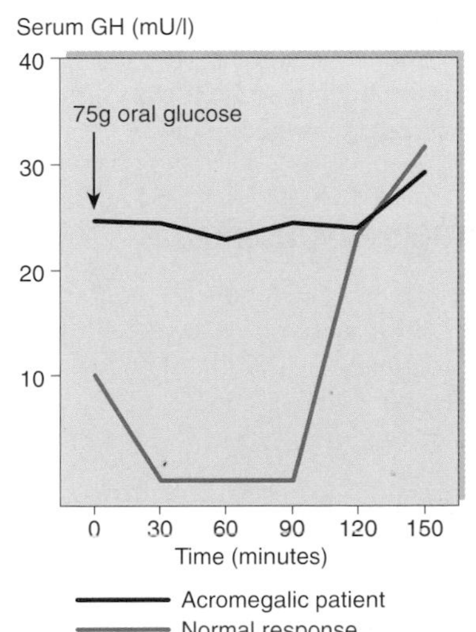

Fig. 4 **The response of GH in a glucose tolerance test in a normal and acromegalic patient.**

Case history 32

James is 5 years old and is much smaller than his classmates at school. His growth rate has been monitored and has clearly dropped off markedly in the past year. He is an active child, and on examination has normal body proportions. His mother and father are of average height. His bone age is that of a 3-year-old child.

- What biochemical tests would be appropriate in the investigation of this boy?

Comment on page 155.

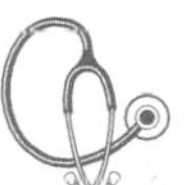

Clinical note

In the investigation of normal looking children with short stature, coeliac disease must always be considered. The diagnosis is frequently overlooked.

Growth disorders and acromegaly

- GH deficiency is a rare cause of short stature in children, and is investigated only after other causes of short stature have been eliminated.
- Diagnosis of GH deficiency is made on the failure of serum GH to rise in response to clonidine.
- Gigantism in children is caused by increased GH secretion, usually from a pituitary tumour. Acromegaly is the consequence of increased GH secretion in adults.
- Lack of suppression of serum GH levels in response to a glucose tolerance test is the diagnostic test for acromegaly.
- Serum IGF 1 concentrations are of value in the diagnosis of acromegaly and the monitoring of treatment.

THYROID PATHOPHYSIOLOGY

INTRODUCTION

Thyroxine (T_4) and tri-iodothyronine (T_3) are together known as the 'thyroid hormones'. They are synthesized in the thyroid gland by iodination and coupling of two tyrosine molecules whilst attached to a complex protein called thyroglobulin. T_4 has four iodine atoms while T_3 has three (Fig. 1).

The thyroid gland secretes mostly T_4 whose concentration in plasma is around 100 nmol/l. The peripheral tissues, especially the liver and kidney, deiodinate T_4 to produce approximately two-thirds of the circulating T_3, present at a lower concentration of around 2 nmol/l. Most cells are capable of taking up T_4 and deiodinating it to the more biologically active T_3. It is T_3 which binds to receptors and triggers the end-organ effects of the thyroid hormones. Alternatively, T_4 can be metabolized to reverse T_3, which is biologically inactive. By modulating the relative production of T_3 and rT_3, tissues can 'fine tune' their local thyroid status. Exactly how this is accomplished is not yet fully understood.

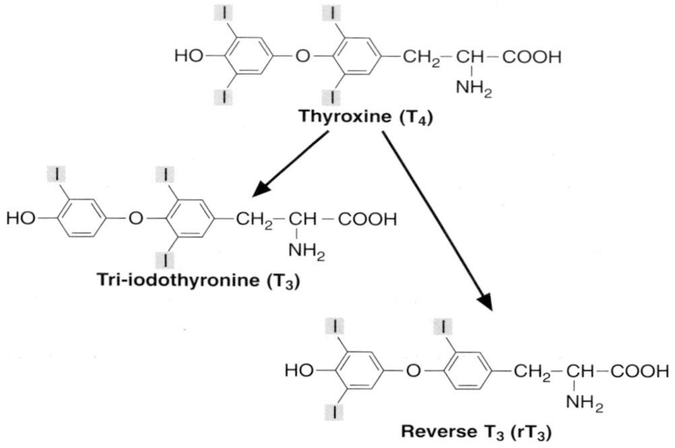

Thyroxine (T_4)

Tri-iodothyronine (T_3)

Reverse T_3 (rT_3)

Fig. 1 **The chemical structures of T_4, T_3 and rT_3.**

THYROID HORMONE ACTION

Thyroid hormones are essential for the normal maturation and metabolism of all the tissues in the body. Their effects on tissue maturation are most dramatically seen in congenital hypothyroidism, a condition which, unless treated within 3 months of birth, results in permanent brain damage. Hypothyroid children have delayed skeletal maturation, short stature and delayed puberty.

Thyroid hormone effects on metabolism are diverse. The rates of protein and carbohydrate synthesis and catabolism are influenced. An example of the effect of thyroid hormones on lipid metabolism is the observation of a high serum cholesterol in some hypothyroid patients. This is a consequence of a reduction in cholesterol metabolism due to down regulation of low-density lipoprotein (LDL) receptors on liver cell membranes, with a subsequent failure of sterol excretion via the gut.

Binding in plasma

In plasma, over 99.95% of T_4 is transported bound to proteins. Thyroxine binding globulin (TBG) carries 70% of T_4, albumin approximately 25% and transthyretin (formerly called prealbumin) around 5%. Over 99.5% of T_3 is transported by the same proteins. It is the unbound, or 'free', T_4 and T_3 concentrations which are important for the biological effects of the hormones, including the feedback to the pituitary and hypothalamus. Changes in binding protein concentration complicate the interpretation of thyroid hormone results, e.g. in pregnancy.

Regulation of thyroid hormone secretion

The components of the hypothalamic–pituitary–thyroid axis are outlined in Figure 2. TRH, a tripeptide, is secreted by the hypothalamus and in turn causes the synthesis of a large glycoprotein hormone, TSH, from the anterior pituitary. This drives the synthesis of thyroid hormones by the thyroid. Production of TSH is regulated by feedback from circulating unbound thyroid hormones. A knowledge of these basics is essential for the correct interpretation of results in the investigation of thyroid disease. Remember:

- If a patient's thyroid is producing too much thyroid hormone, then the circulating TSH will be suppressed.
- If the thyroid is not secreting enough thyroid hormone, the TSH levels will be very high in an attempt to stimulate the gland to secrete more.

THYROID FUNCTION TESTS

Biochemical measurements in the diagnosis of thyroid disease have traditionally been known as 'thyroid function tests'. TSH and some estimate of T_4 status (either total T_4 or free T_4) are the first line tests.

Measurement of TSH is a good example of how better technology has helped in the diagnosis and monitoring of disease. Early assays for TSH were unable to measure low concentrations of the hormone — the detection limits of the radioimmunoassays overlapped significantly with concentrations at the low end of the reference range in healthy subjects. Now, very sensitive TSH assays can detect much lower concentrations and it is possible to tell with a greater degree of certainty whether TSH secretion is really lower than normal.

Knowledge of thyroid hormone binding in plasma, either by measuring the 'free' hormone concentration or by determining TBG levels, may sometimes be needed in the assessment of a patient's thyroid status.

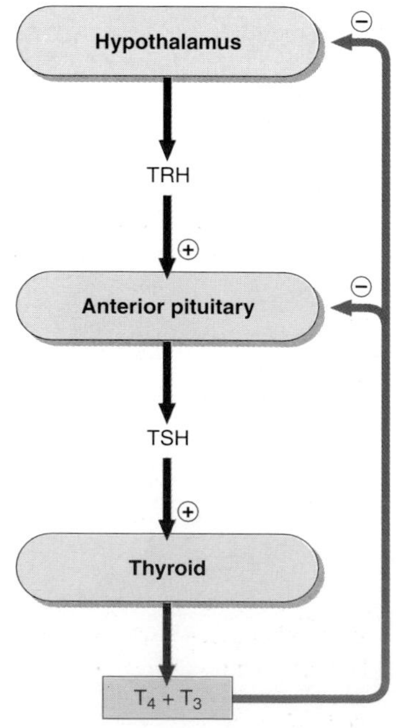

Fig. 2 **Outline of the hypothalamic–pituitary–thyroid axis.**

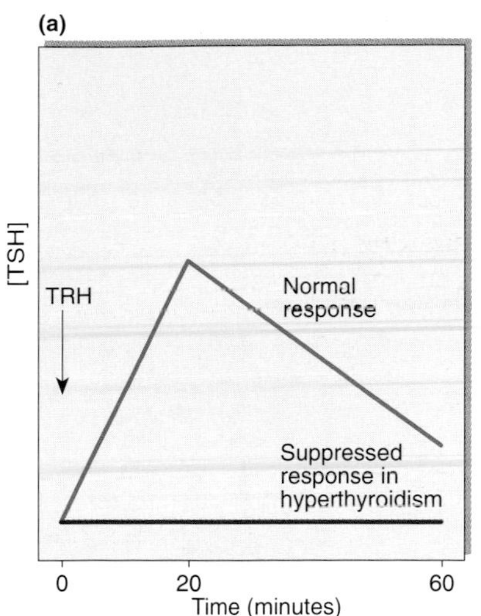

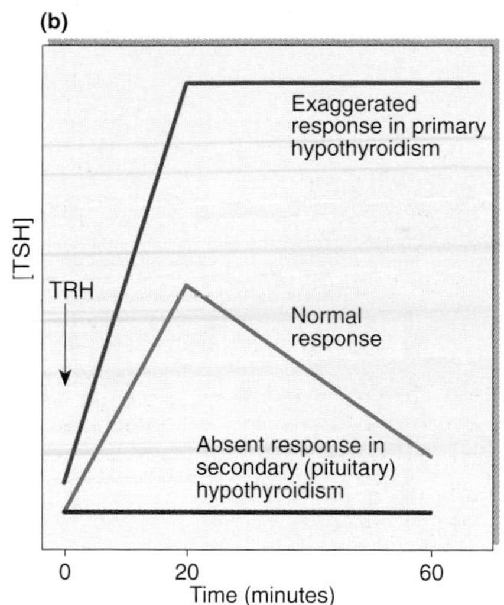

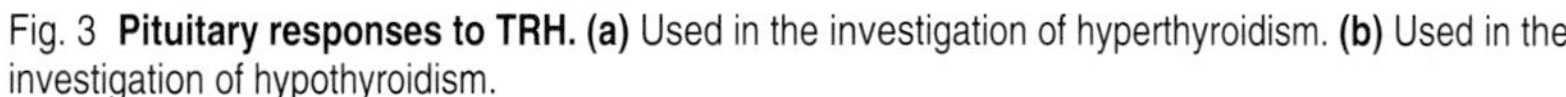

Fig. 3 **Pituitary responses to TRH. (a)** Used in the investigation of hyperthyroidism. **(b)** Used in the investigation of hypothyroidism.

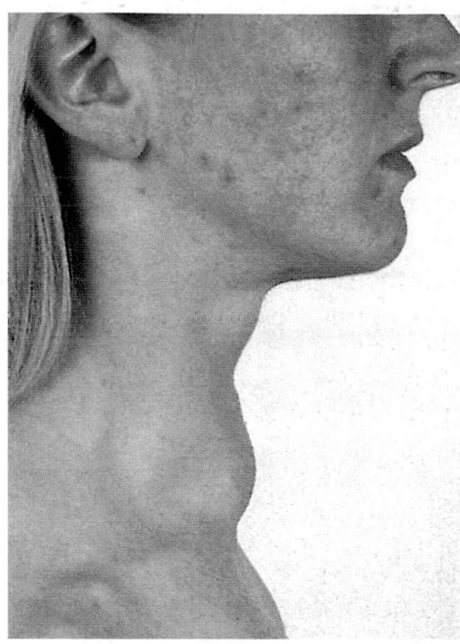

Fig. 4 **A patient with a goitre.**

Knowledge of the T_3 concentration is helpful in some cases of hyperthyroidism, where T_3 is elevated but T_4 is normal.

The TRH test involves intravenous injection of TRH and the measurement of pituitary TSH secreted in response to the stimulation. The test is used in two ways (Fig. 3):

- *Investigation of pituitary disorders* (see pp. 76–77). There will be a subnormal TSH response if the pituitary cannot make TSH.
- *Investigation of hyperthyroidism.* There will be an impaired TSH response if high circulating thyroid hormone levels are supressing the pituitary. The availability of sensitive TSH assays has made the TRH test almost redundant in the diagnosis of hyperthyroidism in all but the most difficult of cases.

The titre of autoantibodies to thyroid tissue antigens can be helpful in the diagnosis and monitoring of autoimmune thyroid disease. Anti-thyroid peroxidase (Anti-TPO) may be useful in hypothyroidism and stimulating anti-TSH receptor antibodies in thyrotoxicosis.

GOITRE

A goitre is an enlarged thyroid gland (Fig. 4). This may be associated with hypofunction, hyperfunction or, indeed, normal concentrations of thyroid hormones in blood. With such a clinical presentation, the biochemistry laboratory can confirm if a patient is hypothyroid, hyperthyroid or euthyroid.

Case history 33

A 49-year-old woman receiving hormone replacement therapy was found to have a thyroid nodule. No lymphadenopathy was detectable and she appeared clinically to be euthyroid. A technetium scan revealed a 'cold' nodule and an ultrasound scan indicated it was cystic.

Biochemistry results in a serum specimen:

T_4 *(nmol/l)*	TSH *(mU/l)*
172	0.40

- Explain why the T_4 is elevated.
- What other investigations should be performed in this patient?

Comment on page 155.

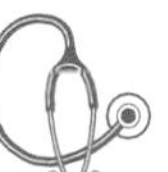

Clinical note

Autoimmune thyroid disorders are relatively common. Their presence should alert the clinician to the possibility that other autoimmune disorders, some of which are uncommon, may have been overlooked. Examples are:

- insulin-dependent diabetes mellitus
- autoimmune hypoparathyroidism
- primary gonadal failure
- autoimmune destruction of the adrenal cortex causing Addison's disease
- pernicious anaemia
- vitiligo.

Thyroid pathophysiology

- The thyroid gland synthesizes, stores, and secretes the thyroid hormones T_4 and T_3 which are important for normal development and metabolism.
- The secretion of thyroid hormones is controlled primarily by TSH from the anterior pituitary.
- Most T_4 and T_3 circulates in plasma bound to protein. Only a small proportion is not bound, yet it is this 'free' fraction which is biologically important.
- Knowledge of TSH, thyroid hormone and binding protein concentrations in serum may all be needed in the assessment of a patient's thyroid status.
- A patient may have severe thyroid disease, such as a large goitre or thyroid cancer, yet have normal concentrations of thyroid hormones in blood.

HYPOTHYROIDISM

CLINICAL FEATURES

The clinical features of hypothyroidism include:

- lethargy and tiredness
- cold intolerance
- weight gain
- dryness and coarsening of skin and hair
- hoarseness
- slow relaxation of muscles and tendon reflexes
- many other associated signs including anaemia, dementia, constipation, bradycardia, muscle stiffness, carpal tunnel syndrome, subfertility and galactorrhoea.

CAUSES

Over 90% of cases of hypothyroidism occur as a consequence of:

- autoimmune destruction of the thyroid gland (Hashimoto's disease)
- radioiodine or surgical treatment of hyperthyroidism.

Rarer causes include:

- transient hypothyroidism due to treatment with drugs such as lithium carbonate
- TSH deficiency which may be a component of panhypopituitarism
- congenital defects such as blocks in the biosynthesis of T_4 and T_3, or end-organ resistance to their action
- severe iodine deficiency.

DIAGNOSIS

Hypothyroidism is caused by a deficiency of thyroid hormones. Primary hypothyroidism is failure of the thyroid gland itself and is one of the most commonly encountered endocrine problems. The demonstration of an elevated TSH concentration is usually diagnostic. Secondary hypothyroidism, failure of the pituitary to secrete TSH, is much less common. Isolated pituitary deficiency of TSH is rare, but impairment of the hypothalamic–pituitary–thyroid axis may happen as a result of any pituitary disease or damage.

Clinical features other than those of hypothyroidism may indicate the need for investigation of pituitary function (see pp. 76–77), and the TRH test will be included in such a protocol.

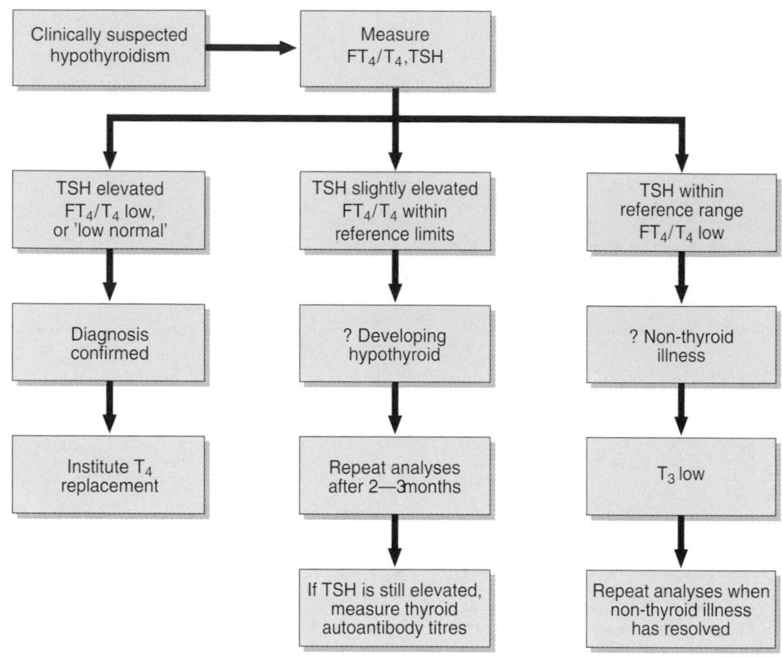

Fig. 1 **Strategy for the biochemical investigation of suspected hypothyroidism.**

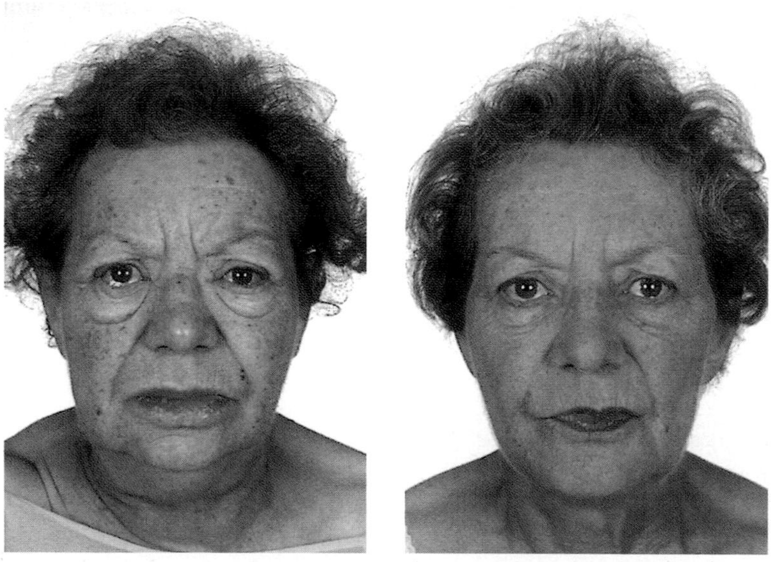

Fig. 2 **A patient before and after successful treatment of primary hypothyroidism.**

A strategy for the biochemical investigation of clinically suspected hypothyroidism is shown in Figure 1.

TREATMENT

Replacement therapy with T_4 is the treatment of choice since the hormone is readily available in a pure stable form, and is inexpensive. Monitoring TSH concentrations can be helpful in assessing the adequacy of treatment. Once the dosage is established, the patient will be required to continue treatment for life (Fig. 2).

Figure 3 shows the need for careful monitoring of treatment. This graph shows the changes in thyroid hormone results as a hyperthyroid woman patient became hypothyroid after radioiodine treatment, and it subsequently proved difficult to stabilize her on a replacement dose of thyroxine.

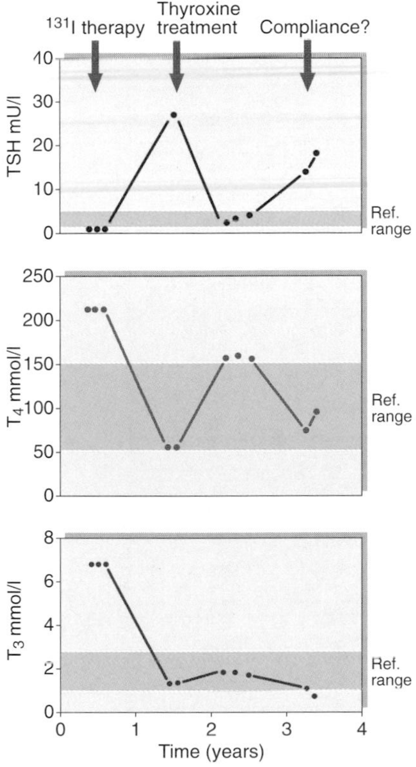

Fig. 3 **Biochemical monitoring of a patient during treatment for thyroid disease.** This 55-year-old woman was first diagnosed as hyperthyroid, and received radioiodine therapy. She became profoundly hypothyroid, and was treated with thyroxine. Her thyroid hormone results at first indicated good replacement, but recently they indicate that she is under replaced. It is possible that she is not taking her thyroxine tablets regularly.

Case history 34

Investigation of a 63-year-old woman with effort angina revealed a serum TSH of 96 mU/l and a serum T_4 of 23 nmol/l. An ECG showed some evidence of ischaemia but was not diagnostic of myocardial infarction. Further biochemical investigation revealed:

Cholesterol *(mmol/l)*	Creatine kinase	AST
	(U/l)	
9.3	290	35

- How should these results be interpreted?

Comment on page 155.

SCREENING FOR NEONATAL HYPOTHYROIDISM

Congenital hypothyroid disorders occur with a frequency of one in every 4000 live births (pp. 144–145). If diagnosed at an early age, replacement thyroid hormone can be given and normal development can occur. Delays in treatment result in cretinism (see p. 144). Elevated TSH, measured in blood spots, is diagnostic of disorders of the thyroid itself, i.e. primary neonatal hypothyroidism. The TSH screening test does not pick up pituitary dysfunction in the newborn.

NON-THYROIDAL ILLNESS

In health the major factor which regulates the serum concentration of TSH is the feedback of thyroid hormone activity on the pituitary, and to a lesser extent on the hypothalamus. Other factors also play a role. There is a diurnal rhythm with the serum TSH peaking around midday when the concentration is approximately 30% higher than at midnight, when it is at its nadir. In systemic illness the normal regulation of TSH, T_4 and T_3 secretion, and the subsequent metabolism of the thyroid hormones, is disturbed. Increased amounts of T_4 are converted to the biologically inactive reverse T_3, rather than to T_3. The resultant reduction in thyroid hormone activity does not result in an increased serum TSH concentration. TSH secretion is also suppressed, and the secretion of T_4 and T_3 by the thyroid gland is therefore decreased.

The concentrations of the transport proteins also decrease. A low serum albumin and transthyretin (pre-albumin) are classic features of the metabolic response to illness, and increased free fatty acid concentrations compete with T_4 and T_3 for their binding sites.

These changes result in sick patients having low serum T_4, T_3 and TSH, and if thyroid function tests are requested the results may well be misinterpreted. A typical non-thyroidal illness pattern might be:

T_4 nmol/l	*T_3 nmol/l*	*TSH mU/l*
44	*0.6*	*5.1*

These results were obtained in a man with acute pancreatitis. In developing hypothyroidism the T_3 would be maintained within the reference range. In decreased TBG states the T_4 and T_3 would fall in parallel. A low T_3 is almost invariably due to the presence of non-thyroidal illness.

This condition is also known as the 'low T_3 syndrome'. The message is simple: thyroid function tests should not be performed in patients during an acute illness unless there are good clinical grounds for suspecting that underlying hypothyroidism is a major feature of their illness. Thyroid function testing should be postponed until after the acute phase has passed. Patients with non-thyroidal illness results should not be given T_4 since there is no evidence that this would benefit them.

Clinical note

Patients with severe hypothyroidism should be initially treated with very small doses of thyroxine — 25 micrograms (i.e. 0.025 mg) daily. At higher doses, patients are at an increased risk of developing angina or suffering a myocardial infarction. The dose should be slowly increased over a number of months until the patient is rendered euthyroid.

Hypothyroidism

- Hypothyroidism is common and is most often due to the destruction of the thyroid gland by autoimmune disease, surgery or radioiodine therapy.
- Primary hypothyroidism is confirmed by an elevated TSH in a serum specimen.
- A TRH test is used to investigate secondary hypothyroidism due to pituitary or hypothalamic causes.
- Hypothyroidism is managed by thyroxine replacement, and therapy is monitored by measuring the serum TSH concentration.
- Patients with severe non-thyroidal illness may show apparent abnormalities in thyroid hormone results, known as the 'low T_3 syndrome' or non-thyroidal illness pattern of results.

HYPERTHYROIDISM

Thyrotoxicosis occurs when tissues are exposed to high levels of the thyroid hormones. Used correctly, the term 'hyperthyroidism' refers to the overactivity of the thyroid gland, but thyrotoxicosis can also occur from ingestion of too much T_4 or, rarely, from increased pituitary stimulation of the thyroid.

CLINICAL FEATURES

The clinical features of hyperthyroidism may be dramatic and include:

- weight loss despite normal appetite
- sweating and heat intolerance
- fatigue
- palpitation — sinus tachycardia or atrial fibrillation
- agitation and tremor
- generalized muscle weakness; proximal myopathy
- angina and heart failure
- diarrhoea
- oligomenorrhoea and subfertility
- goitre
- eyelid retraction and lid lag.

CAUSES

Hyperthyroidism can result from:

- Graves' disease, diffuse toxic goitre
- toxic multinodular goitre
- solitary toxic adenoma
- thyroiditis
- exogenously administered iodine and iodine-containing drugs, e.g. amiodarone
- excessive T_4 and T_3 ingestion.

Graves' disease is the most common cause of hyperthyroidism, and is an autoimmune disease in which antibodies to the TSH receptor on the surface of thyroid cells appear to mimic the action of the pituitary hormone. The normal regulatory controls on T_4 synthesis and secretion are lacking. Pituitary secretion of TSH is completely inhibited by the high concentrations of thyroid hormones in the blood.

Although the eyelid retraction commonly seen in the patient with Graves' disease (Fig. 3) is due to the effects of high thyroid hormone concentration, not all of the eye signs are caused this way. Rather, the thyroid and orbital muscle may have a common antigen which is recognized by the circulating autoantibodies. The inflammatory process in the eye may lead to severe exophthalmos. This may even occur in the euthyroid patient.

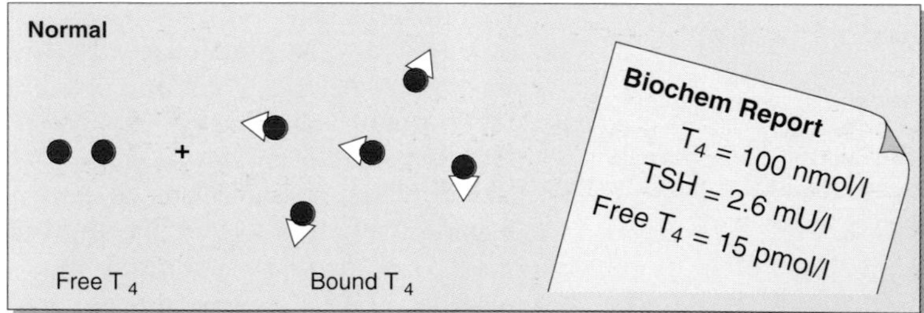

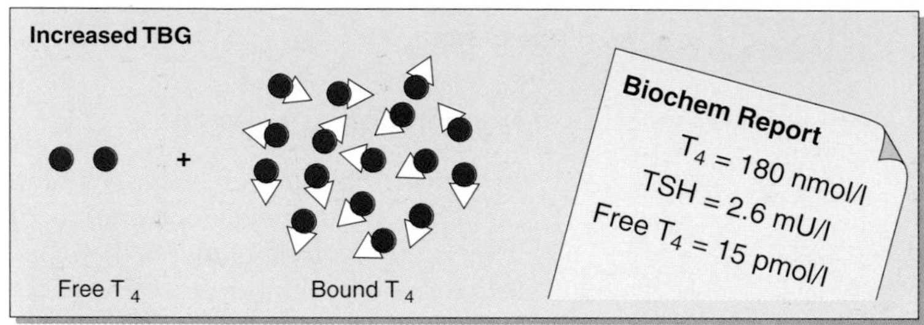

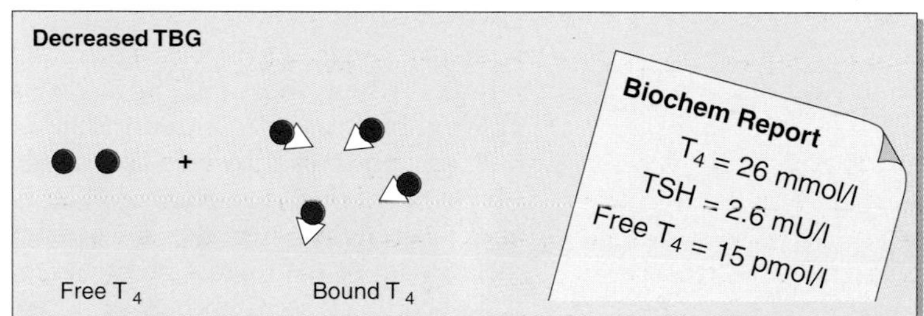

Fig. 1 **The interpretation of thyroid hormone results when TBG concentration changes.**

DIAGNOSIS

The demonstration of a suppressed TSH concentration and raised thyroid hormone concentration will confirm the diagnosis of primary hyperthyroidism. In particular, the finding that TSH is undetectable in one of the modern sensitive assays for this hormone strongly suggests that the symptomatic patient has primary hyperthyroidism.

Occasionally, biochemical confirmation of suspected hyperthyroidism will prove more difficult. The total T_4 concentration in a serum sample does not always reflect metabolic status, because of changes in binding protein concentration. In pregnancy, high circulating oestrogens cause stimulation of TBG synthesis in the liver. Total T_4 concentrations will be above the reference range, although unbound T_4 will be normal (Fig. 1). Congenital TBG deficiency can cause confusion also if a specimen is screened for thyroid hormones, even if thyroid disease is not suspected (Fig. 1). TBG deficiency is encountered much less frequently than increased TBG.

It has been suggested that assays measuring 'free' T_4 could be used as

Table 1 **Thyroid hormone and binding protein results in pregnancy**

Patient	T4 nmol/l (55–144)	T3 nmol/l (0.9–2.8)	TSH mU/l (0.35–5.0)	TBG mg/l (12–30)	Free T4 pmol/l (9–24)	Comment
1	130	2.0	3.4	25	18	Euthyroid
2	175	3.6	1.1	35	14	Euthyroid, pregnant
3	190	5.0	<0.05	36	30	Hyperthyroid, pregnant

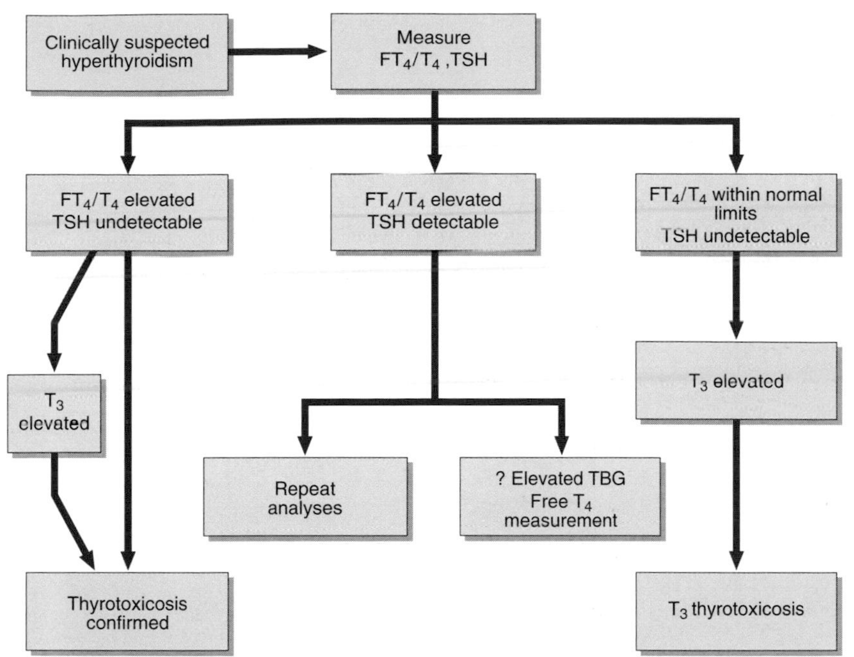

Fig. 2 **Strategy for the biochemical investigation of suspected hyperthyroidism.**

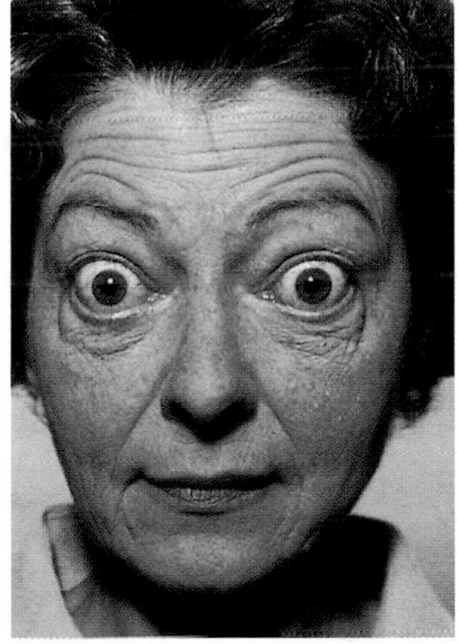

Fig. 3 **Lid retraction and exophthalmos in patient with Graves' disease.**

first-line tests of thyroid dysfunction. However, serum TSH measurement provides a better test because pituitary TSH secretion is very sensitive to changes in free T_4 concentration. Free T_4 analyses are invaluable in diagnoses where binding proteins are altered, e.g. in pregnancy, in women on the oral contraceptive pill and in patients with the nephrotic syndrome (Table 1).

In a few patients with clinical features of hyperthyroidism, total T_4 concentration is found to be within the reference range. Subsequent investigations reveal an elevated T_3 concentration. This is referred to as 'T_3 toxicosis'. TSH is undetectable in these patients.

A strategy for the biochemical investigation of clinically suspected hyperthyroidism is shown in Figure 2.

TREATMENT

There are three methods for the treatment of Graves' disease:

- *Antithyroid drugs* (such as carbimazole and propylthiouracil). These are of most use in the younger patient.
- *Radioiodine.* Therapy with sodium ^{131}I is commonly used in older patients. Most will eventually require replacement thyroxine. Thus 'thyroid function tests' should be checked regularly to detect developing hypothyroidism.
- *Surgery.* Many patients who have subtotal thyroidectomy may later require thyroxine replacement. Occasionally the parathyroids may be damaged and the patient may become hypocalcaemic post-operatively due to lack of PTH.

Thyroid function tests are important in the monitoring of all three treatments. In these circumstances it must be remembered that it takes a number of weeks before the tissue effects of thyroid hormones accurately reflect the concentration in the serum.

Case history 35

A 28-year-old woman with thyrotoxicosis has had two courses of carbimazole. Results from her recent visit to the thyroid clinic now show:

TSH	T_4
mU/l	*nmol/l*
< 0.05	*210*

- What has happened?
- What other biochemistry might be useful here?

Comment on page 155.

Clinical stop

Elderly thyrotoxic patients frequently do not exhibit many of the clinical features of hyperthyroidism. This is called 'apathetic hyperthyroidism'. Isolated idiopathic atrial fibrillation may be the only manifestation in some patients. Others may present with weight loss which may lead to anxiety and a futile search for malignant disease.

Hyperthyroidism

- Autoimmune disease is the commonest cause of hyperthyroidism.
- Diagnosis is confirmed by suppressed TSH and elevated T_4 in a serum specimen, although T_3 concentration, free hormone levels and binding protein status may all be needed in difficult situations.
- The management of hyperthyroidism is by antithyroid drugs, radioiodine therapy or partial thyroidectomy. TSH and T_4 are used to monitor therapy after all of these treatments.

ADRENOCORTICAL PATHOPHYSIOLOGY

The hormones of the adrenal glands are essential for survival. The adrenal cortex is the source of the two important steroid hormones, aldosterone and cortisol (Fig. 1). The adrenal medulla is embryologically and histologically distinct from the cortex and is part of the sympathetic nervous system. Medullary cells synthesize, store and secrete adrenaline, along with noradrenaline and dopamine. The adrenal medullary hormones are discussed further on pages 126–127.

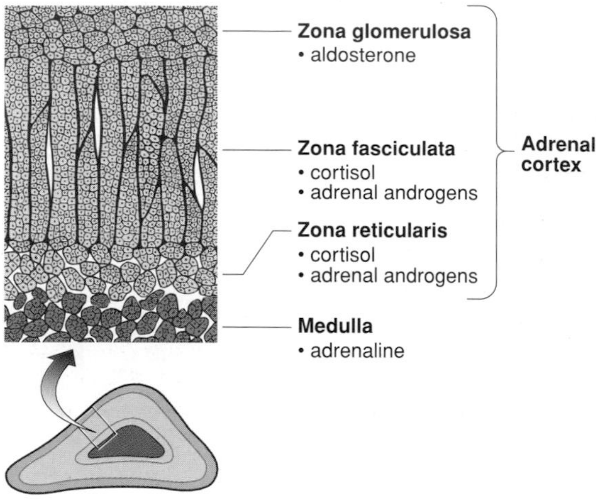

Fig. 1 **The histology of an adrenal gland.**

CORTISOL

Cortisol is produced in the zona fasciculata and zona reticularis of the adrenal cortex, the end product of a cascade of hormones which make up the hypothalamic–pituitary–adrenocortical axis (Fig. 2). Corticotrophin releasing hormone (CRH) is secreted by the hypothalamus under the influence of cerebral factors. Adrenocorticotrophic hormone (corticotrophin, or simply ACTH) is secreted by the anterior pituitary under the control of CRH to maintain the fascicular and reticular zones of the adrenal cortex and to stimulate the secretion of cortisol. Hypothalamic secretion of CRH and pituitary secretion of ACTH are modulated by cortisol in negative feedback loops.

Adrenal cortex cells have many low-density lipoprotein receptors on their surface. This enables them to take up cholesterol rapidly, from which the adrenal steroid hormones are synthesized (Fig. 3). The adrenal glands are also capable of synthesizing cortisol from acetate, though this appears to be of minor importance.

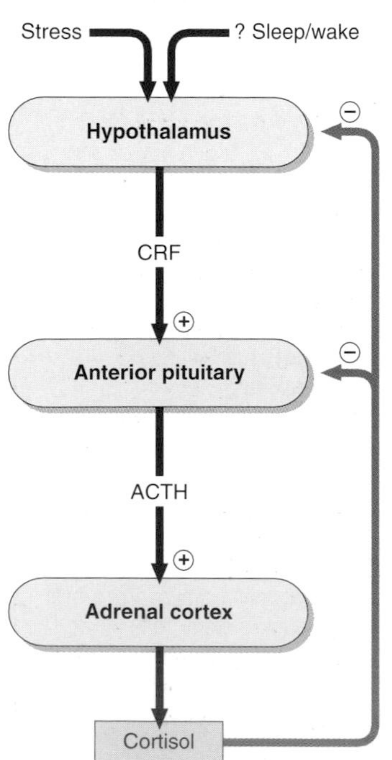

Fig. 2 **The hypothalamic–pituitary–adrenocortical axis.**

The conversion of cholesterol to pregnenolone is the rate-limiting step in the biosynthesis of cortisol; this conversion is stimulated by ACTH. Cortisol biosynthesis from pregnenolone involves the action of a specific reductase/isomerase and three separate hydroxylase enzymes. Inherited defects of all of these enzymes have been characterized.

Cortisol is an important hormone with effects on many tissues in the body. It plays a major role in metabolism by promoting protein breakdown in muscle and connective tissue and the release of glycerol and free fatty acids from adipose tissue. Thus, cortisol provides the substrates necessary for gluconeogenesis which it promotes in the liver.

Natural or synthetic steroids with cortisol-like effects are called glucocorticoids. Such compounds can act as anti-inflammatory or immunosuppressive agents. Synthetic glucocorticoids have found therapeutic applications in a wide range of clinical situations, e.g. asthma and connective tissue disorders.

ADRENAL ANDROGENS

The fascicular and reticular zones of the adrenal cortex also produce androgens — androstenedione, DHA (dehydroepiandrosterone) and DHA sulphate. These compounds probably owe their andro-

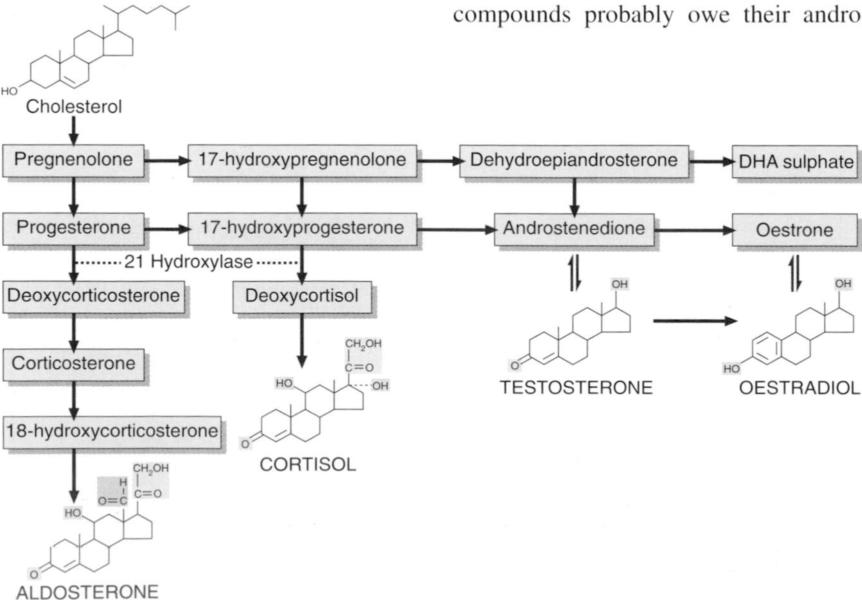

Fig. 3 **Pathways of steroid metabolism.**

genic activity to peripheral conversion to testosterone. In females the adrenal cortex is an important source of androgens, but in adult males this source is insignificant compared with testosterone made by the testes.

ASSESSING THE FUNCTION OF THE HYPOTHALAMIC–PITUITARY–ADRENOCORTICAL AXIS

Cortisol secretion fluctuates widely throughout the day, and single serum measurements are of little value in clinical practice. There is a marked diurnal rhythm. Dynamic tests of cortisol production involving stimulation of the adrenal cortex by synthetic ACTH, or of stimulation or suppression of the whole HPA axis, form an important part of investigations of adrenocortical hyper- or hypofunction and are discussed on the following pages.

ALDOSTERONE

Aldosterone is produced exclusively by the zona glomerulosa and is primarily controlled by the renin–angiotensin system (p. 15). The metabolic pathway for the synthesis of aldosterone has many of the same enzymes involved in cortisol biosynthesis. The glomerular zone lacks the 17-hydroxylase enzyme and has the additional 18-hydroxylase and 18-hydroxysteroid dehydrogenase enzymes necessary for aldosterone synthesis.

Other factors, including ACTH, are also involved in the regulation of aldosterone synthesis. Aldosterone is responsible for promoting sodium reabsorption and potassium excretion in the kidney.

A natural or synthetic steroid with aldosterone-like activity is called a mineralocorticoid. All of the 21-hydroxylated steroids have mineralocorticoid effects to varying degrees.

CONGENITAL ADRENAL HYPERPLASIA (CAH)

CAH is the result of an inherited enzyme defect in corticosteroid biosynthesis. The adrenals cannot secrete cortisol and electrolyte disturbances may involve severe hyponatraemia and hyperkalaemia if aldosterone biosynthesis is also affected. If the condition is not diagnosed quickly the afflicted infant may die.

Because of the lack of cortisol, negative feedback to the pituitary is absent and ACTH secretion continues to drive steroid biosynthesis (Fig. 3). Cortisol precursors are secreted in large amounts, their nature depending on which enzyme is lacking. The 21-hydroxylase is the deficient enzyme in 95% of cases of CAH. Here, large amounts of 17-hydroxyprogesterone are secreted. Elevated plasma concentrations are diagnostic as early as 2 days after birth. Increased stimulation of adrenal androgen production can cause virilization in baby girls, and precocious puberty in boys.

One variant of the condition, the late onset form, presents as menstrual irregularity and hirsutism in young women. This is presumably the result of a partial enzyme defect.

THE RELATIONSHIP OF ADRENAL CORTEX AND ADRENAL MEDULLA

For a multicellular organism to survive it is essential that the extracellular fluid bathing the tissues is continually circulating so that nutrients may be supplied to the cells and waste products removed from their environment. The adrenal medulla and the two separate hormone systems of the adrenal cortex act in harmony to ensure that this occurs. Adrenaline and noradrenaline through their inotropic effects on the heart and their vasoconstrictor actions on the arterioles maintain the blood pressure and facilitate tissue perfusion. Cortisol facilitates the synthesis of adrenaline and potentiates its vasopressor effects. Cortisol is also required for the efficient excretion of water in the kidney. Aldosterone, through its action in promoting sodium reabsorption, maintains the extracellular volume.

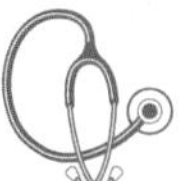

Clinical note

Stress is the most important stimulus for ACTH secretion and it, along with the sleep/wake-induced ACTH rhythm, will override the negative feedback control mechanisms. As a result, when investigating disturbances in ACTH/cortisol secretion, it is essential to eliminate stress (e.g. due to illness or trauma) and to ensure that a normal sleep/wake cycle has been established.

Case history 36

A 40-year-old man was investigated for severe skeletal muscle pains. The following biochemical results in a serum sample were unexpected:

Na^+	K^+	Cl^-	HCO_3^-	Urea	Creatinine
mmol/l					*μmol/l*
130	6.1	90	17	7.6	150

- Suggest a likely diagnosis.
- What other biochemistry tests might be helpful in the investigation of this patient?

Comment on page 156.

Adrenocortical pathophysiology

- The adrenal glands comprise three separate hormone systems
  - the zona glomerulosa which secretes aldosterone
  - the zona fasciculata and reticularis which secrete cortisol and the adrenal androgens
  - the adrenal medulla which secretes adrenaline.
- Steroids with cortisol-like activity are known as glucocorticoids; they are potent metabolic regulators and immunosuppressants.
- Steroids with aldosterone-like activity are called mineralocorticoids; they promote renal sodium retention.
- Adrenal steroid concentrations in serum fluctuate widely. Single measurements are therefore of limited value in clinical investigations, and dynamic tests are widely used in diagnosis.
- Congenital adrenal hyperplasia is an inherited enzyme defect in corticosteroid biosynthesis which can prove fatal unless diagnosed early.
- 21-hydroxylase deficiency is the most commonly encountered form of CAH. The finding of a raised plasma 17-hydroxyprogesterone confirms the diagnosis.

HYPOFUNCTION OF THE ADRENAL CORTEX

ADRENAL INSUFFICIENCY

Acute adrenal insufficiency is a rare condition which if unrecognized is potentially fatal. Because of its low incidence it is often overlooked as a possible diagnosis. It is relatively simple to treat once the diagnosis has been made, and patients can lead a normal life. The clinical features of adrenal insufficiency are shown in Figure 1.

Formerly, adrenal gland destruction was often due to tuberculosis; autoimmune disease is now the main cause of primary adrenal failure. Both cortisol and aldosterone production may be affected. Secondary failure to produce cortisol is more common. Frequently, this is due to long-standing suppression and subsequent impairment of the hypothalamic–pituitary–adrenocortical axis from therapeutic administration of corticosteroids. The causes of adrenal insufficiency are summarized in Figure 2.

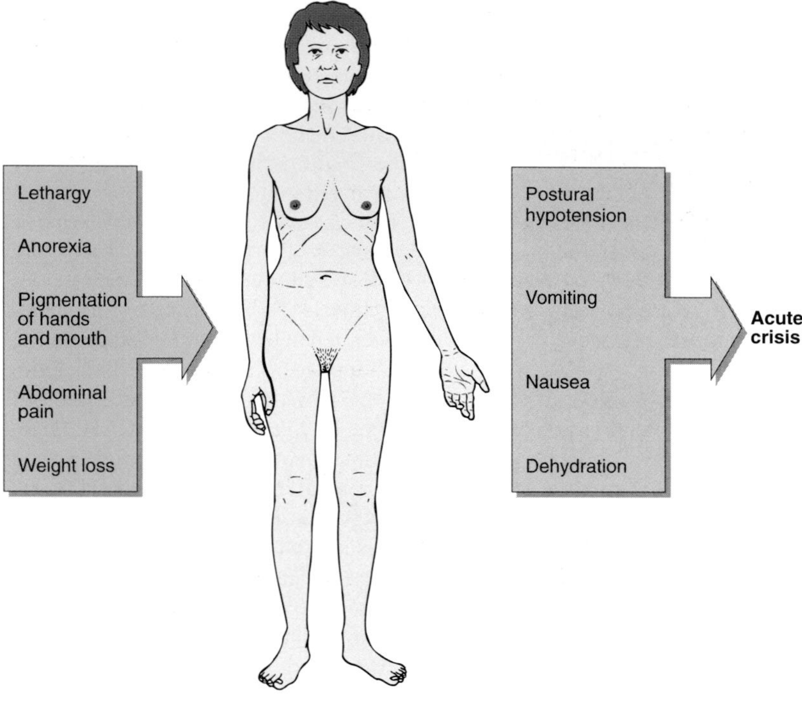

Fig. 1 **Features of adrenocortical insufficiency.**

Biochemical features

In addition to the clinical observations, a number of biochemical results may point towards adrenocortical insufficiency. These are hyponatraemia, hyperkalaemia and elevated serum urea, and may be seen in many patients with Addison's Disease.

In primary adrenal insufficiency, patients become hyponatraemic for two reasons. The lack of aldosterone leads to pathological sodium loss by the kidney which results in a contraction of the extracellular fluid volume, causing hypotension and pre-renal uraemia. Patients may develop life-threatening sodium depletion and potassium retention due to aldosterone deficiency. The hypovolaemia and hypotension stimulate AVP secretion, thus causing water retention. In the absence of cortisol, the kidneys' ability to excrete a water load is impaired, thus leading to hyponatraemia. Overall, however, the total body water is reduced and this is reflected by the increase in the serum urea.

Lack of negative feedback of cortisol on the anterior pituitary results in an excessive secretion of ACTH. The structure of this hormone contains part of the amino acid sequence of melanocyte-stimulating hormone. Where excessive ACTH secretion occurs, patients may show darkening of the skin and mucous membranes.

Diagnosis

If a patient is suspected to be suffering from adrenal insufficiency, it is essential to ensure that they have an adequate sodium intake whilst investigations proceed. Serum aldosterone measurements have no role to play in the initial diagnosis of adrenal insufficiency, nor do random, single serum cortisol measurements, which are frequently misleading.

The short Synacthen test indicates the ability of the adrenal cortex to respond to ACTH (Fig. 3). Synacthen, a synthetic 1–24 analogue of ACTH, is administered intravenously at a dose of 0.25 mg. The increase in plasma cortisol is measured after 30 minutes.

Normally, the resting value is within the reference range (280–720 nmol/l at 08.00–10.00 am). An acceptable basal concentration is >225 nmol/l. There should be an increment of more than 200 nmol/l after Synacthen and the final

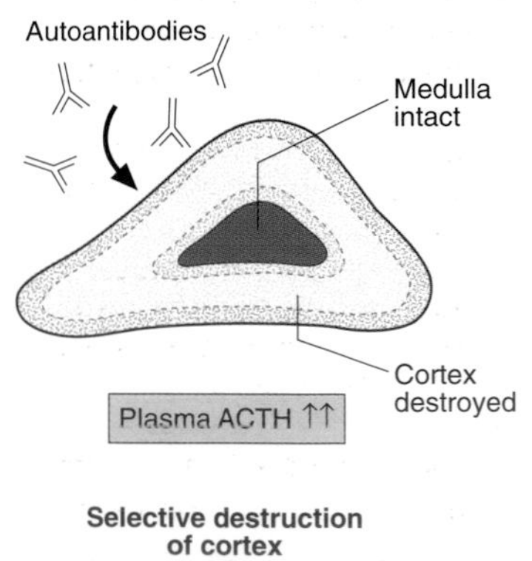

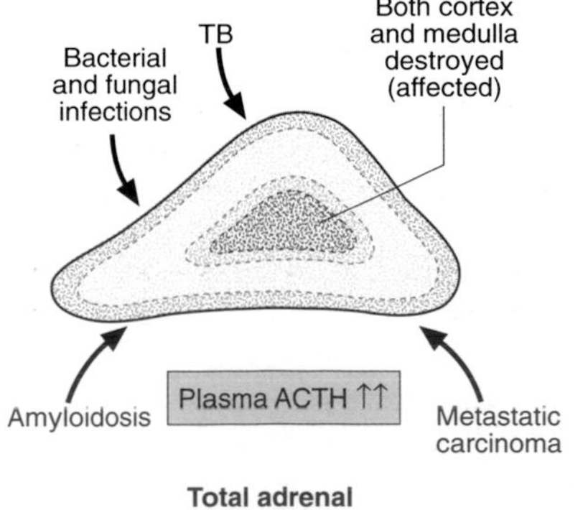

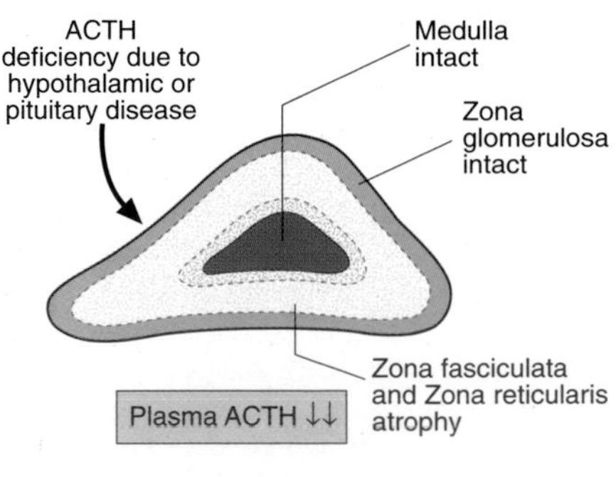

Fig. 2 **Causes of adrenocortical insufficiency.**

value should be greater than 500 nmol/l. All criteria must be met. Failure to meet *any* of the criteria indicates adrenocortical inadequacy. A normal response to the Synacthen test excludes primary hypofunction. An elevated ACTH concentration will confirm the diagnosis of primary adrenal failure in a patient with an impaired response to the Synacthen test.

Patients with equivocal responses to the short Synacthen test may be retested after stimulation of the adrenal cortex with *depot* Synacthen. This longer acting material (1 mg) is given intramuscularly daily for three days. On the fourth day a short Synacthen test is carried out as before. If the normal criteria for the short Synacthen test are fulfilled on the second testing, the adrenal insufficiency is not of primary origin. Such a result points towards secondary adrenocortical insufficiency.

The hypothalmic–pituitary–adrenocortical axis may be investigated by performing an insulin tolerance test (ITT). The details and hazards of this test have been previously described (p. 77).

Management

Once adrenal insufficiency is diagnosed, patients should commence life-long steroid replacement therapy. A standard regimen for adults would consist of 30 mg of hydrocortisone daily in divided doses, with the mineralocorticoid α-fludrocortisone being added as required.

ISOLATED ALDOSTERONE DEFICIENCY

Analdosteronism is rare and may be due to an adrenal lesion, such as an 18-hydroxylase defect, or to primary renin deficiency, as in the anephric patient.

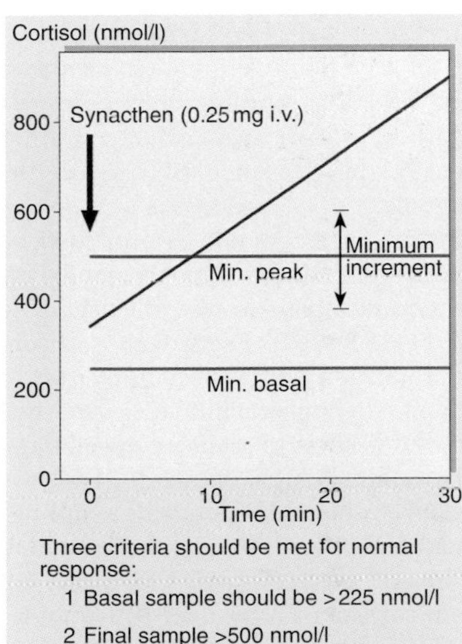

Fig. 3 **Synacthen test responses.** Synacthen is given i.v. after basal blood samples have been taken.

Clinical note

Primary adrenal insufficiency has an insidious onset. Pallor is a characteristic feature, as is dry flaky skin with pigmentation especially in palmar creases and pressure points (Fig. 4). Patients may present asymptomatically with apparently isolated hyperkalaemia or hyponatraemia. Addison's disease must always be considered as a possible diagnosis in patients with raised serum potassium, especially if they do not have renal failure.

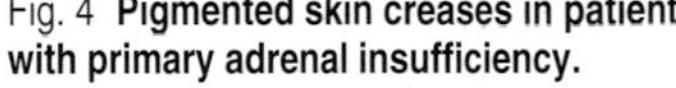

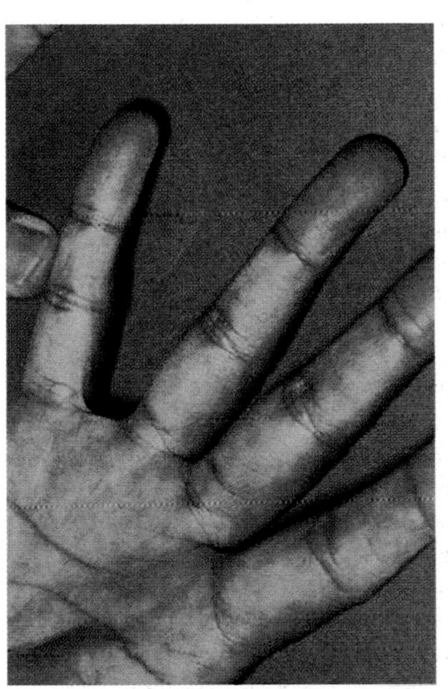

Fig. 4 **Pigmented skin creases in patient with primary adrenal insufficiency.**

Case history 37

A 31-year-old woman was admitted to a surgical ward with a two day history of abdominal pain and vomiting. Her blood pressure was 110/65 mmHg and her pulse 88 beats per minute and regular. A provisional diagnosis of intestinal obstruction was made. On admission, tests showed:

Na^+	K^+	Cl^-	HCO_3^-	Urea	Creatinine
mmol/l					*µmol/l*
128	6.1	92	18	10.8	180

She was given 1.5 litres of 0.9% saline intravenously, overnight, and the following morning her symptoms had resolved. Her serum sodium had increased to 134 mmol/l and her serum potassium had fallen to 4.8 mmol/l. On reviewing her history she had been unwell for a number of months with weight loss and anorexia. She was noted to be pigmented.

A short Synacthen test was performed and the serum cortisol was less than 60 nmol/l both before and after an intravenous injection of 0.25 mg of Synacthen.

- Suggest the diagnosis.
- How could the changes in her sodium and potassium be explained?

Comment on page 156.

Hypofunction of the adrenal cortex

- Adrenocortical insufficiency is rare, but life-threatening.
- Failure of the adrenal cortex to produce cortisol and aldosterone may be due to autoimmune or infiltrative diseases.
- The Synacthen test is used in diagnosis of primary adrenocortical failure.
- The insulin tolerance test is used in diagnosis of pituitary insufficiency which may lead to secondary failure of the adrenal cortex.
- The mainstay of therapy is maintenance of sodium intake and appropriate hormone replacement.

HYPERFUNCTION OF THE ADRENAL CORTEX

Hyperfunction of the adrenal cortex can be conveniently discussed in terms of the overproduction of the three main products:

- cortisol
- adrenal androgens
- aldosterone.

CORTISOL EXCESS

A prolonged excessive exposure of body tissues to cortisol or any other glucocorticoid results in Cushing's syndrome. It is one of the most difficult endocrine diagnoses to make. The condition is relatively rare, and a family practitioner may not experience a case in his or her entire working life. The main clinical features of Cushing's syndrome are shown in Figure 1.

In any investigation of Cushing's syndrome the clinician should ask two questions:

- 'Does the patient actually have Cushing's syndrome?' The possibility that a patient may have Cushing's syndrome frequently arises because they are obese or hypertensive, conditions frequently encountered in the population at large. Initial investigations will in most cases exclude the diagnosis of Cushing's syndrome.
- Once the diagnosis of Cushing's syndrome is established, then a second question may be asked: 'What is the cause of the excess cortisol secretion?' Tests used in the differential diagnosis are different from those used to confirm the presence of cortisol overproduction.

Confirming the diagnosis

Iatrogenic Cushing's syndrome should be diagnosed from the patient history and clinical examination. The steroid may have been taken orally, inhaled or applied topically. Iatrogenic Cushing's syndrome will not be considered further here.

Cortisol, secreted in excess by the adrenal cortex, will rapidly exceed the available capacity of the plasma binding protein, cortisol binding globulin. Unbound cortisol is filtered readily into the urine. 'Urinary free cortisol' in a 24 h collection, or assessed as a cortisol: creatinine ratio in an early morning urine sample, is the initial screening test in a patient suspected of adrenocortical hyperfunction. The latter measurement can be made on a small aliquot of urine. Repeatedly high early morning urine cortisol:creatinine ratios are evidence enough to proceed with further investigations of the patient. If the test is negative on three occasions, Cushing's syndrome may be excluded from the differential diagnosis.

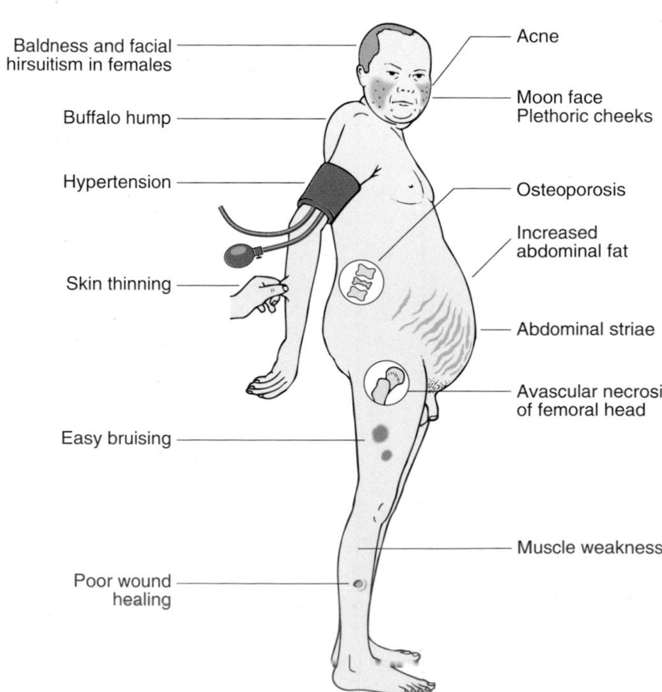

Fig. 1 **Some clinical features of Cushing's syndrome.**

Cortisol concentrations measured at 08:00 and 22:00 normally show a circadian rhythm with the evening sample having a lower value than that in the morning. This difference is usually not apparent in the patient with Cushing's syndrome. It is essential that the patients are not stressed when such measurements are made.

Failure of 1 mg of dexamethasone taken at 23:00 to suppress the serum cortisol level at 08:00 the following morning, or failure to suppress urinary cortisol secretion overnight (as measured by an early morning urine cortisol: creatinine ratio) is another pointer towards the presence of Cushing's syndrome.

Failure of the serum cortisol to rise after insulin-induced hypoglycaemia is also a characteristic feature of Cushing's syndrome. Since patients with cortisol overproduction will be insulin-resistant, adequate hypoglycaemia may not be achieved with 0.15 units of insulin/kg body weight. A higher dose may have to be used. In normal individuals a fall of blood glucose concentration to less than 2.2 mmol/l is accompanied by a rise in serum cortisol of more than 200 nmol/l. A patient who shows such a response in the ITT is unlikely to have a pathological excess of cortisol production.

Determining the cause

The possible causes of Cushing's syndrome are illustrated in Figure 2. These include:

- pituitary adenoma
- ectopic ACTH
- adrenal adenoma
- adrenal carcinoma.

Classically, ACTH is not detectable in the plasma of patients with adrenal tumours. In patients with pituitary-dependent Cushing's syndrome (known somewhat confusingly as *Cushing's disease*) the plasma ACTH may be within the reference range or modestly elevated. The plasma ACTH level is often very high in patients with ectopic ACTH production.

In patients with pituitary-dependent Cushing's disease the serum or urinary cortisol will be partially suppressed after two days of dexamethasone, 2.0 mg q.i.d. (Fig. 3). Failure to suppress suggests either ectopic ACTH prod-

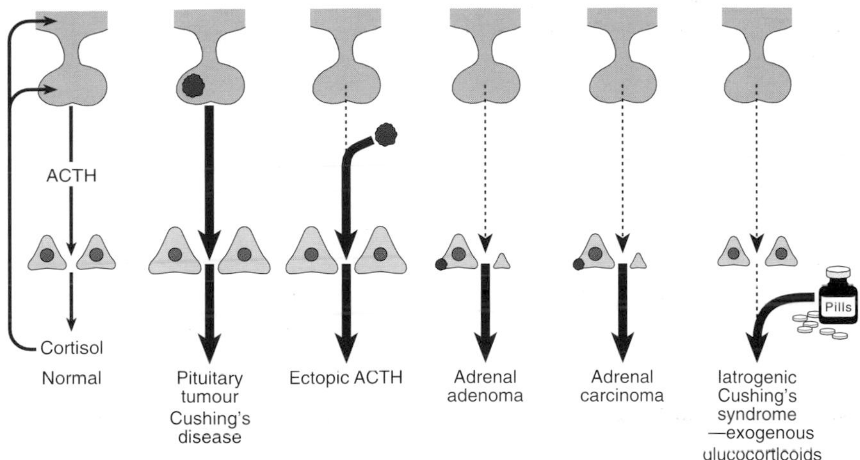

Fig. 2 **The possible causes of Cushing's syndrome.**

uction or the autonomous secretion of cortisol by an adrenal tumour.

The cause of Cushing's syndrome will determine the therapeutic options, and it is therefore essential that a definitive diagnosis is made. CT scans or magnetic resonance imaging of the pituitary may be helpful in detecting a pituitary adenoma in patients with Cushing's disease. Selective venous sampling with ACTH measurement is frequently carried out to locate the ACTH source in difficult cases.

ANDROGEN EXCESS

Adrenocortical tumours, particularly adrenal carcinomas, may produce excess androgens (DHA, androstenedione and testosterone) causing hirsutism and/or virilisation in females (see pp. 92–93).

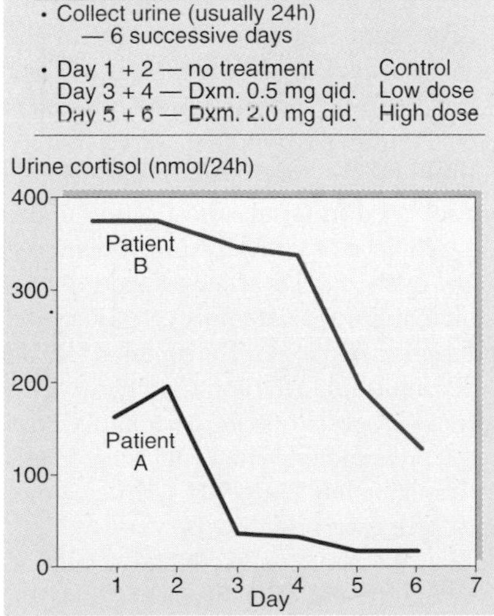

Fig. 3 **The dexamethasone suppression test.** Patient A showed a >75% fall in urinary cortisol excretion on the low dose. This is a **normal response**. Patient B showed some suppression of cortisol secretion on the high dose. This is typical of **pituitary-dependent Cushing's syndrome.**

This may not necessarily be accompanied by cortisol excess, and signs of Cushing's syndrome may be absent. Patients with congenital adrenal hyperplasia (p. 87) may also present with signs of increased androgen production.

ALDOSTERONE EXCESS

Primary hyperaldosteronism (Conn's syndrome) is rare. In most cases, the disease is due to a single adrenocortical adenoma. Patients may present with polydipsia and polyuria, symptoms of neuromuscular abnormalities such as weakness, paraesthesiae and tetany, and hypertension. All symptoms other than hypertension are attributable to potassium depletion.

Preliminary investigations must include determination of serum and urine electrolytes over several days, with adequate sodium intake. Serum potassium will be low, and urinary potassium excretion will be elevated. Documented, careful collection of specimens for assay of aldosterone, renin or 'plasma renin activity', may be made on two consecutive days after 8 h recumbency, and again with the patient ambulatory, to confirm the diagnosis.

The diagnosis of hyperaldosteronism may be made in the hypokalaemic patient if the serum aldosterone level exceeds the upper limit of normal or if the level is persistently inappropriate to the serum potassium. In primary hyperaldosteronism, where the excess aldosterone arises from an adrenal adenoma, the levels of plasma renin will be low.

Secondary hyperaldosteronism is common and is associated with renal, heart or liver disease.

Case history 38

A 31-year-old woman presented with a three-month history of weight gain, hirsutism, amenorrhoea and hypertension. Her urine cortisol: creatinine ratio was increased, and serum cortisol diurnal rhythm was absent. Treatment with 0.5 mg of dexamethasone q.i.d. did not suppress her cortisol, and insulin-induced hypoglycaemia did not cause her serum cortisol to rise.

- What investigations should now be carried out?

Comment on page 156.

Clinical note

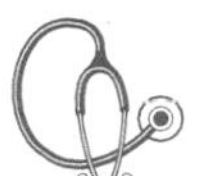

Excessive alcohol intake can cause *pseudo-Cushing's syndrome* when patients may present with hypertension, truncal obesity, plethora or acne. Preliminary investigations may demonstrate hypercortisolism which may fail to suppress with dexamethasone. The biochemical features of Cushing's syndrome will resolve after two to three weeks abstinence.

Hyperfunction of the adrenal cortex

- Cushing's syndrome is a difficult diagnosis to make.
- To confirm hypercortisolism, early morning urinary cortisol:creatinine ratios will be elevated, diurnal rhythm of serum cortisol will be absent, there will be no cortisol rise during an insulin-tolerance test, and serum cortisol will not suppress with a low dose of dexamethasone.
- Once the diagnosis of Cushing's syndrome has been made, the cause can be established by the long dexamethasone suppression test and by measuring ACTH.
- Clinical and biochemical evidence of increased adrenal androgens may be present.
- Primary excess of aldosterone is rare and due usually to an adenoma (Conn's syndrome).

GONADAL FUNCTION

SEX STEROID HORMONES

Testosterone and oestradiol are known as the sex steroid hormones. Testosterone is the principal androgen and is synthesized by the testes in the male. Oestradiol, which is secreted by the ovaries, varies widely in concentration in plasma throughout the female menstrual cycle. Steroids with oestradiol-like action are called oestrogens. Progesterone is a product of the ovary and is secreted when a corpus luteum forms after ovulation. Normal female plasma also contains testosterone, about half of which comes from the ovary and half from peripheral conversion of androstenedione and dehydroepiandrosterone (DHA) sulphate which are secreted by the adrenal cortex. Some oestradiol is present in low concentration in normal male plasma.

Testosterone and oestradiol circulate in plasma mostly bound to plasma proteins, particularly sex hormone-binding globulin (SHBG). SHBG has a higher affinity for testosterone than for oestradiol. Oestradiol stimulates SHBG synthesis by the liver, and testosterone decreases it. The plasma concentration of SHBG in females is twice that in males. Factors which alter SHBG concentration alter the ratio of unbound testosterone to unbound oestradiol. In both sexes the effect of an increase in SHBG is to increase oestradiol-like effects, whereas a decrease in SHBG is to increase androgen effects. As oestradiol itself increases SHBG concentration and testosterone decreases it, this system functions as a biological servo mechanism.

Testosterone and SHBG concentrations are sometimes reported by the laboratory as a ratio (the free androgen index) which gives a clearer indication of androgen status than does serum testosterone alone.

HYPOTHALAMIC–PITUITARY–GONADAL AXIS

The episodic secretion of the hypothalamic hormone, gonadotrophin-releasing hormone (GnRH), stimulates synthesis and release of the gonadotrophins, LH (luteinizing hormone) and FSH (follicle-stimulating hormone), from the anterior pituitary. Despite the names, both gonadotrophins act cooperatively on the ovaries in the woman and the testes in the man to stimulate sex hormone secretion and reproductive processes.

MALE GONADAL FUNCTION

The testes secrete testosterone and manufacture spermatozoa. Before puberty, gonadotrophin and testosterone concentrations in plasma are very low. The development of the Leydig cells and their secretion of testosterone is influenced by LH, whereas Sertoli cell function is influenced by FSH. Stimulation and maintenance of spermatogenesis require that both FSH and LH be present (Fig. 1). Testosterone is responsible for growth and function of the prostate and epididymis, and for the development of the male secondary sex characteristics such as hair growth, deep voice and characteristic musculature.

In some target tissues, the biological activity of testosterone is due to its conversion to dihydrotestosterone by the enzyme 5α-reductase.

Disorders of male sex hormones

Hypogonadism

Hypogonadism may result in deficient sperm production and decreased testosterone secretion. This may be due to a testicular deficiency (primary disorders or hypergonadotrophic hypogonadism) or to a defect in the hypothalamus or pituitary (secondary disorders or hypogonadotrophic hypogonadism). In hypogonadotrophic hypogonadism both gonadotrophins, or only LH, may be absent. There may be a generalized failure of pituitary function.

Causes of primary hypogonadism include:

- congenital defects such as Klinefelter's syndrome or testicular agenesis
- acquired defects due to testicular infections (e.g. mumps), trauma, irradiation, or cytotoxic drugs.

Causes of secondary hypogonadism include:

- pituitary tumours
- hypothalamic disorders such as Kallmann's syndrome.

Dynamic tests such as stimulation with GnRH may help to establish the cause of the hypogonadism in some patients.

Disorders of male sexual differentiation

Disorders of male sexual differentiation are rare. Testosterone production may be impaired. In the testicular feminization syndrome, androgen receptors are inactive and target tissues cannot respond to stimulation by circulating testosterone.

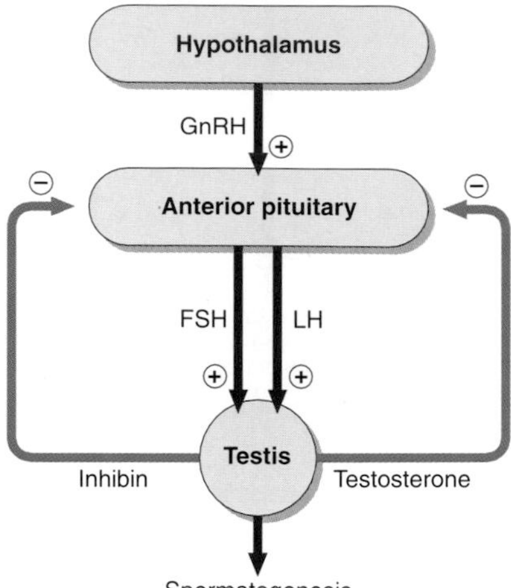

Fig. 1 **Control of testicular function by the gonadotrophins.**

FEMALE GONADAL FUNCTION

Oestradiol is responsible for:

- female secondary sex characteristics
- stimulation of follicular growth
- development of the endometrium.

Concentrations are low before puberty, but then rise rapidly and fluctuate cyclically during reproductive life. After the menopause, plasma oestradiol concentrations fall despite high circulating concentrations of the gonadotrophins.

The normal hormonal control of the menstrual cycle is shown in Figure 2, and depends on the interaction of hormones secreted from the hypothalamus, pituitary and ovary. The pituitary gonadotrophins are released in a pulsatile fashion under the influence of GnRH. At the beginning of the cycle, FSH is released and initiates follicular growth. At mid-cycle a surge of LH triggers ovulation. The ruptured follicle differentiates into the corpus luteum which secretes progesterone and oestradiol whose target is the endometrium which it prepares for implantation. Thus FSH, LH, oestradiol and progesterone levels vary widely through the menstrual cycle, and in addition there may be mid-cycle peaks of prolactin, SHBG and testosterone.

Disorders of female sex hormones

Disorders of female sex hormones include:

- *Subfertility, amenorrhoea and oligomenorrhoea* (see p. 94).

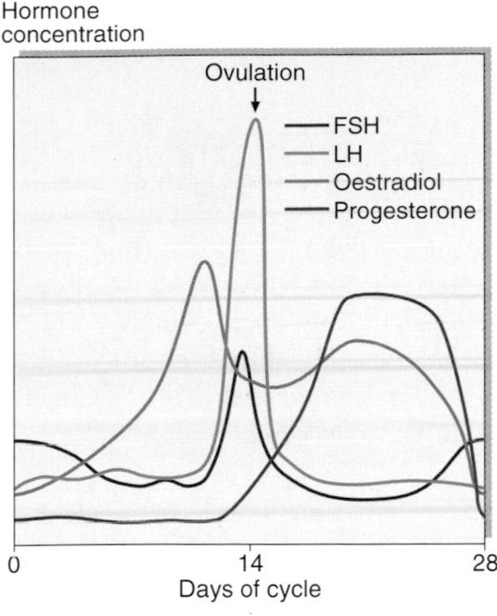

Fig. 2 **Plasma hormone concentrations throughout the female menstrual cycle.**

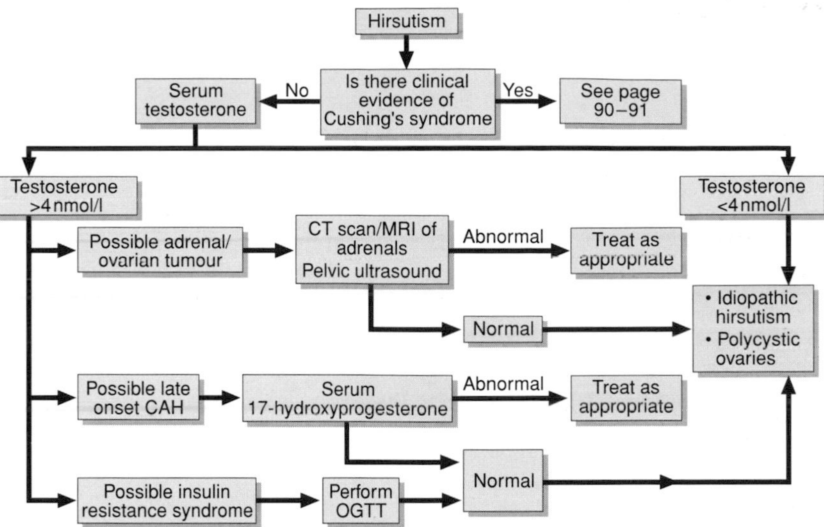

Fig. 3 **Diagnostic decision chart for the investigation of hirsutism.**

- *Hirsutism.* This is an increase in body hair with male pattern distribution. In the majority of cases it is genetic in origin and benign. These cases are frequently termed idiopathic. The commonest pathological cause is polycystic ovarian disease. It is essential when investigating hirsute women that serious disease is excluded. A diagnostic decision chart for the investigation of hirsutism is shown in Figure 3.
- *Virilism.* Although uncommon it is a sign of serious disease. Testosterone concentrations are markedly elevated in the virilised patient and there is evidence of excessive androgen action such as clitoral enlargement, hair growth in a male pattern, deepening of the voice and breast atrophy. Tumours of the ovary or of the adrenal are the likely cause.

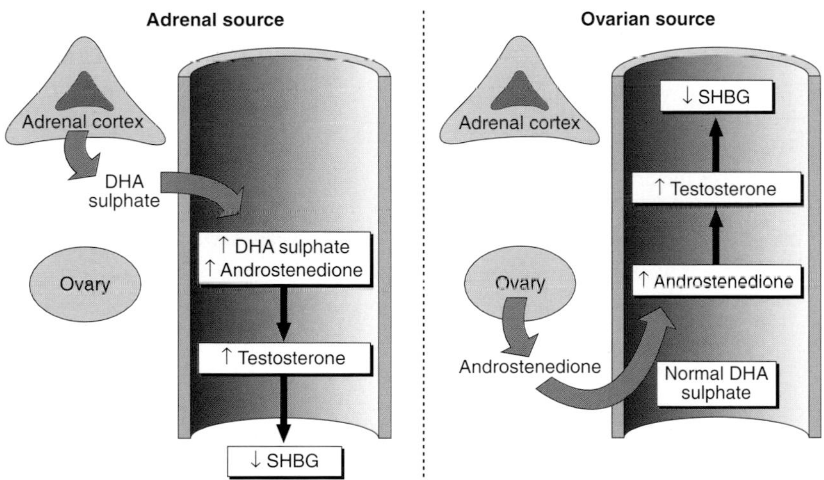

Fig. 4 **Investigation of an elevated testosterone concentration in a woman.**

Case history 39

A 29-year-old woman complained of acne and irregular periods. On examination she was overweight and moderately hirsute.

Initial investigations showed a slightly elevated testosterone of 3.7 nmol/l. LH was 15 U/l and FSH 5.6 U/l.

- What other investigations should be undertaken to make a diagnosis in this patient?

Comment on page 156.

The androgen screen in women

The observation of an elevated testosterone in a woman should always be investigated further. A decreased SHBG concentration is evidence of elevated androgen, as the synthesis of this protein in the liver is depressed by testosterone. It may not be immediately apparent whether the source of the testosterone is the ovary or the adrenal cortex. By measuring the concentration of other androgens such as androstenedione and DHA sulphate (an 'androgen screen'), the source of the testosterone can be pin-pointed (Fig. 4). An elevated DHA sulphate suggests that the adrenal, or an adrenal tumour, is overproducing androgens. If the ovary is the source then only androstenedione will be raised.

Gonadal function

- Testosterone is the main hormone secreted by the testes in the male and is regulated by pituitary LH. Testosterone is responsible for the male secondary sex characteristics.
- Oestradiol is the main product of the ovary and is responsible for the female secondary sex characteristics, development of the ovarian follicle and proliferation of the uterine epithelium.
- Hypogonadism in the male may be primary (where the cause is a failure of testosterone synthesis or of spermatogenesis in the testes) or secondary where the problem is in the hypothalamus or pituitary.
- Gonadal dysfunction in women may present as primary or secondary amenorrhoea, infertility, hirsutism or virilism.

SUBFERTILITY

Subfertility is defined as the failure of a couple to conceive after one year of regular, unprotected intercourse. A full clinical history obtained prior to physical examinations should seek information about previous pregnancies, contraceptive practice, serious illnesses, past chemotherapy or radiotherapy, congenital abnormalities, smoking habits, drug usage, sexually transmitted disease and the frequency of intercourse. Physical examination should look for indications of hypothalamic–pituitary or thyroid disorders, Cushing's syndrome, galactorrhoea and hirsutism. In the male, semen analysis should detail volume, sperm density, motility and the presence of abnormal spermatozoa.

In the female, endocrine abnormalities are found in one third of patients. Hormone dysfunction is a very rare cause of male subfertility. In some couples no cause can be identified.

ENDOCRINE INVESTIGATIONS IN THE SUBFERTILE WOMAN

The investigation of the infertile female depends on the phase of the menstral cycle. If there is a regular menstrual cycle, serum progesterone should be measured in the middle of the luteal phase (day 21). If progesterone is high (>30 nmol/l), the patient has ovulated and there is no need for further endocrine investigations. Other causes of subfertility should be sought. If progesterone is low (<10 nmol/l), ovulation has not occurred.

In women who present with irregular or absent menstruation (oligomenorrhoea or amenorrhoea) or who are not ovulating, hormone measurements may be diagnostic. A protocol for investigation is shown in Figure 1. Measurement of oestradiol and gonadotrophin concentrations may detect primary ovarian failure or polycystic ovarian disease. Measurement of prolactin, and androgens may also assist.

Endocrine causes of subfertility in women include:

- *Primary ovarian failure.* This is indicated by elevated gonadotrophins and low oestradiol concentration (a postmenopausal pattern). Hormone replacement therapy assists libido and prevents osteoporosis, but does not restore fertility.
- *Hyperprolactinaemia* (pp. 76–77).
- *Polycystic ovarian disease.* This is indicated by an elevated LH and normal FSH. Oestradiol measurements are often unhelpful. Hirsutism, a feature of this condition, is associated with raised testosterone and subnormal sex hormone binding protein concentrations.
- *Cushing's syndome* (pp. 90–91).
- *Hypogonadotrophic hypogonadism.* Rarely, subnormal gonadotrophin and oestradiol concentrations suggest the presence of a hypothalamic–pituitary lesion such as interference from a pituitary tumour. The mechanisms responsible for the amenorrhoea or oligomenorrhoea in women with normal gonadotrophin and oestradiol concentrations remain to be elucidated.

ENDOCRINE INVESTIGATIONS IN THE SUBFERTILE MAN

In the eugonadal male with normal sperm analysis, no endocrine investigations are required. In the hypogonadal male, testosterone and the gonadotrophins should be measured first (Fig. 2). Causes of subfertility in the male include:

- *Primary testicular failure.* Where both the interstitial cells and tubules are damaged, FSH and LH will be elevated and testosterone reduced. Where tubular function only is impaired, FSH is selectively increased and androgen levels may be normal.
- *Hypothalamic–pituitary disease.* Decreased testosterone with low or normal gonadotrophins suggests hypogonadotrophic hypogonadism.
- *Hyperprolactinaemia.* This is a rare cause of infertility in the male (pp. 76–77).

Subfertility

- Endocrine problems are a common cause of subfertility in the female but are rare in the male.
- An elevated serum progesterone in a specimen at day 21 of the menstrual cycle indicates that ovulation has occurred.
- In both men and women a serum FSH concentration greater than 25 U/l indicates primary gonadal failure.
- Hyperprolactinaemia is a common cause of female subfertility.

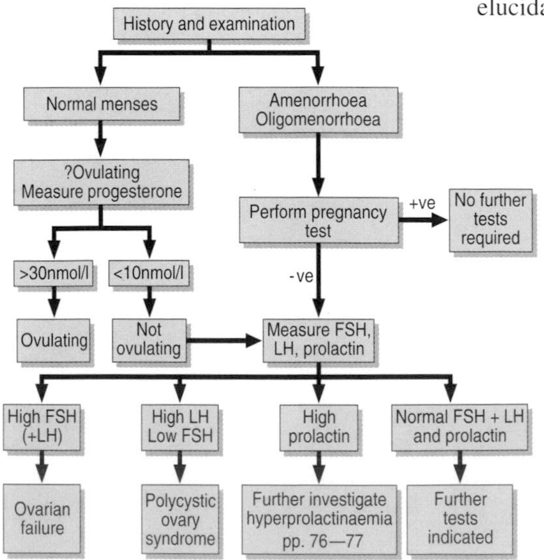

Fig. 1 **Diagnostic approach to subfertility in the woman.**

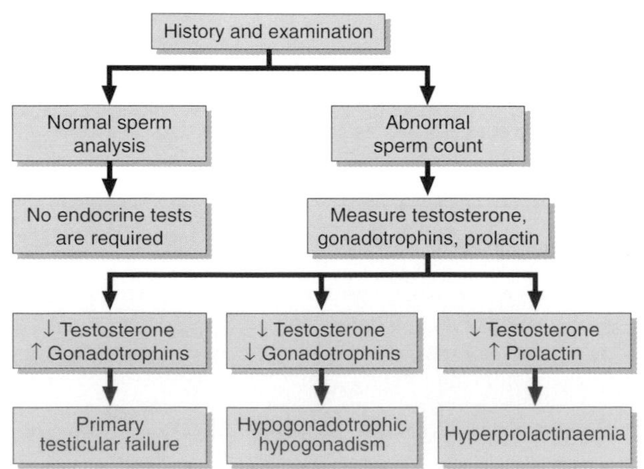

Fig. 2 **Diagnostic approach to subfertility in the man.**

SPECIALIZED INVESTIGATIONS

NUTRITIONAL ASSESSMENT

Malnutrition is a common problem worldwide, and in developed countries it is associated particularly with poverty and alcoholism. It is also encountered among patients in hospital. Various studies have shown that patients may have evidence, not only of protein-calorie malnutrition, but also of vitamin and mineral deficiencies, especially after major surgery or chronic illness.

Malnutrition to the layman usually means starvation, but the term has a much wider meaning encompassing both the inadequacy of any nutrient in the diet as well as *excess* food intake. The pathogenesis of malnutrition is shown in Figure 1.

Malnutrition related to surgery or following severe injury occurs because of the extensive metabolic changes that accompany these events: the 'metabolic response to injury' (pp. 102–103).

The assessment of a patient suspected of suffering from malnutrition is based on:

- history
- examination
- laboratory investigations including biochemistry.

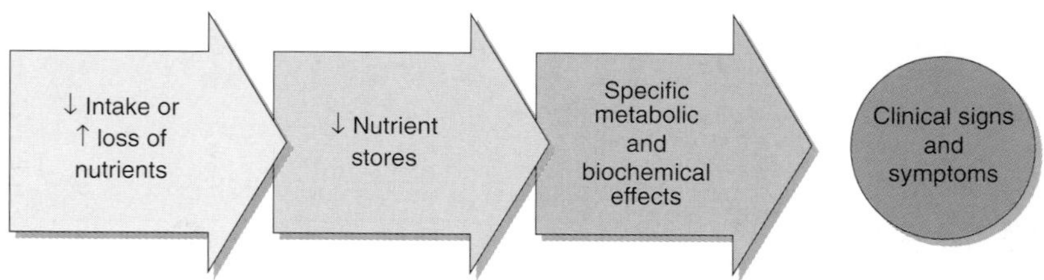

Fig. 1 **The development of malnutrition.**

HISTORY

Past medical history may point to changes in weight, poor wound healing or increased susceptibility to infection. The ability to take a good *dietary* history is one of the most important parts of a full nutritional assessment. Taking a dietary history may involve recording in detail the food and drink intake of the patient over a 7 day period. More usually, however, a few simple questions may yield a lot of useful information about a person's diet. Depending on the background to the problem, different questions will be appropriate. For example, in the wasted patient, questions about appetite and general food intake may suggest an eating disorder such as anorexia nervosa, but in the patient presenting with a skin rash, details of the specific food groups eaten will be required to help exclude a dietary cause. In the patient at increased risk of coronary heart disease, questions on saturated fat intake may be most revealing.

EXAMINATION

Simple anthropometric measurements will include height, weight, arm circumference and skin-fold thickness.

Body mass index (weight in kg divided by the height squared in metres) is a reasonable indicator of nutritional state, except when the patient is oedematous. Arm circumference is an indicator of skeletal muscle mass, while skin fold thickness is proportional to body fat levels. In addition, general physical examination may reveal signs of malnutrition in the skin, nails, hair, teeth and mucous membranes.

BIOCHEMISTRY

A number of biochemical tests are used to complement the history and examination in assessing the general nutritional status of a patient. None are completely satisfactory and should never be used in isolation. The most common tests include:

- *Protein.* Serum albumin concentration is a widely used but insensitive indicator of protein nutritional status. It is affected by many factors other than nutrition, e.g. hepatic and renal diseases and the hydration of the patient. Serum albumin concentration rapidly falls as part of the metabolic response to injury, and the decrease may be mistakenly attributed to malnutrition.
- *Blood glucose concentration.* This will be maintained even in the face of prolonged starvation. Ketosis develops during starvation and carbohydrate deficiency. Hyperglycaemia is frequently encountered as part of the metabolic response to injury.
- *Lipids.* Fasting plasma triglyceride levels provide some indication of fat metabolism, but are again affected by a variety of metabolic processes. Essential fatty acid levels may be measured if specific deficiencies are suspected. Faecal fat may be measured both qualitatively and quantitatively in the assessment of malabsorption (pp. 104–105).

Table 1 **Classification of vitamins**

Vitamins	Deficiency state	Lab assessment
Water soluble		
C (Ascorbate)	Scurvy	Plasma or leucocyte levels
B_1 (Thiamin)	Beri-Beri	Plasma levels or RBC transketolase activation
B_2 (Riboflavin)	Rarely single deficiency	Plasma levels or RBC glutathione reductase activation
B_6 (Pyridoxine)	Dermatitis / Anaemia	Plasma levels or RBC AST activation
B_{12} (Cobalamin)	Pernicious anaemia	Serum B_{12}, full blood count
Folate	Megaloblastic anaemia	Serum folate, RBC folate, full blood count
Niacin	Pellagra	Urinary niacin metabolites
Fat Soluble		
A (Retinol)	Blindness	Serum vitamin A
D (Cholecalciferol)	Osteomalacia / rickets	Serum 25–hydroxycholecalciferol
E (Tocopherol)	Anaemia / Neuropathy	Serum vitamin E
K (Phytomenadione)	Defective clotting	Prothrombin time

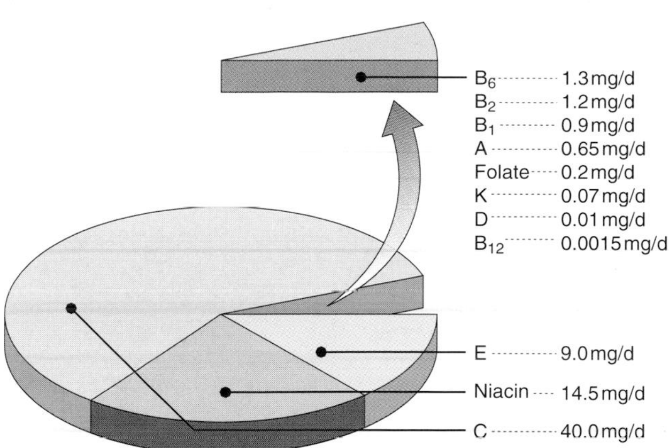

Fig. 2 **Average adult daily requirements of vitamins.**

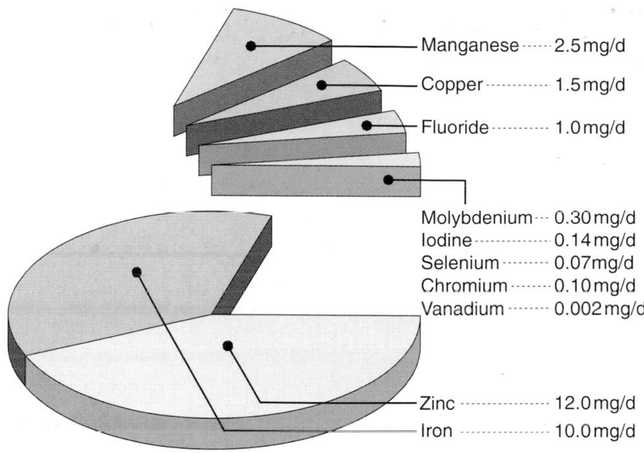

Fig. 3 **Average adult daily requirements of essential trace elements.**

Unlike the assessment of overall status, biochemical measurements play a key role in identifying excesses or deficiencies of specific components of the diet. Both blood and urine results may be of value. Such assays include:

- *Vitamins***.** These organic compounds are not synthesized by the body but are vital for normal metabolism. Usually they are classified by their solubility; they are listed in Table 1 and their average adult daily requirements shown in Figure 2. Some assays are available to measure the blood levels of vitamins directly, but often functional assays that utilize the fact that many vitamins are enzyme cofactors are used. These latter assays may help identify gross abnormalities. However, to detect subtle deficiencies and the increasing problem of excess intake, quantitative measurements are required.
- *Major minerals.* These inorganic elements are present in the body in quantities greater than 5g. The main nutrients in this category are sodium, potassium, chloride, calcium, phosphorus and magnesium. All of these are readily measurable in blood and their levels in part reflect dietary intake.
- *Trace elements.* Inorganic elements present in the body in quantities less than 5g are often found in complexes with proteins. The essential trace elements are shown in Figure 3.

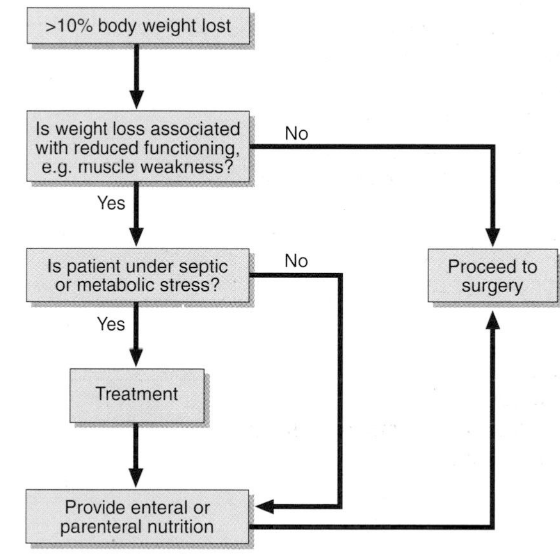

Fig. 4 **Selection of patients for preoperative nutritional support .**

PRE-OPERATIVE NUTRITIONAL ASSESSMENT

Nutritional assessment is not only necessary following surgical procedures. Patients need to be in good nutritional condition before an operation and the assessment should be done well in advance to allow build up of reserves before surgery (Fig. 4).

Clinical note

Accurate measurement of height and weight are the most important features of global nutritional assessment at all stages of life—from the neonatal period to old age. These are also often very poorly recorded in patient notes.

Case history 40

A 68-year-old male with motor neurone disease is admitted because of severe anorexia and weight loss. Suspecting malnutrition, the house officer requests a battery of biochemical tests including serum vitamin E and selenium.

- How useful will these be in the management of this patient?

Comment on page 156.

Nutritional assessment

- Nutritional assessment is important in every patient.
- Malnutrition is common and usually reflects the inadequacy of any nutrient or nutrients in the diet.
- History, examination and laboratory investigations are complementary.
- A variety of biochemical investigations may assist in the diagnosis of nutritional deficiencies and in the monitoring of patients undergoing nutritional support.

NUTRITIONAL SUPPORT

Nutritional support may range from simple dietary advice to long-term total parenteral nutrition (TPN). In between is a whole spectrum of clinical conditions and appropriate forms of nutritional support (Fig. 1). As we move to the right, climbing the scale of severity of disease, we increase the level of support and in so doing increase the need for laboratory back-up. The clinical biochemistry laboratory plays an important role in the diagnosis of some disorders that require specific nutritional intervention, e.g. diabetes mellitus, iron deficiency anaemia and hyperlipidaemia, but a much greater role is played in the monitoring of patients receiving the different forms of nutritional support.

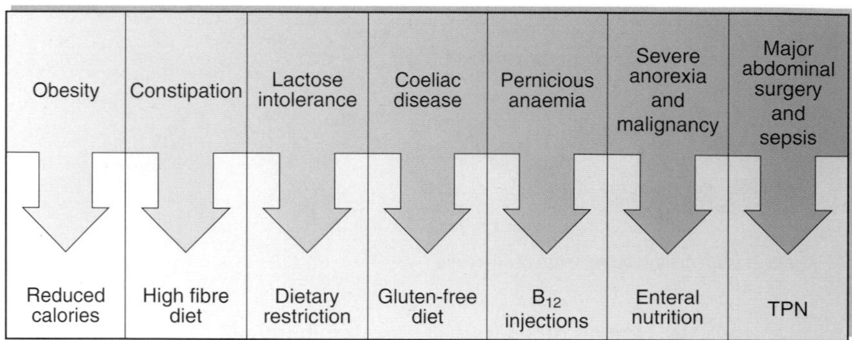

Fig. 1 **The spectrum of nutritional support.**

WHAT DO PATIENTS NEED?

Assessing the dietary needs of some patients is a highly specialized task, but some general guidelines can be considered. A balanced mix of nutrients must contain adequate provision for growth, healing and pathological losses, e.g. a draining fistula. Where patients are able to eat a mixed diet, the detailed consideration of their specific dietary intakes is seldom an issue. However, for those patients where the clinical team has to assume the responsibility of providing the balance of nutrients, much greater care must be taken.

Energy

Patients require energy, the amount of which can be roughly calculated from the Harris–Benedict equation (Fig. 2). This formula provides the basal energy requirements of an individual, and these must be adjusted to take account of increased requirements or losses as described above.

The principal energy sources in the diet are carbohydrates and fats. Glucose provides 4 kcal/g while fat provides 9 kcal/g. The entire calorie load may be administered using carbohydrates, but prescribing a mixture of carbohydrates and lipids is more physiological and serves to reduce the volume of the diet. This is important in tube feeding as well as in parenteral nutrition.

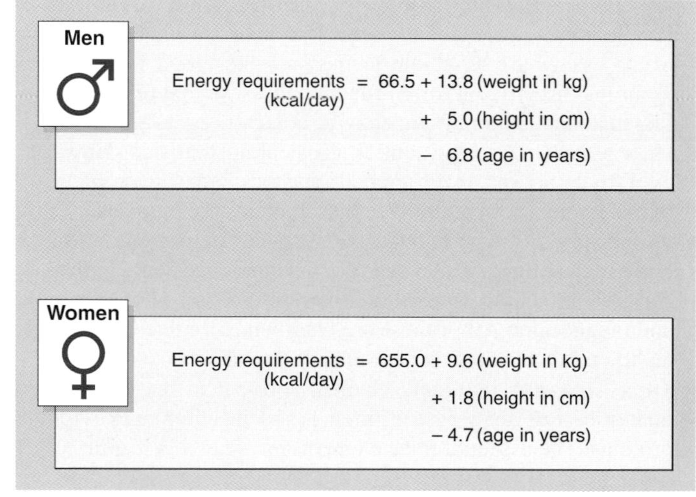

Fig. 2 **The Harris–Benedict equation.**

Nitrogen

Proteins and the amino acids provide nitrogen and also yield energy at 4 kcal/g. Amino acids are essential both for protein synthesis and for the synthesis of other nitrogen-containing compounds. Usually it is recommended that protein intake should constitute 10–15% of the total calorie requirement. Positive nitrogen balance can only be achieved if the energy intake is at least adequate to cover the resting energy expenditure. The energy needs can be calculated from knowledge of urinary urea excretion (Fig. 3). This dictates amino acid needs as well as the energy requirements to ensure that protein synthesis takes place.

Vitamins and trace elements

Vitamins and trace elements are collectively described as 'micronutrients', not because they are of limited importance but because they are required in relatively small amounts. Recommended dietary allowances (RDAs) have been defined for most nutrients and these are used in the make up of artificial diets.

HOW SHOULD THEY RECEIVE IT?

Patients may be fed in the following ways:

- oral feeding
- tube feeding into the gut
- parenteral feeding.

Oral feeding should be used whenever possible. Tube feeding (Fig. 4) involves the use of small bore nasogastric, nasoduodenal and gastrostomy tubes. Defined diets of homogeneous composition can be continually administered. Tube feeding in this way bypasses problems with oral pathology,

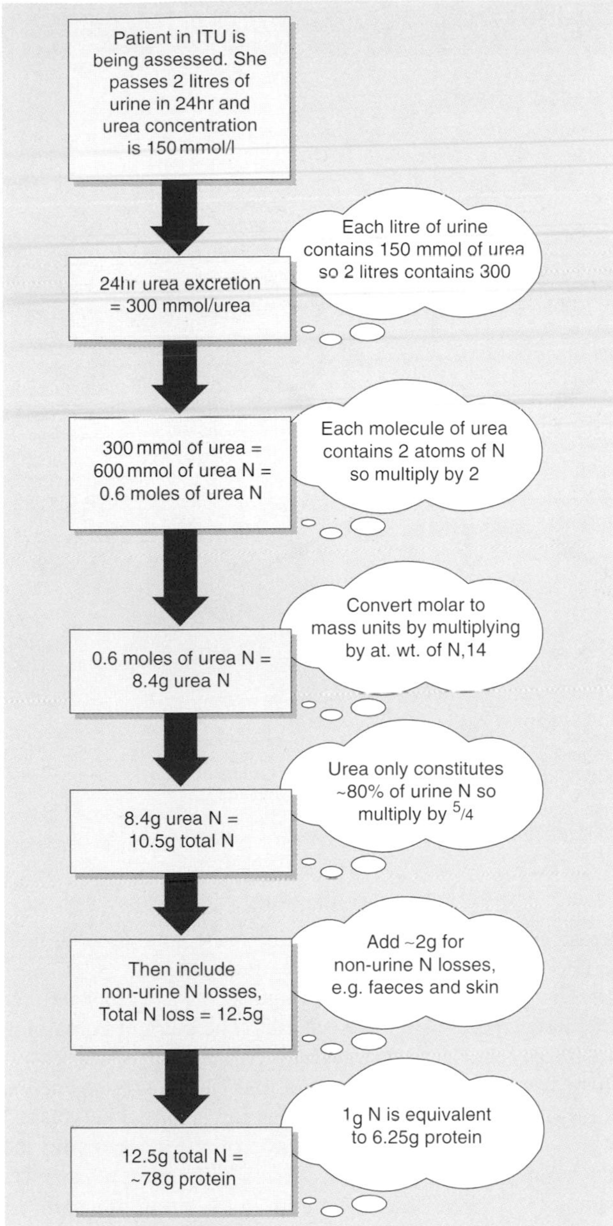

Fig. 3 **Urine urea measurements over 24 hr may be used to assess nitrogen balance.**

swallowing difficulties (e.g. after a stroke) and anorexia. Even patients who have had gastric surgery can be tube fed post-operatively if a feeding jejunostomy is fashioned during the operation distal to the lesion. However, tube feeding also presents mechanical problems in terms of blockage or oesophageal erosion. Gastrointestinal problems such as vomiting and diarrhoea, and metabolic problems can be minimized by the gradual introduction of the feeds and rarely are contraindications to enteral feeding. The problems associated with parenteral nutrition are even more severe and are discussed on pages 100-101. It should be noted, however, that the vast majority of patients can be fed very successfully either orally or with enteral tube feeds.

MONITORING PATIENTS

Clinical and biochemical monitoring should always go hand in hand in the assessment of any form of nutritional support. In some circumstances the contribution of the laboratory may be the simple measurement of blood glucose, while in other situations the measurements and advice provided by the lab may dictate the regimen in a patient receiving parenteral nutrition.

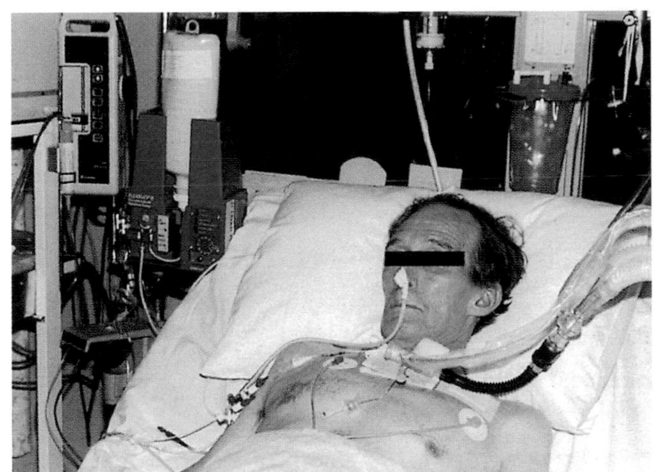

Fig. 4 **Patient on tube feeding in ITU.** Note this patient is also being ventilated via a tracheostomy and has a central line in place.

Case history 41

A patient with pernicious anaemia is being treated with parenteral vitamin B_{12}. Because she has recently been feeling tired and 'run down', her physician sends a sample to the clinical biochemistry lab requesting a serum B_{12} level.

- Is this the most appropriate way to monitor the patient?

Comment on page 156.

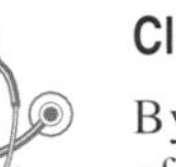

Clinical note

By far the most effective route of supplying nutrients to a patient is via the gut. By using nasogastric tubes and electively inserted stoma tubes to the stomach or small intestine, only a small minority of patients will require to be fed parenterally.

Nutritional support

- Nutritional support is required in a wide spectrum of conditions.
- It consists of a variety of approaches, from simple dietary advice to total parenteral nutrition.
- The route of first choice for nutritional support is oral followed by enteral followed by parenteral.
- Careful clinical and laboratory monitoring is required to some extent in all forms of nutritional support.
- Most laboratory support is needed for those patients receiving parenteral nutrition.

PARENTERAL NUTRITION

The provision of nutrients to the body's cells is a highly complex physiological process involving many endocrine, exocrine and other metabolic functions. Total parenteral nutrition (TPN) completely bypasses the gastrointestinal tract, delivering processed nutrients directly into the venous blood. It is more physiological to feed patients enterally and parenteral nutrition should only be considered once other possibilities have been deemed unsuitable. The institution of TPN is never an emergency and there should always be time for consultation and for baseline measurements to be performed. A team approach is desirable (Fig. 1).

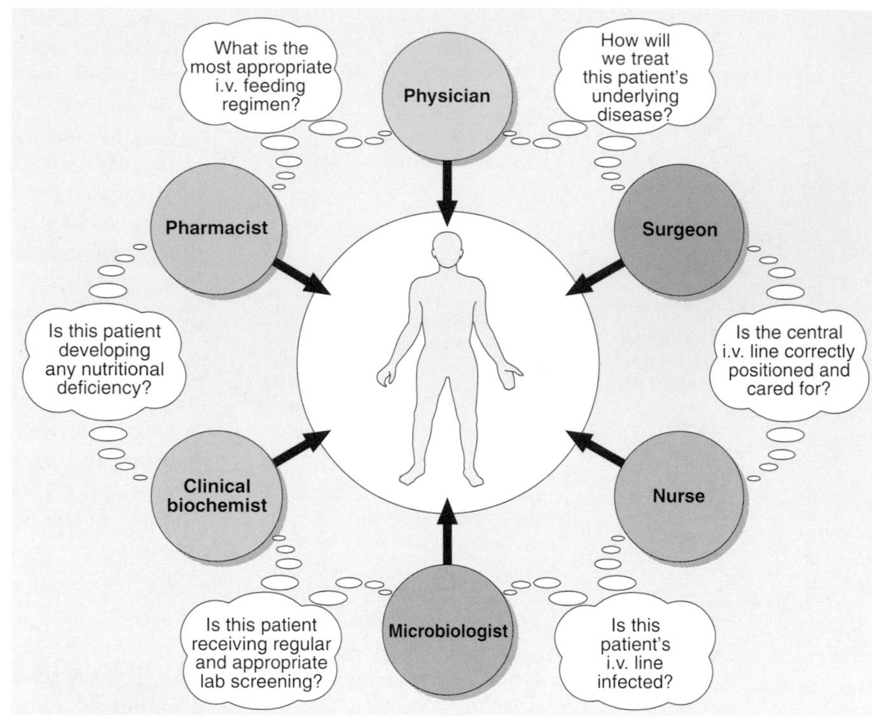

Fig. 1 **Team approach to TPN.**

INDICATIONS FOR PARENTERAL NUTRITION

Patients who are unable to eat or absorb food adequately from the gastrointestinal tract should be considered for parenteral nutrition. The circumstances where this occurs include:

- inflammatory bowel disease, e.g Crohn's disease
- short bowel syndrome, e.g. mesenteric artery infarction.

ROUTE OF ADMINISTRATION

Parenteral nutrition may be given in the following ways:

- *Via peripheral veins.* This route may be successfully used for a short period of 1-2 weeks.
- *Via a central venous catheter.* This route is used where long-term i.v. feeding is anticipated. Central vein catheters may remain patent for years if cared for properly.

Although most recipients of TPN are in-patients, many individuals who require long-term TPN have successfully managed to administer TPN in the home. These patients have permanent central catheters through which pre-packaged nutrition fluids are administered, usually at night.

COMPONENTS OF TPN

TPN should, as its name suggests, provide complete artificial nutrition. An appropriate volume of fluid will contain a source of calories, amino acids, vitamins and trace elements (Fig. 2). The calorie source is a mixture of glucose and lipid. Many patients who receive TPN are given standard proprietary regimens of pre-packaged solutions. These have made TPN much easier, but as with any such approach in medicine there are some patients who require more tailored regimens.

COMPLICATIONS

Total parenteral nutrition is the most extreme form of nutritional support and can give rise to considerable difficulties. In order to pre-empt these, consistent careful nursing care and biochemical monitoring are required.

Catheter site sepsis is a constant fear in these patients. The nutrient-containing infusion fluids are, of course, also excellent bacterial and fungal growth media, and risk of infection is further heightened by the presence of a foreign body, the catheter. Strict attention to aseptic technique both in the siting of a catheter and in its maintenance will serve to avoid many of these problems.

Misplacement of a catheter and infusion of nutrient solutions extravascularly can be very serious. Central catheters should

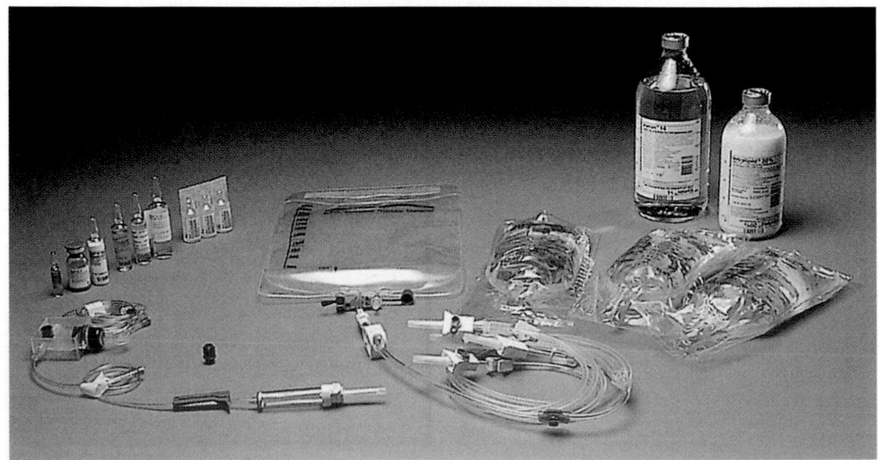

Fig. 2 **TPN preparations.**

be placed under X-ray control. The possibility of embolism, either thrombotic or air should be easily avoided as long as their potential is recognized.

The most common metabolic complication is that of hyperglycaemia. Against a background of increased stress hormones, especially if there is infection, there may be marked insulin resistance and consequently an increased glucose level. The use of insulin to correct these metabolic effects is best avoided. The composition of the i.v. regimen should be adjusted if metabolic disorders occur. Many other biochemical abnormalities have been reported in association with TPN. These include:

- hypokalaemia
- hypomagnesaemia
- hypophosphataemia
- hypercalcaemia
- acid–base disorders
- hyperlipidaemia.

If patients are properly monitored both clinically and biochemically during their TPN these potential disorders should be avoided.

MONITORING PATIENTS ON TPN

In addition to baseline assessment of patients receiving TPN, there should also be a strict policy for careful clinical and biochemical monitoring of these patients (Fig. 3). This is especially important if the TPN is medium to long-term. The tests described on pages 96–97 have particular relevance here.

Special attention must be paid to the micronutrients in long-term TPN patients as any imbalance here may result in a single nutrient deficiency state. Such situations are increasingly rare except in those patients relying solely on artificial diets for their nutrients.

Because biochemical changes may precede the development of any clinical manifestation of a nutritional deficiency, careful laboratory monitoring should be instituted.

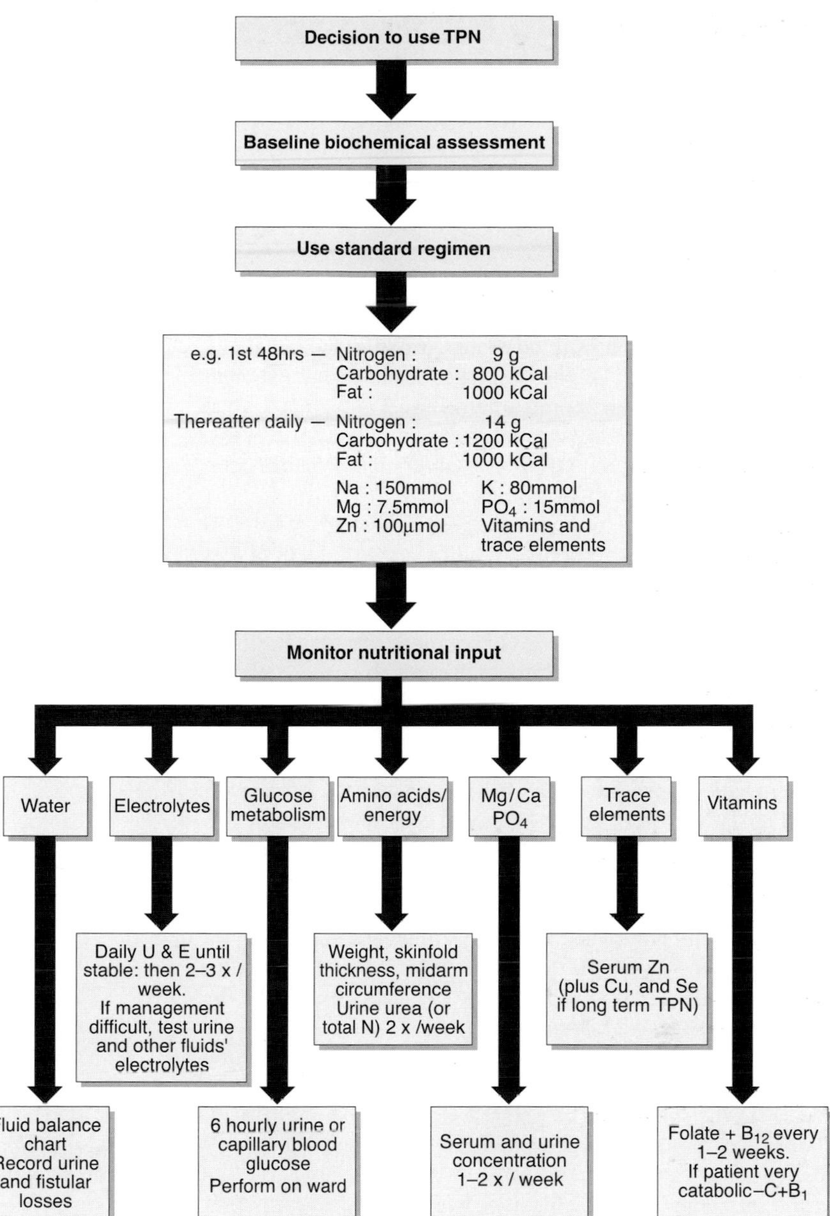

Fig. 3 **Intravenous nutrition and its monitoring.**

Clinical note

Patients often receive lipid emulsions as part of their i.v. regimen. Visible lipidaemia in a blood sample usually suggests that the patient is unable to clear the lipid from the plasma.

Case history 42

A 54-year-old man was admitted with a superior mesenteric artery thrombosis. He had gross bowel ischaemia and necrosis. Subsequently he had only 15 cm of viable small bowel.

- What form of feeding would be appropriate in this man?
- What assessment should be made before commencing treatment?

Comment on page 156.

Parenteral nutrition

- TPN is never an emergency procedure and should be carefully planned.
- A multidisciplinary team approach to TPN is the most effective.
- The main problems are due to sepsis, and mechanical and metabolic complications.
- The use of commercial preparations has made the incidence of deficiency states much less common.
- Patients receiving TPN require careful clinical and biochemical monitoring.

THE METABOLIC RESPONSE TO INJURY

The body reacts to all forms of noxious stimuli with an inflammatory response. This is a complex series of events which varies from mild hyperaemia due to a superficial scratch to major haemodynamic and metabolic responses to a severe injury. Trauma is the major cause of death in those under the age of 40 in the Western world and is the largest single cause of hospital admission. A number of important biochemical changes take place in the traumatized individual as part of the metabolic response to injury (Fig. 1). These changes occur to some extent in all forms of injury but will only attain clinical importance when the degree of injury is severe, i.e. following extensive burns, multiple injuries and fractures. Major surgery or severe infection give rise to similar metabolic consequences.

The problems faced by the traumatized individual are listed in Table 1.The metabolic response to injury can be thought of as a protective physiological response designed to keep the individual alive until healing processes repair the damage that has been done. It is mediated by a complex series of neuroendocrine and cellular processes, all of which contribute to the overall goal—survival.

THE PHASES OF THE METABOLIC RESPONSE TO INJURY

The metabolic response to injury has two phases, the *ebb* and the *flow* (Fig. 2). The ebb phase is short and corresponds roughly to clinical shock. The physiological changes which occur here restore adequate vascular volume and maintain essential tissue perfusion. The ebb phase may progress either to death or to the flow phase, which may last from days to weeks depending on the extent of the injury. In this phase, metabolism is altered to ensure that energy is available for dependent tissues at the expense of muscle and fat stores.

These biochemical changes (Table 2) are mediated by the hormones cortisol, glucagon and the catecholamines. They ensure survival in the short term but exact a penalty from the patient. Whereas loss of body fat is acceptable and easily reversed, loss of muscle tissue is a serious concern.

The inflammation subsequent to injury or infection is mediated by paracrine regulators; cytokines such as tumour necrosis factor and the interleukins, and lipid mediators such as platelet-activating factor and thromboxane A_2.

THE ACUTE PHASE PROTEIN RESPONSE

The acute phase protein response leads to greatly increased de novo synthesis (principally by the liver) of a number of plasma proteins along with a decrease in the plasma concentration of some others. This response is stimulated by the release of cytokines such as interleukin 1 and 6 and tumour necrosis factor, and raised concentrations of the hormones cortisol and glucagon. The major human acute phase proteins are listed in Table 3.

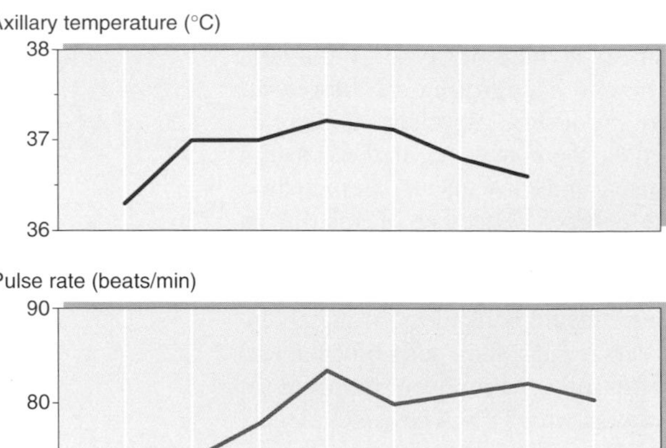

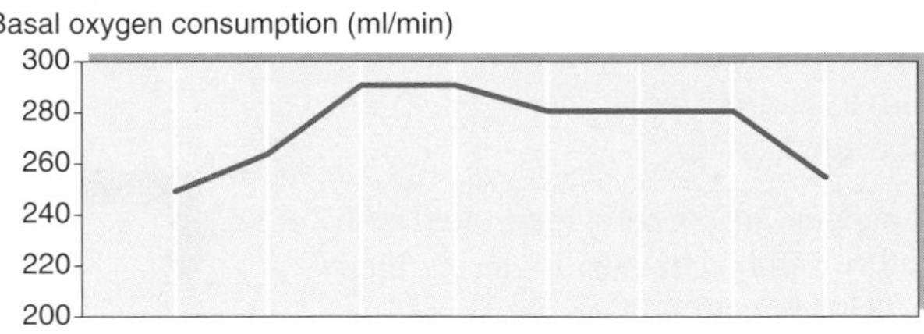

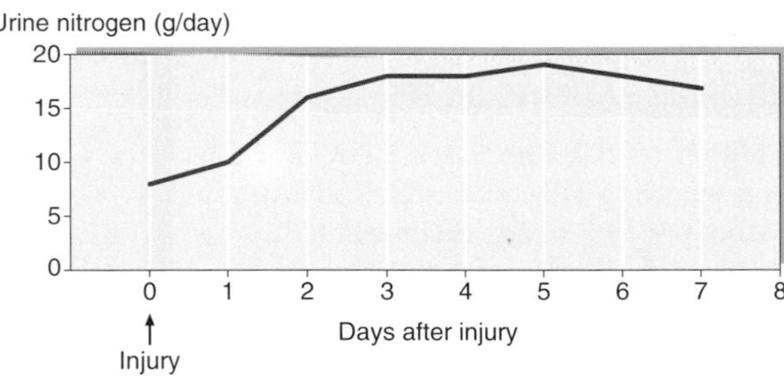

Fig. 1 **The changes in body temperature, pulse rate, oxygen consumption and urinary nitrogen excretion which accompany injury.**

The acute phase protein response is an adaptive response to disease. Its role is not fully understood but certain aspects can be seen to be of benefit to the individual. The increases in C-reactive protein (CRP) and complement will contain and eliminate infection; increased coagulation factors will aid and prevent excess blood loss; protease inhibitors will prevent the spread of tissue necrosis when lysosomal enzymes are released by damaged cells at the site of injury. The precise role of other proteins in this response such as caeruloplasmin and serum amyloid A remains to be established.

Table 1 **Major problems faced by traumatized individuals**

Bleeding and circulatory collapse
Pain
Major tissue damage
Food and water deprivation
Immobilization
Infection

Table 2 **Biochemical changes in the metabolic response to injury**

Metabolic change	Consequence
Increased glycogenolysis	Leads to increased circulating blood glucose to be used as an energy substrate
Increased gluconeogenesis	Leads to increased circulating blood glucose to be used as an energy substrate
Increased lipolysis	Leads to increased free fatty acids which are used to provide energy and increased glycerol which may be converted to glucose
Increased proteolysis	Leads to increased amino acids which may be catabolized to provide energy or used for tissue synthesis and wound healing

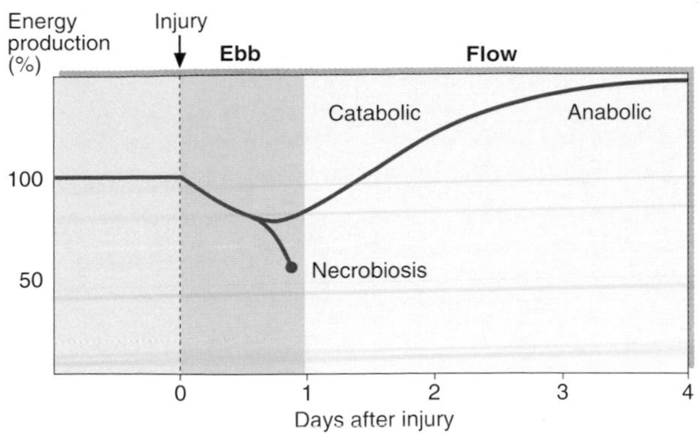

Fig. 2 **The phases of the metabolic response to injury.**

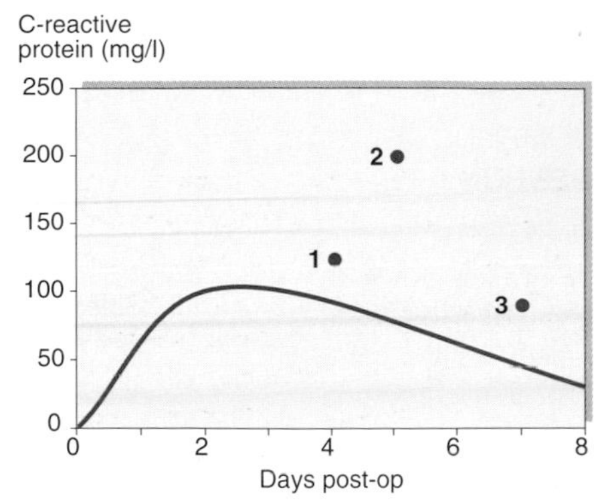

Fig. 3 **CRP concentration in a patient who developed an occult abscess following abdominal surgery.**

Clinical uses

In practice the major use of the acute phase response is to monitor the course of the inflammatory process in the patient. This is done in two ways:

- *By measuring serum CRP.* CRP concentrations change very rapidly and can be used to monitor changes on a daily basis (Fig. 3).
- *By monitoring the erythrocyte sedimentation rate (ESR).* This reflects fibrinogen and immunoglobulin concentration. ESR changes slowly, and is used to monitor the inflammatory process over weeks rather than days.

Table 3 **The acute phase protein response**

Protein types	Increased	Decreased
Protease inhibitors	α_1-Antitrypsin α_2-macroglobulin	
Coagulation proteins	Fibrinogen Prothrombin Factor VIII Plasminogen	
Complement proteins	C1s C2, B C3, C4, C5 C56 C1 INH	Properdin
Miscellaneous	Haptoglobin Caeruloplasmin C-reactive protein Serum Amyloid–A Protein	 Albumin HDL LDL

Clinical note

Antibiotic therapy for an infection, perhaps indicated by increased CRP concentration, should be started only after appropriate specimens have been taken for bacteriological investigation.

In neonates and immunosuppressed patients, bacterial infection can be difficult to diagnose in its early stages. Failure to make the diagnosis may have fatal consequences. In practice, a serum CRP concentration of >100 mg/l (normal <10 mg/l) is frequently taken to indicate the presence of infection.

STARVATION AND THE METABOLIC RESPONSE TO INJURY

The metabolic responses to injury and to starvation are quite different. After injury the body is at war, defences are mobilized, metabolic activity increases and resources are directed to the site of action. In starvation, the body is in a state of famine, resources are rationed and metabolic activity is limited to the minimum for survival. The two situations are quite distinct, but in the clinical situation both can occur together. The severely injured patient is often not fed as a priority. Where starvation and the metabolic response to injury occur together, a good clinical outcome becomes less likely. If a seriously traumatized patient is also nutritionally depleted he or she may be exposed to:

- immunosuppression
- decreased wound healing
- delayed tissue repair
- muscle weakness.

All of these work together to prolong convalescence, increase morbidity and cloud the outcome.

The importance of prompt nutritional support for severely injured patients cannot be overemphasized. In the catabolic state, large amounts of energy and amino acids are required to replace the losses. The nutritional workup and assessment appropriate in the trauma patient are discussed on pages 97–99.

In addition to ensuring adequate nutrition, some investigators believe that other therapies may enhance patient recovery following trauma, burns or severe infection. Strategies which reduce the inflammatory response and enhance protein synthesis and tissue repair are being evaluated.

Case history 43

A 28-year-old man was admitted to the intensive therapy unit after a serious road traffic accident in which he sustained multiple injuries. After initial resuscitation and surgery to his injuries he was considered stable but in coma.

- What is the role of biochemical measurements in this patient's management?

Comment on page 156.

The metabolic response to injury

- The metabolic response to injury is a protective physiological response.
- The ebb phase corresponds to clinical shock, and the physiological changes restore circulating blood volume and maintain tissue perfusion.
- The flow phase involves changes in metabolism to ensure that energy is made available to dependent tissues.
- The flow phase persists until the inflammatory response provides for tissue healing and/or eradication of infection.
- C-reactive protein (CRP) measurements are useful in monitoring day-to-day changes in the inflammatory response.

MALABSORPTION

PHYSIOLOGY OF DIGESTION AND ABSORPTION

Having been initially broken down in part by cooking and mastication, food is assimilated by the body by the combined action of two processes: digestion and absorption. The major nutrients (carbohydrate, protein and fat) are broken down enzymatically to low molecular weight compounds. Digestive enzymes are secreted by the stomach, pancreas and small intestine.

The transport of the products of digestion into gut epithelial cells and from there to the portal blood is termed absorption. The absorption of some nutrients is passive while others require active transport.

MALABSORPTION

Failure of digestion is properly called maldigestion. The term 'malabsorption' describes impairment of the absorptive mechanisms, but in practice is used to encompass both disorders. Malabsorption is a condition which can occur at any stage of life from a variety of causes (Fig.1).

The clinical effects of malabsorption result from the failure to absorb nutrients. The major consequences of generalized malabsorption arise from inadequate energy intake which results in weight loss in adults and growth failure in children.

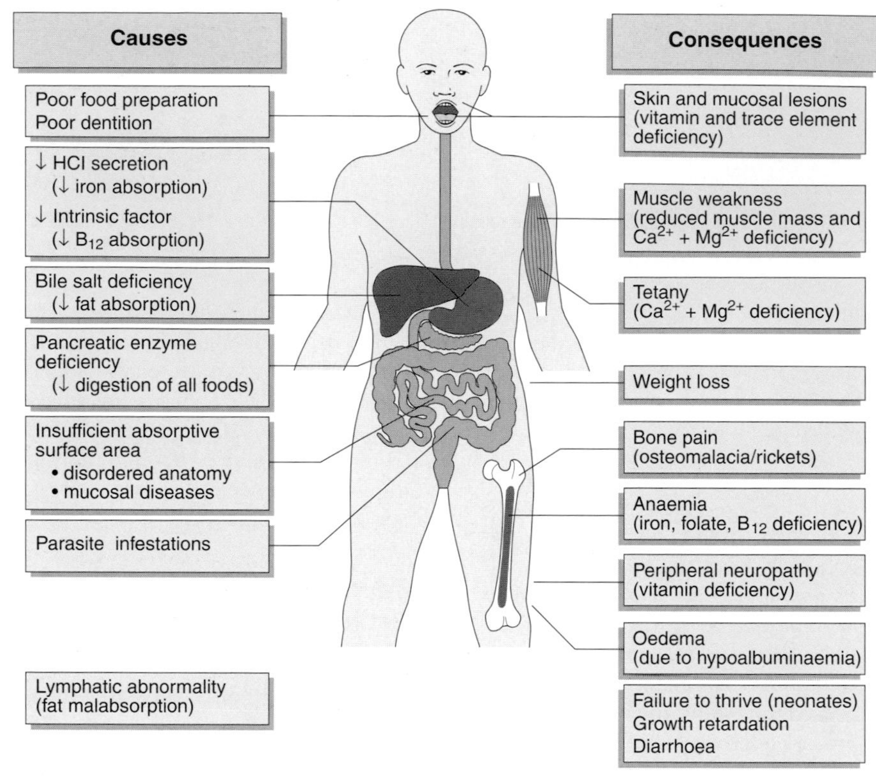

Fig. 1 **Causes and consequences of malabsorption.**

Diagnosis

In suspected malabsorption a detailed dietary history is essential to establish eating patterns and habits. Endoscopy and biopsy are by far the most important tools available for the investigation of gastrointestinal tract disorders. They allow macro- and microscopic study of the intestinal mucosa and are the standard techniques used to diagnose major causes of malabsorption such as coeliac disease. Radiological tests are of assistance when detecting abnormal anatomy of the bowel and motility. Though not usually investigated, it is important to assess the state of teeth and gums, and the adequacy of salivary secretion, as they play an important role in initiating digestion.

Provided that dietary input is adequate, the presence of malabsorption from the small bowel will often be indicated by changes in the faeces, in particular by diarrhoea. Diarrhoea due to malabsorption can be assumed only if other causes, such as infection and laxative abuse, have been excluded. Laxative abuse is an important diagnosis which may be missed. A laxative screen is readily performed in cases of suspected abuse.

In the case of fat malabsorption, the faeces will contain fat which can be detected by microscopic examination of the stools or by quantitative analysis. Where small molecules such as monosaccharides are not absorbed, they exert an osmotic effect which will prevent water absorption in the large intestine, giving rise to a large volume of watery stools.

Biochemical investigations

Laboratory tests in the investigation of gastrointestinal disorders fall into one of two groups: tests which identify malabsorption and tests of pancreatic function. The most frequently performed tests are outlined below. There is little agreement amongst investigators as to the best tests to use.

Tests of malabsorption

- *Faecal fat.* The presence of fatty stools is an important sign of malabsorption. Faecal specimens over a five day period may be collected and total fat content measured.
- *Faecal microscopy.* The presence of fat globules can be observed directly.
- *Butterfat test.* Chylomicrons detected in the plasma of patients after a standard fat load indicate that some fat digestion and absorption has occurred.
- *^{14}C-triglyceride breath test.* An oral dose of radiolabelled triglyceride (e.g. ^{14}C-triolein in which the fatty acid contains the label) is absorbed and metabolized. The $^{14}CO_2$ in expired air is a measure of the effectiveness of digestion and absorption.
- *Xylose absorption test.* Serum measurements of this 5-carbon sugar are made after an oral dose and provide an indication of intestinal ability to absorb monosaccharides.

Tests of pancreatic function

- *Lundh test.* Duodenal contents are collected after a meal and the activity of a pancreatic enzyme, such as trypsin or amylase, is measured.

Table 1 **Additional biochemical tests used in the investigation of gastrointestinal disease**

Test	Purpose
Urea breath test	Used to identify patients with *Helicobacter pylori* infection which is strongly associated with peptic ulcer disease
Hydrogen breath test	Assesses bacterial overgrowth in the intestine
Lactose tolerance test	Different disaccharides may be used to detect specific functional enzyme defects such as lactase or sucrase
Faecal chymotrypsin or elastase function	Indirect pancreatic function tests used in the assessment of pancreatic mainly in cystic fibrosis
Intestinal permeability	Biologically inert polymers are used to assess mucosal permeability by measuring their excretion in urine after an oral load
Schilling test	Assesses vitamin B_{12} absorption

- *Secretin test*. An intravenous injection of secretin stimulates pancreatic secretion which is assessed by aspiration of duodenal contents and measurement of trypsin or amylase activity.
- *Pancreolauryl test*. Fluorescein dilaurate is hydrolysed by cholesterol esterase in pancreatic secretion. The water-soluble fluorescein is absorbed and excreted in urine where its fluorescence gives an indirect measure of pancreatic function.

Other tests which may be employed in the investigation of malabsorption and gastrointestinal disease are shown in Table 1.

Gastrointestinal disease

There are many disorders associated with malabsorption. Generalized malabsorption occurs for a number of reasons. These include:

- Inadequate digestion, which is seen in chronic pancreatitis as a consequence of insufficient pancreatic enzyme release.
- Inadequate intestinal mucosal surface (Fig. 2) as occurs in coeliac disease.
- Inflammation affecting the mucosa, sub mucosa and frequently the entire bowel structures as occurs in Crohn's disease.
- Infections of the bowel causing intestinal hurry. These may be acute as in salmonella, or chronic as in tropical sprue.
- Abnormal bowel anatomy or insufficient bowel. This may occur after repeated surgery for chronic disorders such as Crohn's disease or after bowel infarction and removal of the necrotic bowel.

Malignant disease is not usually associated with malabsorption unless there is abnormal bowel motility which allows bacterial flora to proliferate, or if the tumour secretes a hormone such as VIP, which causes diarrhoea (p. 132).

Inadequate bile salt secretion occurs in many forms of liver disease and gives rise to fat malabsorption. Patients may present with the clinical features of generalized malabsorption on top of the underlying liver disease. Inadequate fat absorption is associated with impaired absorption of vitamin D (a fat-soluble vitamin). In the absence of adequate sunlight exposure, patients may become vitamin D deficient and unable to absorb calcium from the gut. This may lead to the development of osteomalacia or rickets.

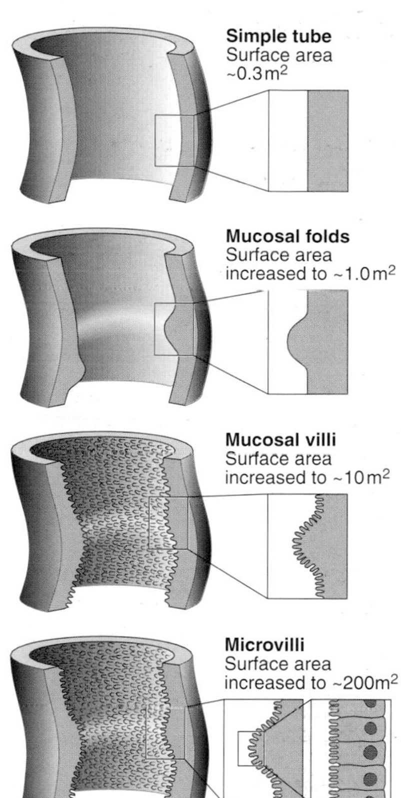

Fig. 2 **Effects of mucosal structure on absorptive surface area of the small intestine.**

The malabsorption of specific substances tends to occur in certain well-defined conditions such as vitamin B_{12} malabsorption which leads to pernicious anaemia. This occurs when intrinsic factor production is lost due to gastric mucosal atrophy. Patients may also have inherited deficiencies of intestinal saccharidases such as lactase which cause malabsorption when the patient drinks milk or eats milk products. This is known as lactose intolerance.

Case history 44

A 69-year-old woman, who had made an excellent recovery after local excision of a breast tumour 8 years previously, presented with weight loss, bone tenderness and weakness. Her symptoms had developed over a number of months. Her family were concerned that she was not caring for herself nor eating adequately. There was no clinical evidence of recurrence of breast cancer. LFTs showed only an elevated alkaline phosphatase (430 U/l).

- What other biochemical tests would be of assistance in making a diagnosis?

Comment on page 156.

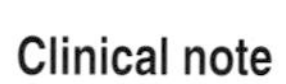

Clinical note

Many patients with malabsorption recognise that certain things in their diet—usually fatty foods—cause diarrhoea. They avoid these foods and reduce their fat intake. As a result, faecal fat excretion may be normal because of this low dietary fat intake.

Malabsorption

- In suspected malabsorption, a detailed dietary history is essential to establish eating patterns and habits.
- Endoscopy and biopsy are the most important tools and frequently allow a specific diagnosis to be made.
- Laboratory tests in the investigation of gastrointestinal disorders fall into one of two groups: tests of malabsorption and tests of pancreatic function.

IRON

Iron is an essential element in humans, being the central ion in haem, the non-protein constituent of haemoglobin (Fig. 1). Haemoglobin is responsible for the transport and delivery of oxygen from the lungs to the tissues. Iron deficiency causes a failure of haem synthesis, leading to anaemia which results in tissue hypoxia. Haem is also a constituent of myoglobin in muscle tissue.

Cytochromes and many other intracellular enzymes also contain iron, but are largely unaffected in all but the most severe cases of iron deficiency.

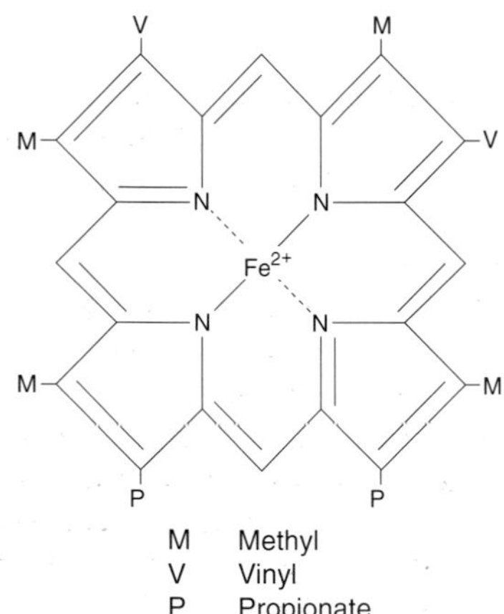

Fig. 1 **Structure of haem.**

IRON PHYSIOLOGY

There are 50–70 mmol (3–4 g) of iron in the body. Three–quarters are present as the molecular complex with haem. Most of the remainder is in tissue stores bound to the iron storage proteins, ferritin and haemosiderin. Less than one per cent of total body iron is in the plasma, where it is associated with the iron-binding protein, transferrin. Body iron is efficiently reutilized. Dietary intake is about 0.35 mmol (20 mg) per day. The factors which regulate intestinal absorption of iron are poorly understood (Fig. 2).

Serum iron concentrations vary with age and sex. Normal adult concentrations are 18–45 μmol/l in males and 14–32 μmol/l in females. In both groups there is a marked circadian rhythm in serum iron concentration.

Iron is transported in plasma bound to the specific glycoprotein, transferrin, each molecule of which binds two Fe^{3+} ions together with bicarbonate as an anion. A number of factors can lower serum iron independently of iron status. These include the acute phase response to infection, trauma and malignant disease.

LABORATORY INVESTIGATIONS OF IRON DISORDERS

Various laboratory investigations are helpful in the diagnosis of iron deficiency and iron overload:

- *Serum iron determinations* are of limited routine value, being of most assistance in the diagnosis of iron overload and acute iron poisoning.
- *Total iron binding capacity* (TIBC) of a serum specimen is an indirect measure of transferrin concentration, although in some laboratories transferrin can be measured directly. Normally transferrin is around 30% saturated with iron. When this falls to less than 15%, iron deficiency is likely and some degree of clinical effect can be expected. A high percent saturation is the most sensitive marker for iron overload. Like serum iron, transferrin is decreased as part of the acute phase response. Protein-energy malnutrition also decreases transferrin synthesis by the liver and hence its serum concentration.
- *Serum ferritin* is the best indicator of body iron stores. It is normally greater than 12 μg/l. The acute phase response to infection, injury or malignant disease can result in increases in serum ferritin, making the diagnosis of marginal iron deficiency difficult in these circumstances.
- *Red cell protoporphyrin* is usually less than 1 μmol per litre of red cells. This haem precursor is markedly increased in iron deficiency. Levels are also affected in porphyria and by exposure to inorganic lead compounds.

IRON DEFICIENCY

Iron deficiency anaemia is the commonest of all single-nutrient deficiences. Millions of people worldwide are affected, with seriously impaired quality of life and work efficiency. The principal causes are chronic blood loss and poor dietary intake of bioavailable iron, e.g. the uptake of iron from the diet can be decreased by a number of dietary constituents such as phytic acid and fibre. Iron deficiency can also occur in coeliac disease and other intestinal disorders where malabsorption is a feature.

In all cases of iron deficiency anaemia it is important to diagnose the underlying condition, especially malignant disease, the presence of intestinal parasites or any other intestinal pathology which may cause chronic blood loss. Iron deficiency may also develop during pregnancy, even in well-nourished women, due to the increased iron requirements of the developing fetus.

Iron deficiency anaemia develops in three stages:

1. *A depletion of iron stores with no functional impairment.* Serum ferritin concentrations of less than 12 μg/l confirm this.
2. *Deficient erythropoiesis.* Haemoglobin levels remain normal, but red cell protoporphyrin is increased. The synthesis of transferrin is increased and percent saturation is decreased.

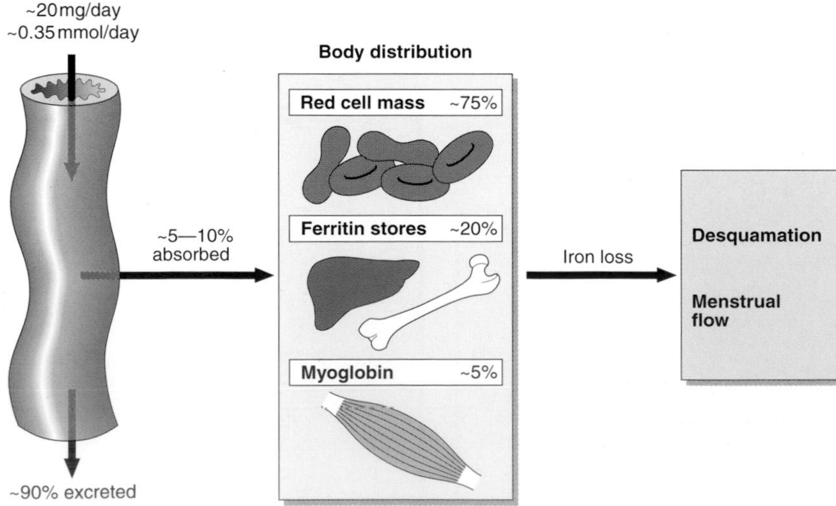

Fig. 2 **Iron balance.**

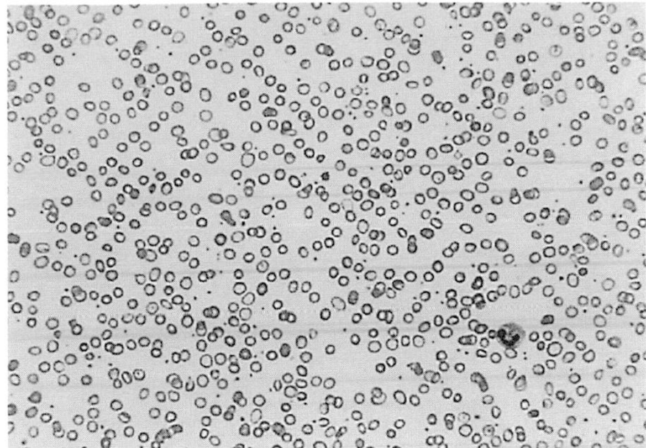

Fig. 3 **Photomicrograph of an iron deficient blood film.**

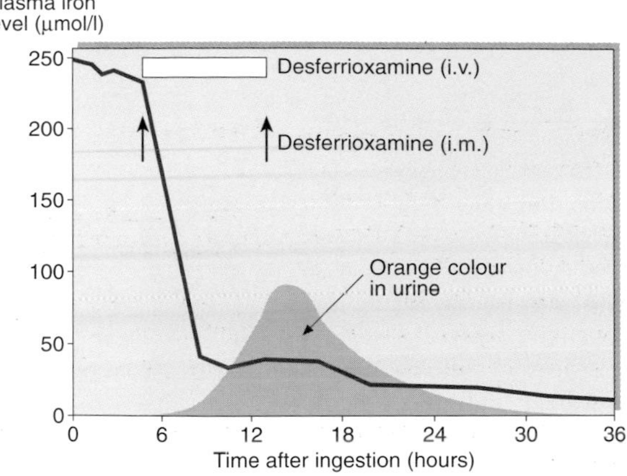

Fig. 4 **The effect of desferrioxamine on iron excretion in overdose.**

When 15% or less saturation is reached, work capacity is impaired.

3. *Iron deficiency anaemia.* There is low haemoglobin resulting in a microcytic hypochromic anaemia (Fig. 3). Low stainable iron is seen in bone marrow. Only in the late stages of iron deficiency anaemia are low concentrations of serum iron observed.

Treatment

Oral therapy with iron salts is widely used to treat iron deficiency anaemia. It can take up to 6 months to replete the body stores. Compliance is a problem since side effects such as nausea, diarrhoea and other intestinal complaints may be encountered. These are all lessened if the iron salts are taken with food. A combination of iron and folate is widely prescribed during pregnancy.

Haemachromatosis

Haemachromatosis (bronze diabetes) is a relatively common inherited disease characterized by increased iron absorption and iron deposition in various organs which leads to fibrosis and organ failure. The clinical presentation varies widely depending upon dietary iron intake, alcohol abuse or the presence of hepatotoxins. Women are less severely affected than men, being protected by physiological loss of iron during menstruation and in pregnancy. Whole body iron content may be increased to ten times normal.

Clinical features include chronic fatigue and, in extreme cases, skin pigmentation, diabetes mellitus, hypogonadism, liver cirrhosis and hepatoma. Serum iron is increased, with almost complete saturation of transferrin. The serum ferritin is markedly increased to greater than 500 μg/l. Chronic iron overload is usually treated by repeated venesection.

Iron poisoning

Accidental ingestion of iron tablets by children is common and may be life threatening. Symptoms include nausea and vomiting, abdominal pain, diarrhoea and haematemesis. In severe cases, hypotension, liver damage and coma can result. Serum iron is increased and transferrin is saturated (>70%).

Acute iron poisoning is treated by chelating the iron in the stomach and in the plasma with desferrioxamine (Fig. 4). The chelated iron is excreted in the urine as a deep orange-coloured complex. This should not be confused with myoglobinuria.

IRON OVERLOAD

Since there is no major mechanism for excretion of iron except by cell desquamation and occult blood loss, iron overload is always a possibility when iron therapy is prescribed. Iron overload may also be caused by chronic blood transfusions. Two other conditions may be encountered: haemachromatosis and iron poisoning.

Clinical note

A microcytic hypochromic anaemia, with the absence of stainable iron in a bone marrow biopsy, are the best diagnostic indices of established iron deficiency.

Case history 45

A 42-year-old woman presented with a history of increasing lethargy, dizziness and breathlessness. She had brittle hair and nails. She complained of heart palpitation on exercise and reported particularly heavy periods. Biochemical investigation revealed the following results:

Serum iron	4 μmol/l
Transferrin saturation	10%
Ferritin	<5 μg/l

- What is the diagnosis and what other investigations should have been done first?

Comment on page 157.

Iron

- Iron deficiency is commonly caused by the combination of blood loss and low dietary intake.
- Iron deficiency can be diagnosed by finding a hypochromic microcytic anaemia.
- Serum ferritin is the most reliable single biochemical test of iron deficiency.
- Iron overload may arise following repeated blood transfusions.
- Iron overload is diagnosed by finding an increased serum iron concentration and percent saturation, and increased serum ferritin.
- Accidental iron poisoning in children is an important medical emergency.

COPPER AND ZINC

COPPER

Copper is an essential trace metal which is a component of a wide range of intracellular metalloenzymes, including cytochrome oxidase, superoxide dismutase, tyrosinase, dopamine hydroxylase and lysyl oxidase. Most of the copper in plasma is associated with the specific copper-binding protein, caeruloplasmin.

COPPER PHYSIOLOGY

About 50% of the average daily dietary copper of around 25 μmol (1.5 mg) is absorbed from the stomach and the small intestine (Fig. 1). Although copper is present in most foodstuffs, there is evidence that not all modern diets contain sufficient copper, especially when large amounts of refined carbohydrate are consumed. Absorbed copper is transported to the liver in portal blood bound to albumin and is exported to peripheral tissues mainly bound to caeruloplasmin and, to a lesser extent, albumin.

Copper is present in all metabolically active tissues. The highest concentrations are found in liver and in kidney, with significant amounts in cardiac and skeletal muscle and in bone. The liver contains 10% of the total body content of 1200 μmol (80 mg). Excess copper is excreted in bile into the gut, and the faecal copper output (12.5 μmol/24 h) is the sum of unabsorbed dietary copper and that re-excreted into the gut.

LABORATORY ASSESSMENT

A number of different investigations are needed to diagnose disorders of copper metabolism. These are:

- *Serum copper.* Normal concentrations are usually between 10–22 μmol/l, of which 90% is bound to caeruloplasmin. Total copper concentration may vary either due to changes in copper itself or to changes in the concentration of caeruloplasmin.
- *Serum caeruloplasmin.* The normal adult levels are 200–600 mg/l. Caeruloplasmin is increased greatly in the acute phase reaction, and in some cases may be so high as to raise the total copper concentration to 30-45 μmol/l. Caeruloplasmin levels may be helpful in the interpretation of serum copper concentrations.
- *Urinary copper.* Normal excretion is <1.0 μmol/24 h.

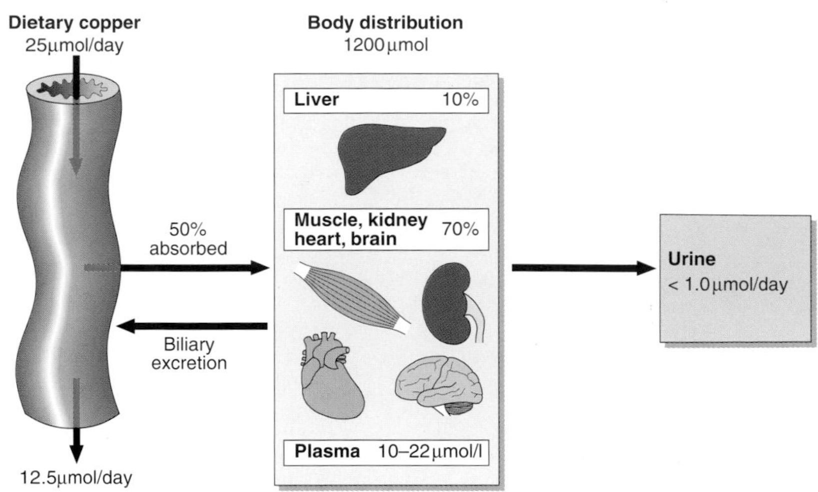

Fig. 1 **Copper balance.**

COPPER DEFICIENCY

Both children and adults can develop symptomatic copper deficiency. Premature infants are the most susceptible since copper stores in the liver are laid down in the third trimester of pregnancy. In adults, deficiency is usually found following intestinal bypass surgery or in patients on parenteral nutrition. Symptoms range from bone disease to an iron-resistant microcytic hypochromic anaemia.

COPPER TOXICITY

Copper toxicity is uncommon and is most usually due to administration of copper sulphate solutions. Oral copper sulphate may lead to gastric perforation. Serum copper concentrations may be greatly elevated. Copper is toxic to many organs, but renal tubular damage is the major concern. Treatment is by chelation with penicillamine.

INBORN ERRORS OF COPPER METABOLISM

There are two inborn errors of copper metabolism: Menkes syndrome and Wilson's disease.

Menkes syndrome

Menkes syndrome is a very rare but fatal condition which presents in infants as growth failure and mental retardation, with lesions of the major blood vessels and bone disease. A characteristic sign is 'steely hair' (pilo torti).

Wilson's disease

All adolescents or young adults with otherwise unexplained neurological or hepatic disease should be investigated for Wilson's disease, since this condition is fatal if not diagnosed and treated. Symptoms are a result of copper deposition in liver, brain, and kidney. Copper deposits in the eye can sometimes be seen as a brown pigment around the iris (the Kayser–Fleischer ring).

The inherited defect in Wilson's disease is believed to be in the gene coding for an enzyme involved in copper excretion into bile and reabsorption in the kidney. Urinary copper excretion is high and serum concentrations low (Table 1). Just what causes the low caeruloplasmin concentrations in these patients remains unclear. Confirmation is by measurement of copper in a liver biopsy which is usually greater than 250 μg/g dry weight in patients with the disease.

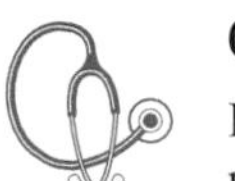

Clinical note

In the general population, marginal copper deficiency may be a cardiovascular disease risk factor, since both experimental animal and human studies show that a low copper diet combined with high carbohydrate intake may lead to hypercholesterolaemia and cardiac abnormalities.

Treatment is by administration of a chelating agent, penicillamine, to promote urinary copper excretion. Patients are maintained on oral penicillamine for life and require regular monitoring to ensure compliance and to check for side effects. Liver transplantation may also be considered, particularly in young patients with severe disease.

Table 1 **Biochemistry determinations in patients with Wilson's disease**

Investigation	Normal adult	Wilson's disease
Serum copper µmol/l	10–22	<10
Caeruloplasmin mg/l	200–600	< 200
Urinary copper µmol/24h	<1	5–15
Liver copper µg/g dry weight	20–50	>250

Case history 46

A 15-year-old girl presented with abdominal pain and diarrhoea for 3 days. She became jaundiced and a presumptive diagnosis of infective hepatitis was made, but serological tests were negative. She subsequently died of fulminant liver failure. At post mortem her liver copper concentration was found to be grossly increased.

- What investigations should be carried out on this patient's younger sister?

Comment on page 157.

ZINC

Zinc is an essential element present in over 200 metalloproteins with a wide range of functions. Carbonic anhydrase, alcohol dehydrogenase, alkaline phosphatase and steroid hormone receptors are examples.

ZINC PHYSIOLOGY

The average daily dietary intake of zinc is around 150 µmol (10 mg) (Fig. 2). It is present in all protein-rich foods. Around 30% is absorbed. Absorption is reduced in the presence of phytates. In the liver, zinc is incorporated into metalloenzymes, while in blood the majority of the zinc is contained in the erythrocytes. In plasma, 90% of zinc is bound to albumin and 10% to α_2-macroglobulin. Zinc reserves in the body are small and are located mainly in muscle and bone. Zinc is excreted in urine, in bile, in pancreatic fluid and in milk in lactating mothers.

LABORATORY ASSESSMENT

The repeated finding of a zinc concentration in a serum specimen of less than 5 µmol/l is suggestive of impending zinc deficiency and requires investigation. Unlike copper, serum zinc falls during the acute phase response to injury or infection.

Marginal zinc deficiency is best demonstrated by a positive clinical response to supplementation. Oral or intravenous zinc reverses the signs and symptoms of zinc deficiency within weeks.

ZINC DEFICIENCY

Zinc deficiency occurs in both adults and children through lack of dietary zinc. In children, the rate of growth during rehabilitation from famine has been clearly related to the dietary supply of bioavailable zinc. Zinc deficiency is known to occur in patients on intravenous nutrition and causes a characteristic skin rash (Fig. 3) and hair loss. Wound breakdown and delayed healing are other complications. Acrodermatitis enteropathica, a rare inherited disorder of zinc metabolism, manifests itself in infancy as skin rash. Untreated, the prognosis is poor, but oral zinc therapy leads to complete remission. Zinc is antagonized by cadmium, and zinc deficiency can be a consequence of chronic cadmium poisoning.

ZINC TOXICITY

Zinc toxicity is uncommon. It is usually due to exposure to high levels of zinc fumes. It is difficult to induce toxicity by dietary means. However, in cases of self poisoning with zinc salts, the symptoms are fever, vomiting, stomach cramps and diarrhoea.

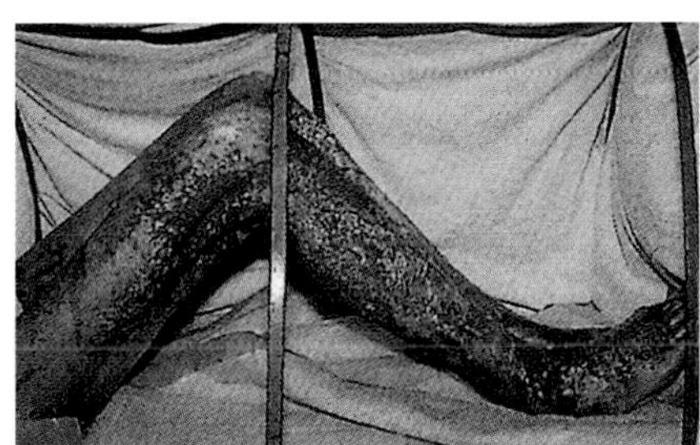

Fig. 3 **Skin lesions in zinc deficiency.**

Fig. 2 **Zinc balance.**

Copper and zinc

- Diagnosis of severe copper deficiency can be made by measurement of serum copper. Values of <10 µmol/l in adults and of <5.0 µmol/l in neonates require investigation.
- The major inborn error of copper metabolism is Wilson's disease.
- Wilson's disease is treatable and requires prompt diagnosis.
- Adequate zinc is needed for growth in children.
- Symptomatic zinc deficiency in the adult causes dermatitis, hair loss and poor wound healing.
- Serum zinc concentrations persistently below 5 µmol/l warn of impending clinical deficiency.

THERAPEUTIC DRUG MONITORING

The effect of most drug therapy is assessed by observing the change in the patient's clinical state. Therapeutic drug monitoring (TDM) is the measurement of drug concentrations in plasma or saliva as a means of assessing the adequacy of dosage. This is particularly important with those drugs for which there is no good objective measure of effectiveness and there is serious risk of toxicity. For TDM to be of value, there must be a proven relationship between the plasma drug concentration and the clinical effect.

Following the administration of a drug, the graph of plasma concentration against time will show a curve rather like that in Figure 1. Such a curve, usually plotted on semi-logarithmic graph paper, can give useful information such as the half-life of the drug ($t^1/_2$) and the volume of distribution. These can be used to estimate the correct dose to give once a plasma concentration has been determined. After several similar doses have been given, the pattern reaches a steady state, at which the plasma concentration will oscillate between a peak and a trough level. It usually takes about five half lives for the steady state to be attained. In the steady state, there is a stable relationship between dose and effect, and decisions about dosage changes can be made with confidence. For most drugs there is a linear relationship between dose and plasma concentration. However, phenytoin shows non-linear kinetics (Fig. 2).

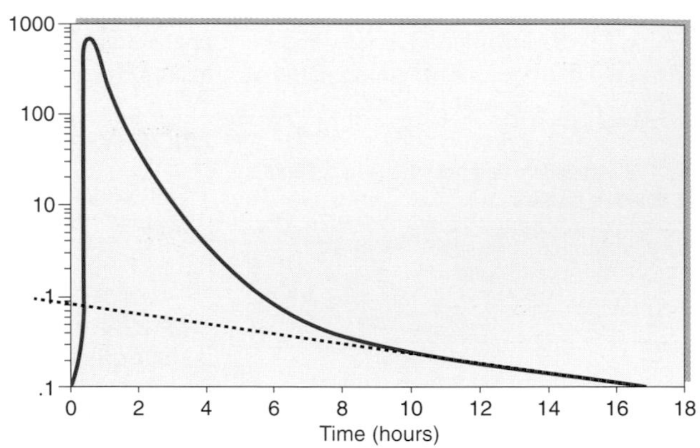

Fig. 1 **Plasma concentration of a drug following administration.**

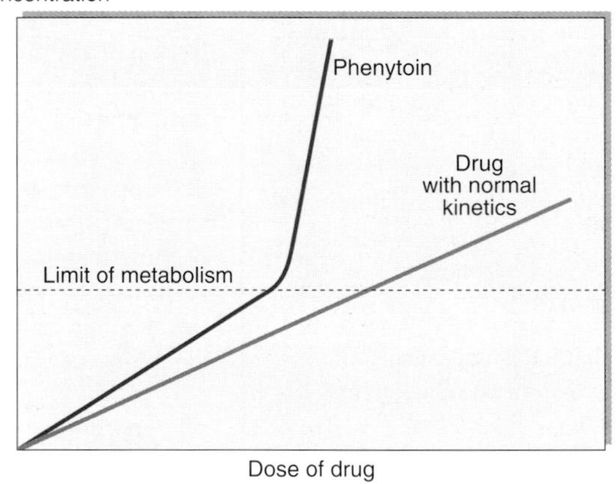

Fig. 2 **Non-linear kinetics of phenytoin.**

SAMPLING FOR TDM

The concentration of a drug in plasma or saliva changes constantly over the period of treatment, and in order to compare one treatment with another, some standardization must be introduced. When taking a sample for TDM it is important to:

- ask the patient about compliance
- check for interacting drugs
- note the dose, and the time since the last dose
- take the sample at an appropriate time.

The best time to take a sample is just before a dose. This is known as a 'trough' concentration.

INTERPRETATION OF DRUG LEVELS

A great deal of information is required in order to interpret drug concentrations correctly. Where concentrations are lower than expected, the most likely cause is non-compliance. In the absence of an increase in dose, higher than expected concentrations indicate that a change has taken place either in other drug therapy or in hepatic or renal function. It is much easier to interpret results if cumulative reports are available, since these allow comparison between levels achieved, provided that dosing details are given.

Each drug has a population reference range which indicates the limits within which most patients will show maximum therapeutic effect with minimum toxicity. However, this is only a rough guide. What may be a therapeutic level in one patient may give rise to toxicity in another (Fig. 3). The most likely reasons for the plasma concentration falling above or below the reference range are given in Table 1.

Although many drugs are monitored in specialist units such as cardiology, neurology and oncology, only a small group of drugs is required to be measured in most laboratories. Examples of drugs for which TDM is appropriate, and the reasons why, are shown in Table 2. Many of these drugs have a low therapeutic

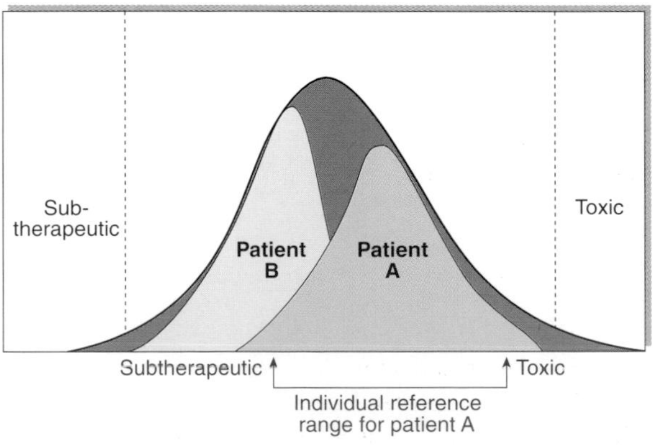

Fig. 3 **A population reference range for a common drug.**

Table 1 **Common reasons for sub-therapeutic or toxic levels**

Sub-therapeutic levels
Non-compliance
Dose too low
Malabsorption
Rapid metabolism
Toxic levels
Overdose
Dose too high
Dose too frequent
Impaired renal function
Reduced hepatic metabolism

index. This means that the concentration at which toxicity occurs is not much higher than that which is required for therapeutic effect.

DRUG INTERACTIONS

Some drugs interfere with the metabolism and excretion of others, and as a result the addition of one drug will alter the plasma concentration of another (Fig. 4). In such circumstances, rather than try to establish a new steady state, it may be appropriate when a patient is receiving a short course of a drug, temporarily to discontinue or lower the dose of the drug it potentiates. For example, a chronic asthmatic, well controlled on theophylline, developed a severe chest infection. The patient was prescribed erythromycin (which can interfere with theophylline) and later presented to her GP complaining of tachycardia and dizziness. Her plasma theophylline concentration was found to be 140 μmol/l, much higher than the therapeutic range of 55–110 μmol/l. Since the erythromycin treatment was still required, her theophylline was stopped for two days and restarted at a lower dose. Once the infection was clear, she was restarted on her original dose of theophylline.

PHARMACOKINETICS

Although there is considerable variation between patients in the rate at which they metabolize and excrete drugs, predictions can be made based on population averages. These allow the calculation of loading and maintenance doses which are better than the rough guidance given by manufacturers. Once a patient with good compliance has been stabilized and the plasma drug concentration at steady state measured, it is possible to adjust plasma concentrations accurately.

Table 2 **Drugs for which TDM is appropriate**

Drug	Reason for TDM: Toxicity	Reason for TDM: Interactions	Reason for TDM: Compliance	Notes
Phenytoin	✓	✓	✓	Has saturable kinetics
Digoxin	✓	✓	✓	Is highly dependent on renal function
Theophylline	✓	✓	✓	Has a low therapeutic index: toxicity is common
Methotrexate	✓			If slowly excreted, patients need folate
Cyclosporin	✓			Is nephrotoxic: creatinine should be measured
Carbamazapine	✓	✓	✓	
Primidone	✓			Is metabolized to phenobarbitone: both should be measured
Phenobarbitone	✓			
Gentamicin and other aminoglycosides	✓			Both peak and trough concentrations should be measured

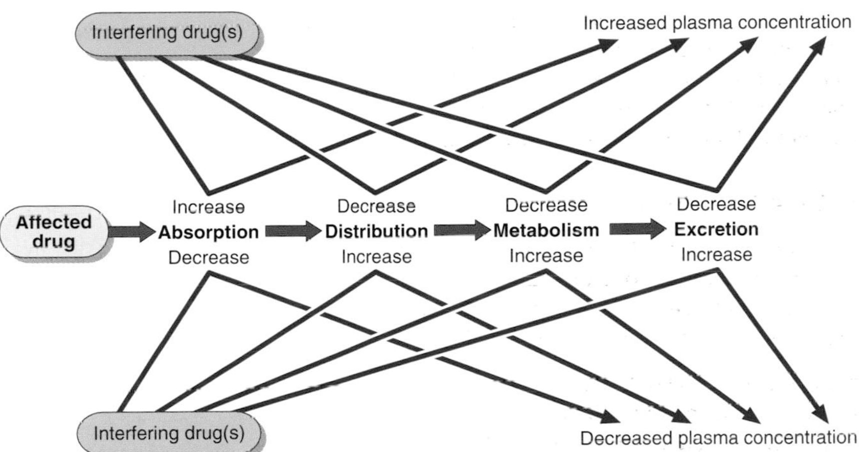

Fig. 4 **Common mechanisms of drug interactions.**

Case history 47

Mrs CG, who has been receiving digoxin for mild heart failure, presented at the geriatric day hospital complaining of nausea. On examination she was found to have bradycardia and appeared dehydrated. Her digoxin concentration, taken 6 hours after her morning dose of 0.125 mg, was found to be 3.1 nmol/l (therapeutic range 0.7 – 2.5). On questioning it emerged that she had been vomiting for three days. Her serum creatinine was elevated.

- Explain the digoxin result.

Comment on page 157.

Therapeutic drug monitoring

- TDM is of use only where the plasma concentration of a drug relates to its clinical effect.
- For a meaningful interpretation of a drug level, full details of the patient's dosing history should be obtained.
- Poor compliance is the commonest cause of inadequate plasma drug concentration.
- The sample should be taken at the correct time following the dose.
- Used correctly, TDM can identify non-compliance and can avoid iatrogenic toxicity.

TOXICOLOGY

Toxicology is the science which involves the investigation of the poisoned patient. In the symptomatic patient, the diagnosis of poisoning is made more often on clinical rather than laboratory findings. In all cases of suspected poisoning, the following biochemical determinations should be requested:

- serum U & Es and LFTs to assess kidney and liver function
- blood glucose to exclude hypoglycaemia
- blood gases to assess acid–base status.

Other biochemical tests which are of value in specific poisonings are given in Table 1.

CONFIRMING POISONING

Few of the signs or symptoms which may be present are specific for any one drug or poison. Patients may well present in coma. A drug screen on a urine specimen can be readily carried out, but this indicates only that a drug has been taken and may give no indication of the severity of the overdose. However, there is frequently no need to know the blood or urine concentration of the drug as this information will not alter the treatment of the patient.

MEASUREMENT OF DRUG LEVELS

Drugs for which measurement is useful include carbon monoxide, digoxin, ethanol, iron, lithium, paracetamol, paraquat, phenobarbitone, phenytoin, quinine, salicylate and theophylline. The main reason for drug analyses is to assess the prognosis. The concentration in a blood or plasma specimen gives a good indication of the severity of poisoning. The length of time which will elapse before the patient recovers consciousness may depend on the half-life of the drug (Fig. 1).

Other reasons for drug analyses include:

- differential diagnosis of coma
- confirmation of brain death
- monitoring drug abuse
- investigation of suspected non-accidental poisoning (e.g. in children).

TREATMENT

Most cases of poisoning are treated conservatively, i.e. the symptoms are treated and the drug is eliminated by normal metabolism and renal excretion. When there is hepatic or renal insufficiency, active measures such as haemodialysis or charcoal haemoperfusion may be attempted. Such measures are normally restricted to a small group of drugs and poisons including salicylate, phenobarbitone, theophylline, ethanol, methanol, ethylene glycol and lithium. Where active measures are used to eliminate drugs, plasma concentrations should be monitored.

For a few drugs there are antidotes (Table 2). These should not normally be given unless it is certain that the drug or poison is present.

COMMON CAUSES OF POISONING

Four examples of poisonings where patients may present with few clinical features are salicylate, paracetamol, theophylline and methanol and ethylene glycol. However, if action is not taken in these cases, the consequence is severe or fatal illness.

Table 1 **Drugs and poisons for which biochemical tests are useful**

Drug / Poison	Biochemical test
Carbon monoxide	Blood carboxyhaemoglobin
Cocaine	Serum creatine kinase, urine myoglobin
Digoxin	Digoxin and serum potassium
Ethylene glycol	Blood gases, serum calcium
Insulin	Blood glucose
Iron	Serum iron
Methanol	Blood gases
Organophosphorus compounds	Serum cholinesterase
Dapsone, oxidizing agents	Blood methaemoglobin
Paracetamol	Paracetamol and liver function tests
Salicylate	Salicylate and blood gases
Theophylline	Theophylline and serum potassium

Table 2 **Commonly used antidotes**

Poison	Antidote
Beta blockers	Glucagon
Cyanide	Dicobalt edetate
Digoxin	Antidigoxin antibody
Ephedrine / theophylline	Propranolol
Fluorides	Calcium gluconate
Heavy metals	Chelating agents
Nitrates / dapsone	Methylene blue
Opiates	Naloxone
Organophosphorus poisons	Atropine / pralidoxime
Ethylene glycol	Calcium gluconate, ethanol
Paracetamol	N-acetyl cysteine
Salicylate	Sodium bicarbonate
Anticoagulants, e.g. warfarin	Vitamin K

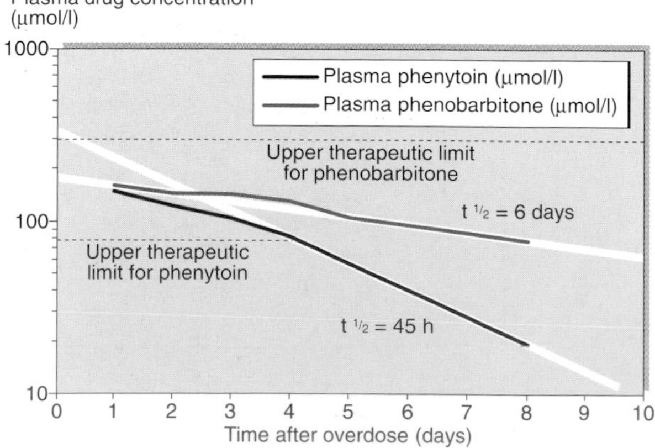

Fig. 1 **Elimination of phenytoin and phenobarbitone from plasma at different rates.**

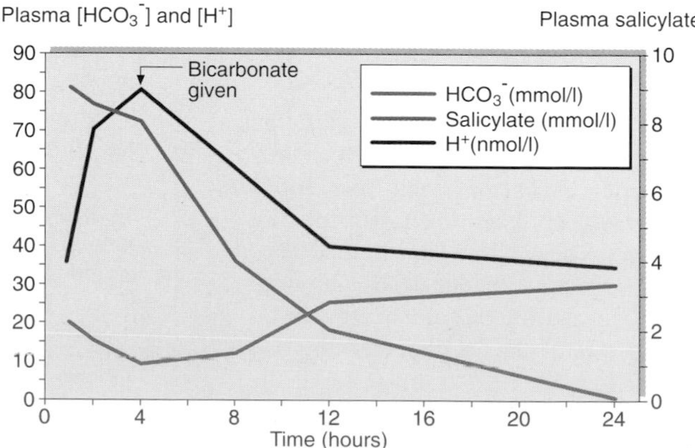

Fig. 2 **Bicarbonate administration in salicylate overdose.**

Salicylate

In salicylate poisoning, failure to detect a large overdose early leads to severe metabolic acidosis from which the patient may not recover. It is therefore important to exclude this common drug if there is any likelihood that it has been taken. A simple qualitative test is available in all hospitals with acute admissions. The treatment for salicylate poisoning is sodium bicarbonate, which both enhances excretion and helps correct the acidosis (Fig. 2).

Paracetamol

In paracetamol poisoning, the plasma paracetamol concentration, related to time of ingestion, is prognostic (Fig. 3). Patients are often asymptomatic when they present at hospital. A specific therapy, N-acetylcysteine given intravenously, can prevent all of the hepatotoxic and nephrotoxic effects of paracetamol poisoning. Therapy should be started within 12 h of admission before any clinical symptoms or biochemical and haematological changes develop. Paracetamol poisoning causes serious liver damage, and severely affected patients may die. Patients who abuse alcohol are at particular risk from paracetamol poisoning.

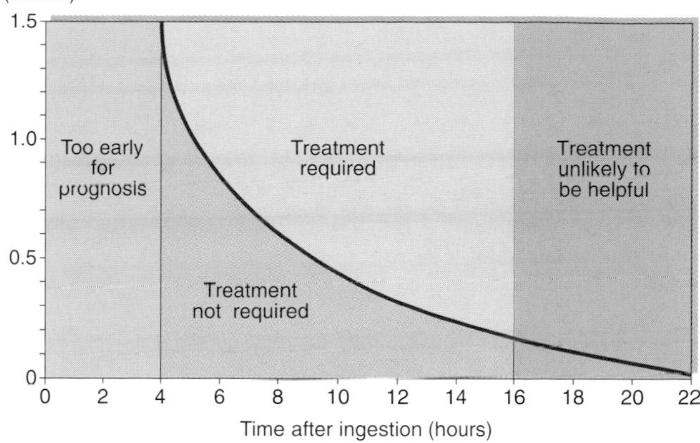

Fig. 3 **Prognosis chart for paracetamol.**

Theophylline

Poisoning with slow-release theophylline preparations can lead to development after 24–48 h of severe arrhythmias, hypokalaemia and death. In cases of suspected poisoning, the theophylline concentration should be measured and its rise or fall monitored. Measures to aid elimination are of limited effect.

Methanol and ethylene glycol

Methanol and ethylene glycol are metabolized to formic acid and oxalic acid respectively. Poisoning with these is not uncommon. Patients develop a severe metabolic acidosis and in the case of ethylene glycol a severe hypocalcaemia, due to precipitation of calcium by the oxalate. Measurement of the serum concentrations of ethylene glycol and methanol are not required. The treatment is to give ethanol and maintain the plasma concentration around 20 mmol/l. The ethanol is preferentially metabolized and the unchanged alcohols are gradually eliminated in the urine.

CHRONIC POISONING

Chronic poisoning occurs when there is a gradual build-up in drug concentration over a period of time, and is usually iatrogenic. Patients may present with a history only of taking their usual medication. In such cases plasma drug concentrations can be of great assistance in assessing the degree of toxicity. Once the drug has been withdrawn, plasma levels fall and treatment with a lower dose should be reinstated.

Poisoning due to the interaction of drugs whose effects are additive is not uncommon. An example is that of alcohol and benzodiazepines, both of which may not be lethal when taken alone but are responsible for numerous deaths when taken together in overdose.

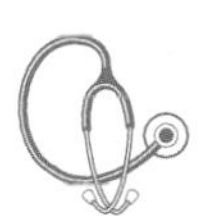

Clinical note

If the plasma drug concentration is rising then drug is still being absorbed. The most likely causes are:

- the presence of a bolus of drug in the GI tract
- correction of hypotension has led to increased absorption via the portal system.

Case history 48

A man aged 38 presented at A&E late one afternoon, claiming to have taken 100 aspirin tablets early in the day. He was hyperventilating and complaining of ringing in his ears. He felt anxious, but his pupils were of normal size and no other abnormalities were observed. He was given gastric lavage and blood was taken for measurement of salicylate, urea and electrolytes, and blood gases. The results were as follows:

Na^+	K^+	Cl^-	HCO_3^-	Urea	Creatinine	H^+	PCO_2	PO_2
mmol/l					*μmol/l*	*nmol/l*	*kPa*	*kPa*
140	3.7	102	20	8.1	110	35	3.7	13.3

Salicylate 4.6 mmol/l

- Comment on these results.
- What other information would be useful in determining treatment?

Comment on page 157.

Toxicology

- Diagnosis of poisoning is often made clinically. Symptoms may be specific or non-specific.
- Serum urea and electrolytes, blood glucose, blood gases and LFTs should be requested in every suspected poisoning.
- Analysis of specific drugs and poisons is required infrequently and only after consultation with the laboratory.
- For salicylate and paracetamol, plasma drug concentrations are used in prognosis and should *always* be requested.
- Poisoning may require general supportive therapy or specific treatment.

METAL POISONING

Poisoning with metals is one of the oldest forms of toxicity known to man. However, it is only recently that the mechanisms of toxicity have become known. More importantly, the means of diagnosis and treatment are now available. The symptoms of poisoning are related to the amount ingested or absorbed and to the duration of exposure. In general, the elemental metals are less toxic than their salts. Organic compounds, where the metal is covalently bound to carbon, may also be toxic.

METALS ASSOCIATED WITH POISONING

The metals which give rise to clinical symptoms in man are shown in Table 1. Apart from the occasional suicide or murder attempt, most poisonings are due to environmental contamination or administration of drugs, remedies or cosmetics which contain metal salts. There are three main clinical effects of exposure to toxic metals. These are:

- renal tubular damage
- gastrointestinal erosions
- neurological damage.

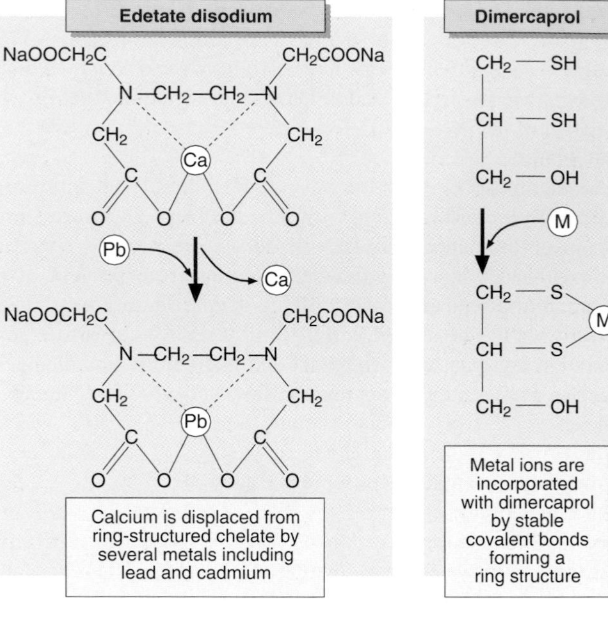

Fig. 1 **Structures and actions of chelating agents.**

DIAGNOSIS

Metal poisoning may be suspected in cases where it is not present and missed in cases where it is the cause of the symptoms. Diagnosis may be made by measuring:

- plasma or blood levels of the metal
- urinary excretion of metals
- an associated biochemical abnormality related to the toxicity.

Blood, plasma, serum or urine can all be used for measurement, and in some cases it may also be helpful to measure the metal concentration in other tissues such as hair. The action limits for metals in plasma and urine are shown in Table 1.

TREATMENT OF METAL TOXICITY

As with most poisons, treatment consists of removal of the source of the metal and increasing the elimination from the body, while correcting deranged physiological or biological mechanisms. Removal of the source may require that a person be removed from a contaminated site or workplace or that the use of a medication or cosmetic be discontinued. Elimination of heavy metals is achieved by treatment with chelating agents which bind the ions and allow their excretion in the urine. The binding in plasma will, by equilibrium, remove some metal ions from tissues. However, removal from brain and bone may take some time.

The structures and mechanisms of action of two chelating agents are shown in Figure 1.

COMMON SOURCES OF METAL POISONING

Aluminium

Aluminium is poorly absorbed from the GI tract, which is just as well since antacid preparations used by dyspeptic patients may contain as much as 500 mg of aluminium per tablet. Aluminium levels in water supplies are variable and may contain from less than 50 to more than 1000 µg/l. This is a potential hazard to renal dialysis patients when the aluminium can enter the body across the dialysis membrane, thus bypassing intestinal absorption. The water used in dialysis is now treated to remove contaminating metals. Acute aluminium toxicity is extremely rare. Aluminium toxicity in patients with renal dysfunction causes bone disease (aluminium osteodystrophy) and gradually failing cerebral function (dialysis dementia).

Diagnosis is by measurement of aluminium in a plasma specimen (Table 1). Aluminium content of bone biopsy material is also used, with levels greater than 100 µg/g dry weight indicating accumulation.

Treatment of aluminium toxicity is by prevention. In cases of toxicity, aluminium excretion may be enhanced by using the chelating agent desferrioxamine.

Arsenic

Arsenic never occurs as the free element, but as the ions As^{3+} and As^{5+} and may be found in some insecticides. Acute ingestion gives rise to violent gastro-

Table 1 **Reference and action ranges for toxic metals**

Metal	Action limits / Indices of toxicity	Clinical sequelae
Arsenic	>0.5 µg/g hair	Diarrhoea, polyneuropathy, gastrointestinal pain, vomiting, shock, coma, renal failure
Aluminium	>3 µmol/l in plasma—chronic >10 µmol/l in plasma—acute	Encephalopathy, osteodystrophy
Cadmium	>90 nmol/l in blood or >90 nmol/24 h in urine	Renal tubular damage, bone disease, hepatocellular damage
Lead	>2.0 µmol/l in blood >0.72 µmol/l in urine	Acute: colic, seizures and coma Chronic: anaemia, encephalopathy
Mercury	>120 nmol/mmol creatinine in urine	Nausea and vomiting, nephrotoxicity, neurological dysfunction
Bismuth	>5 nmol/l in blood	Acute: renal failure Chronic: encephalopathy

intestinal pain and vomiting, with shock developing. Chronic ingestion is evidenced by persistent diarrhoea, dermatitis and polyneuropathy. The best indicator of chronic arsenic exposure is hair analysis. The arsenic content will vary with time along the length of the hair. A level of >0.5μg/g arsenic in hair indicates significant exposure. Urine arsenic measurements are also of value in assessing occupational exposure.

Treatment of acute and chronic arsenic poisoning is by supportive treatment and enhancement of excretion using initially a dimercaprol-type chelating agent and, once symptoms have subsided, N-acetyl-penicillamine. In cases of renal failure, arsenic may be removed by haemodialysis.

Cadmium

Chronic cadmium toxicity occurs in industrial workers exposed to cadmium fumes. The symptoms are those of nephrotoxicity, bone disease and, to a lesser extent, hepatotoxicity. Renal stone formation may be increased.

In diagnosis, indicators of renal damage, in particular β_2 microglobulin in urine, can be used to monitor the effects. Blood and urine cadmium estimates (Table 1) will give an objective index of the degree of exposure, and, in some cases, the cadmium content of renal biopsy tissue may be useful.

Treatment of chronic cadmium toxicity is by removal from exposure. The use of chelating agents is not recommended because mobilization of cadmium may cause renal damage.

The major source of cadmium exposure in the general population is in tobacco smoke, with smokers having blood cadmium levels twice that of non-smokers.

Lead

Inorganic lead has long been known to be toxic, but acute lead poisoning is rare. Chronic toxicity is related to industrial exposure, lead leached from water pipes, the eating of lead-containing paints or dirt by children (pica). There is also concern over the contamination of air by organic lead constituents of petrol. Only 5–10% of lead is absorbed from the gastrointestinal tract in adults but this proportion is higher in children.

Lead poisoning causes anaemia as well as hepatic, renal and neurological sequelae. In general, the consequences of organic lead poisoning are neurological, whereas inorganic lead poisoning results in constipation, abdominal colic, anaemia and peripheral and motor neurone deficiencies. Severe cases develop encephalopathy with seizures and coma.

Biochemical evidence of lead poisoning is by the finding of raised protoporphyrin levels in the erythrocytes due to the inhibition of a number of the synthetic enzymes of the haem pathway by lead (Fig. 2). A clinical sign is the appearance of a blue line on the gums.

Lead is measured in whole blood or in urine (Table 1). Excretion can be enhanced using any of the chelating agents NaCaEDTA, dimercaprol or N-acetyl-penicillamine, but may require to be prolonged in order to deplete bone stores.

Mercury

Mercury poisoning may be acute or chronic and is related to exposure to elemental mercury vapour, inorganic salts or organic forms such as methylmercury. Metallic mercury is relatively non-toxic if ingested, but mercury vapour can give rise to acute toxicity. The symptoms are respiratory distress and a metallic taste in the mouth.

Mercurous salts, notably calomel, have been known to cause chronic toxicity following skin absorption from powders and other forms, but are less toxic than mercuric salts, notably mercuric chloride. This is highly toxic when ingested. The symptoms are nausea and vomiting, muscular tremors, CNS symptoms and renal damage.

Diagnosis is by estimation of blood and urine mercury concentrations (Table 1). Long-term monitoring of exposure, such as may be necessary with those working with dental amalgam, may be carried out using hair or nail clippings.

Treatment of acute mercury poisoning is by use of the dimercaprol chelating agents which leads to excretion via both bile and urine. Chronic exposure is best treated with N-acetyl-penicillamine, unless renal function is compromised.

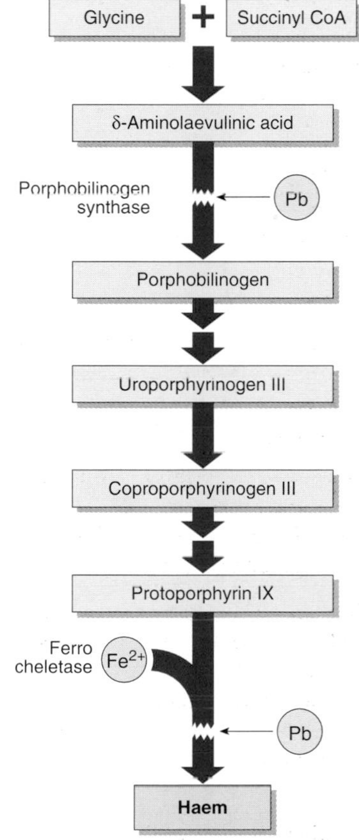

Fig. 2 **Effects of lead on haem synthesis.** Lead (Pb) inhibits porphobilinogen synthase and Fe^{++} incorporation into haem, resulting in increased levels of δ-aminolaevulinic acid and coproporphyrin in urine and protoporphyrin in erythrocytes.

Case history 49

A 12-year-old Asian girl presents with nausea and vomiting and non-localizing neurological signs. She has been using brightly coloured facial cosmetics obtained abroad.

- What biochemical investigations would be appropriate?

Comment on page 157.

Clinical note

Often associated in the past with murders, arsenic poisoning may still be encountered as an industrial disease. The features are abdominal pain, headache, confusion, peripheral neuropathy and coma.

Metal poisoning

- Heavy metals are an insidious cause of gastrointestinal, renal and neurological disease.
- Measurement of blood and urine levels are used in diagnosis of poisoning.
- Treatment of acute exposure is with chelating agents.

ALCOHOL

Abuse of alcohol (ethanol) is a major contributor to morbidity and mortality in the UK, far outstripping other drugs in its effects on the individual and on society. Alcohol is a drug with no receptor. The mechanisms by which it exerts its detrimental effect on cells and organs are not well understood, but the effects are summarized in Table 1.

For clinical purposes alcohol consumption is estimated in arbitrary 'units'— one unit representing 200–300 mmol of ethanol. The ethanol content of some common drinks is shown in Figure 1. The legal limit for driving in the UK is a blood alcohol level of 17.4 mmol/L (80mg/dL) but there is pressure to reduce this to 10.9 mmol/L (50mg/dL).

Table 1 **Effects of ethanol on organ systems**

System	Condition	Effect
CNS	Acute Chronic Withdrawal	Disorientation → coma Memory loss, psychoses Seizures, delirium tremens
Cardiovascular	Chronic	Cardiomyopathy
Skeletal muscle	Chronic	Myopathies
Gastric mucosa	Acute Chronic	Irritation, gastritis Ulceration
Liver	Chronic	Fatty liver → cirrhosis, decreased tolerance to xenobiotics
Kidney	Acute	Diuresis
Blood	Chronic	Anaemia, thrombocytopaenia
Testes	Chronic	Impotence

1 pint beer
= 500 mmol
~ 2 units
1/5 gill whisky
= 250 mmol
~ 1 unit
1 glass sherry
= 325 mmol
~ 1 unit
1 glass wine
= 200 mmol
~ 1 unit

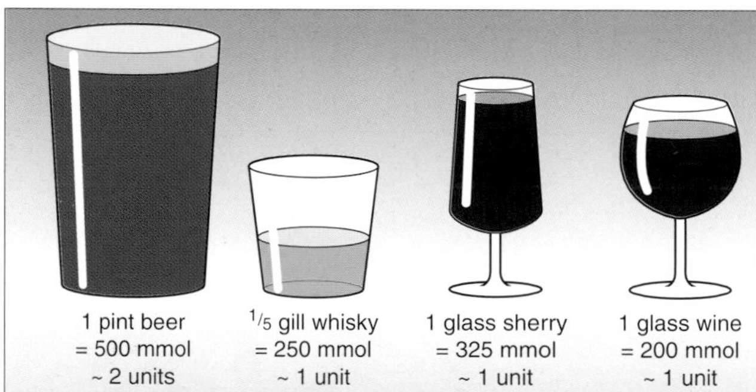

Fig.1 **Alcohol content of common drinks.**

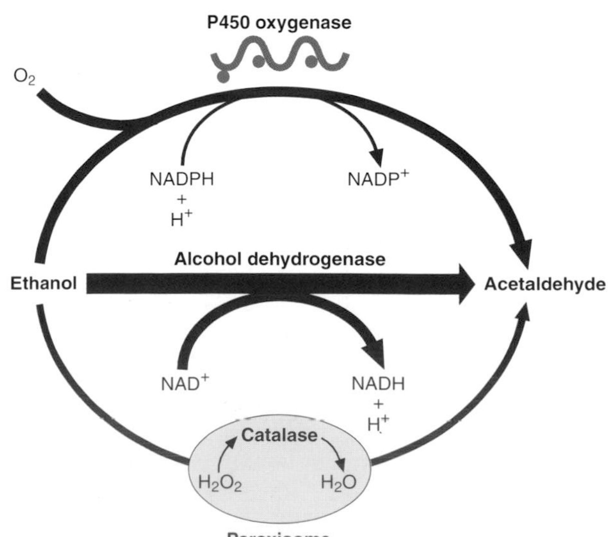

Fig. 2 **The metabolism of ethanol.**

METABOLISM OF ETHANOL

Ethanol is metabolized to acetaldehyde by two main pathways (Fig. 2). The alcohol dehydrogenase route is operational when the blood alcohol concentration is in the range 1–5 mmol/l. Above this most of the ethanol is metabolized via the microsomal P450 system. Although the end product in both cases is acetaldehyde, the side effects of induced P450 can be significant. Ethanol metabolism and excretion in a normal 70 kg man is summarized in Figure 3.

ACUTE ALCOHOL POISONING

The effects of ethanol excess fall into two categories:

- those which are directly related to the blood alcohol concen-tration at the time, such as coma
- those which are caused by the metabolic effects of continued high ethanol concentrations.

The relative contribution of ethanol in cases of coma, especially where other drugs and/or head injury are present, may be difficult to distinguish. Blood ethanol determinations are the best guide. Where these are not available, plasma osmolality measurement and calculation of the osmolal gap may help.

Recovery from acute alcohol poisoning is usually rapid in the absence of renal or hepatic failure, and is speeded up if hepatic blood flow and oxygenation is maximized. The elimination rate of ethanol is dose-related; at a level of 100 mmol/l it is around 10–15 mmol/h. Ethanol concentrations in a group of chronic alcoholics admitted in coma with acute alcohol poisoning are shown in Figure 4.

Alcohol inhibits gluconeogenesis and some patients are prone to develop hypoglycaemia 6 – 36 hours after alcohol ingestion, especially if they are malnourished or fasted. A small number of these malnourished patients develop alcoholic ketoacidosis.

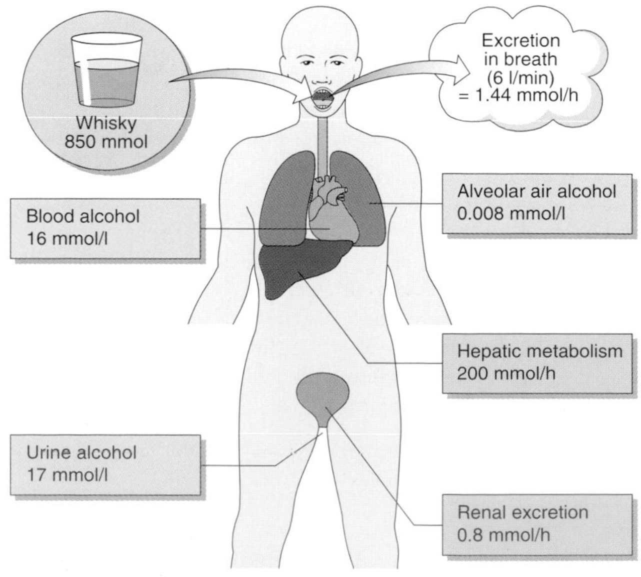

Fig. 3 **Metabolism and excretion of alcohol.**

CHRONIC ALCOHOL ABUSE

Many of the effects of chronic alcohol abuse are due either to the toxicity of acetaldehyde and/or the failure of one or more of the many homeostatic and synthetic mechanisms in the liver. One of the earliest signs of chronic alcohol abuse is hepatomegaly. This results from the accumulation of triglyceride due to increased synthesis from the carbohydrate load and reduced protein synthesis. Continued high ethanol intake may cause the following sequelae:

- impaired glucose tolerance and diabetes mellitus
- hypertriglyceridaemia
- cirrhosis of the liver with resultant decreased serum albumin concentration
- portal hypertension with resultant oesophageal varices
- coagulation defects
- cardiomyopathy
- peripheral neuropathy.

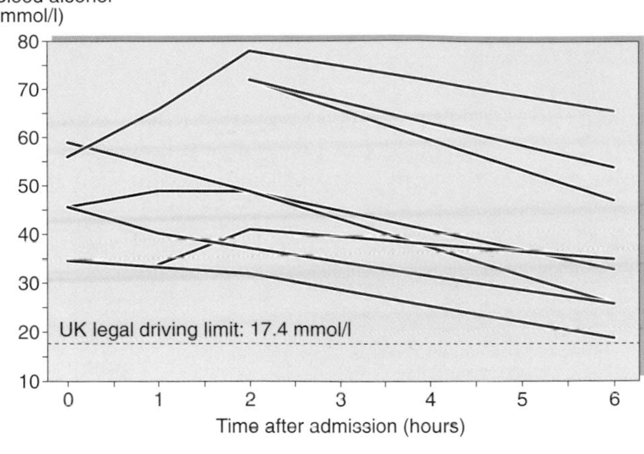

Fig. 4 **Alcohol concentrations in comatose patients.**

Diagnosis of chronic alcohol abuse

Chronic alcohol abuse can be very difficult to detect, and is usually determined from the patient's history. In order to be more objective, there has been a continued search for markers of ethanol abuse. As yet there is no highly sensitive and specific marker. However, a number of blood components are altered and these can give an indication of chronic alcohol ingestion. The most commonly used are:

- Hyperuricaemia.
- Elevated γGT. This enzyme is increased in 80% of alcohol abusers. It is not a specific indicator as it is increased in all forms of liver disease and is induced by drugs such as phenytoin and phenobarbitone.
- Elevated serum triglyceride.

There are a number of other potentially useful markers, notably isoforms of transferrin which are deficient in the carbohydrate linked to the protein. This carbohydrate-deficient transferrin is present in more than 90% of patients with chronic alcohol abuse. Such assays are not yet widely available.

Once the diagnosis of chronic alcohol abuse is made, these markers are of use in monitoring behaviour, since a single 'binge' will lead to their derangement. γGT is used regularly in this manner.

Chronic alcohol abuse exposes the individual to increased risk of damage from other substances. Chronic alcoholics have higher rates of smoking-related disease, and are more susceptible to poisoning with hepatotoxic substances. They also have different rates of metabolism of therapeutic drugs and care needs to be taken in treating them with drugs which are metabolized by the cytochrome P450 system.

Admission rates to hospital with alcohol-related diseases are high, and since the diagnosis is sometimes unsuspected, it should always be considered when carrying out an initial examination (Fig. 5).

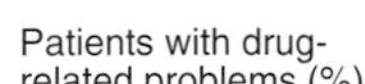

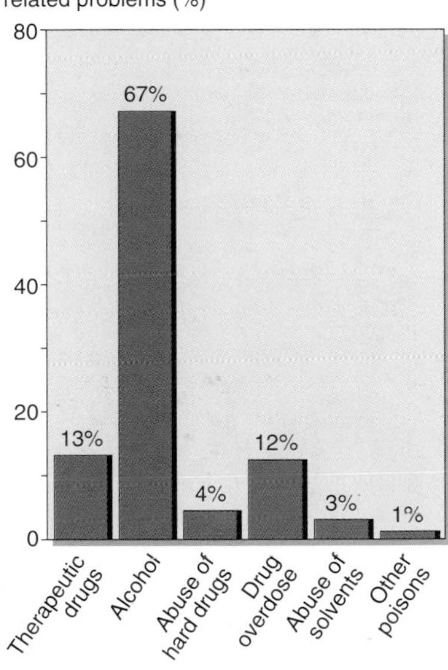

Fig. 5 **Admissions of drug-related problems to one UK hospital.**

Case history 50

A 16-year-old boy whose epilepsy had recently become poorly controlled was found to have a raised γGT of 82 U/l. Because of his troublesome behaviour his parents suspected he was drinking.

- How might alcohol abuse be confirmed or excluded?
- His serum alkaline phosphatase was 520 U/l. Does this support a diagnosis of alcoholic liver disease?

Comment on page 157.

Clinical note

Methanol and ethylene glycol (antifreeze) are both metabolized by alcohol dehydrogenase to formic and oxalic acids, which are toxic. In order to prevent this metabolism, ethanol is infused to a concentration of 20 mmol/l until the alcohols, methanol and ethylene glycol, are excreted unchanged. Alcoholics who drink ethanol as well as methanol in fact protect themselves against the worst effects of methanol poisoning.

Alcohol

- Ethanol abuse is a common clinical problem.
- An elevated serum osmolality and an increased osmolal gap can be of diagnostic value in acute ethanol poisoning.
- Chronic ethanol abuse can be difficult to detect.
- Serum γGT is of limited value for diagnosis of ethanol abuse but good for monitoring abstinence.
- The effects of chronic alcohol abuse are not limited to the liver.

COMA

The comatose patient presents a number of problems to the physician, some in relation to initial diagnosis and some later during treatment.

Best motor response

6 Carrying out request
5 Localized response to pain
4 Flexor response to pain
3 Extensor posturing to pain
2 Flexor posturing to pain
1 None

Best verbal response

5 Orientated
4 Confused conversation
3 Inappropriate speech
2 Incomprehensible speech
1 None

Eye opening

4 Spontaneous eye opening
3 Eye opening in response to speech
2 Eye opening in response to pain
1 No eye opening

Fig. 1 **The Glasgow Coma Scale.**

The depth of coma can be defined following clinical examination using a scale such as that in Figure 1. This allows clinical staff to establish the severity of the coma and to monitor changes. Obtaining the correct diagnosis is paramount. To this end the most valuable information is usually obtained from the clinical history, but frequently a reliable history is not available.

Patency of airway, blood pressure, temperature, pupillary reflex and blood glucose concentration need to be monitored repeatedly and a search should be made for evidence of trauma or needlemarks at the time of admission. A careful history and physical examination will give the correct diagnosis in over 90% of cases. Other biochemical tests can help in diagnosis or for the continued monitoring of comatose patients.

DIFFERENTIAL DIAGNOSIS OF COMA

A helpful mnemonic in the diagnosis of the unconscious patient is given in Figure 2. However, within each of these categories described there are many possible causes. The first priorities in treating an unconscious patient are to ensure that airways are clear and that breathing and circulation are satisfactory.

Cerebrovascular accident

Where coma of cerebrovascular origin is suspected a CSF examination (Fig. 3) will show the presence of blood and will help to differentiate a subarachnoid haemorrhage from cerebral infarction. When available, imaging with a CT scan is preferable.

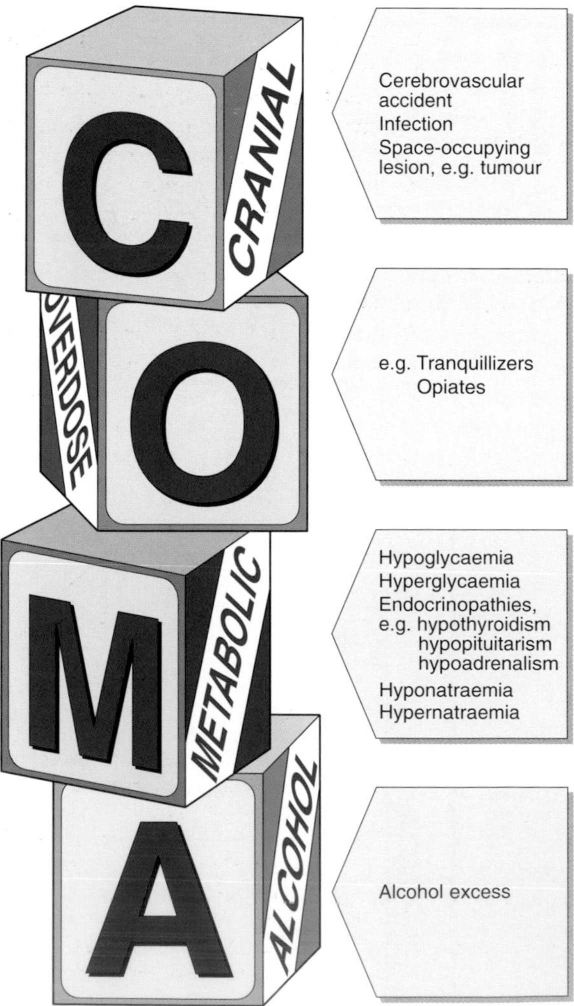

Fig. 2 **Differential diagnosis of a coma patient.**

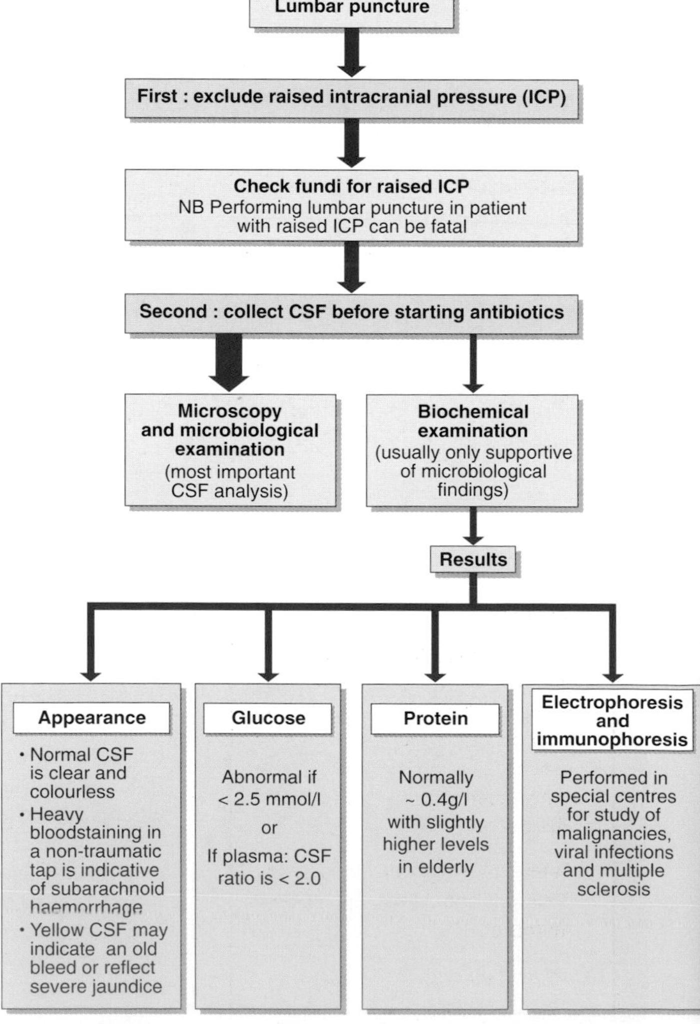

Fig. 3 **Investigation of the cerebrospinal fluid.**

Infectious causes

Meningitis (bacterial and viral) and encephalitis (viral) can both lead to coma. Meningococcal meningitis has a high mortality, especially in children. Diagnosis is of great importance and CSF specimens should be obtained *before* antibiotic therapy is commenced. The usual findings are:

- *In bacterial meningitis* CSF protein is increased and glucose is low or absent. There is a leucocytosis which may be visible as cloudiness in severe cases.
- *In viral meningitis* glucose is normal or only slightly depressed and protein may be normal.

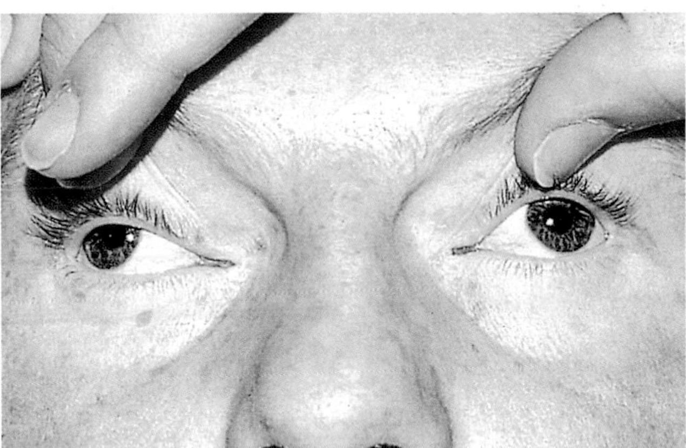

Fig. 4 **Divergent strabismus.**

Metabolic causes

The brain is acutely sensitive to failure in metabolic homeostasis, and a wide range of disorders can give rise to disorientation and later coma. Many of these cases can be corrected rapidly by treatment and thus their early diagnosis is mandatory. The most common forms are shown in Figure 2.

Hypoglycaemic and hyperglycaemic comas must always be considered. Diagnosis is by measurement of blood glucose, which should be carried out on admission. Glucose can be safely given to any diabetic in coma outside hospital, but insulin must not be administered until hyperglycaemia is confirmed. Over 99% of hypoglycaemic episodes encountered in Accident and Emergency Departments will be in patients with known diabetes mellitus.

Drugs and poisons

A wide variety of drugs and poisons can give rise to coma if taken in sufficient dose. In very few cases are there specific clinical signs. Exceptions are the pinpoint pupils of opiate poisoning for which the specific antagonist naloxone is effective in restoring consciousness, and the divergent strabismus (Fig. 4) associated with tricyclic antidepressant overdose. In most cases of drug or poison-induced coma, conservative therapy is all that is required to maintain vital functions until the substance is eliminated by metabolism and excretion. The best specimen to analyze for diagnosis is urine. Where drugs such as phenytoin or theophylline are suspected, plasma levels should be measured on admission and thereafter until they fall to therapeutic levels (see pp. 110–111).

Alcohol

Alcohol is a common cause of coma in all age ranges. Coma depth and length is associated with the amount of alcohol ingested, and this shows wide inter-patient variation. Alcoholic coma can be associated with head injuries, hypothermia and the presence of other drugs with which its action may be additive. In most cases, coma caused by ethanol will resolve relatively rapidly, the exception being when there is hepatic insufficiency. In cases where the blood alcohol level exceeds 80 mmol/l, haemodialysis may be required. The fact that alcohol can be detected on the breath is not sufficient for diagnosis, and a full clinical examination should be made in all cases of alcoholic coma. If acidosis is present, methanol or ethylene glycol poisoning should also be suspected.

Carbon monoxide poisoning

Carbon monoxide poisoning accounts for a large number of deaths in the UK each year. Coma can occur with carboxyhaemoglobin concentration above 30% of haemoglobin. Carbon monoxide poisoning may be insidious due to a faulty heater or poor ventilation and may be presaged by headaches and confusion. Treatment with oxygen restores oxyhaemoglobin. This is a dangerous form of poisoning which requires careful aftercare.

Hepatic coma

Acute or chronic hepatic failure may result in coma. This is believed to be due to the failing liver's inability to remove neurotoxins such as ammonia from the blood.

Case history 51

A 20-year-old insulin-dependent diabetic was found unconscious beside his bicycle. An hour or so earlier he had left a party where he had been drinking. He was brought to the Accident and Emergency Department.

- What investigations and interventions would be appropriate in this case?

Comment on page 157.

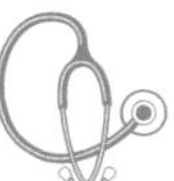

Clinical note

Coma associated with a cerebrovascular accident will have an abrupt onset and give rise (in most cases) to unilateral signs. Coma caused by metabolic or toxic causes will usually affect all parts of the body equally and will develop over a period of time.

Coma

- The first priority is to ensure clear airways and satisfactory breathing and circulation.
- Lateralizing neurological signs should always be sought as evidence of a cerebrovascular accident.
- Hypoglycaemia in the known diabetic patient is the commonest metabolic cause of coma.
- A high percentage of patients in coma from all causes will have alcohol as a complicating factor.

LIPOPROTEIN METABOLISM

The lipoprotein system evolved to solve the problem of transporting fats around the body in the aqueous environment of the plasma. A lipoprotein is a complex spherical structure which has a hydrophobic core wrapped in a hydrophilic coating (Fig. 1). The core contains triglyceride and cholesteryl esters, while the surface contains phospholipid, free cholesterol and proteins—the apolipo-proteins (Table 1). Cholesterol is an essential component of all cell membranes and is the precursor for steroid hormone and bile acid biosynthesis. Triglyceride is central to the storage and transport of energy within the body.

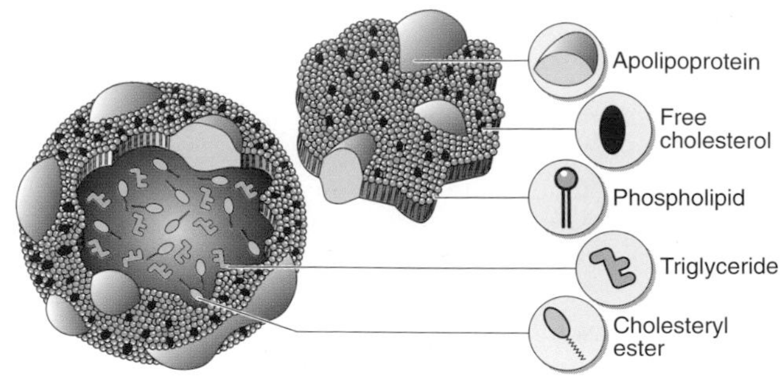

Fig. 1 **Structure of a lipoprotein.**

NOMENCLATURE

Several different classes of lipoproteins exist whose structure and function are closely related. Apart from the largest species, the chylomicron, these are named according to their density, as they are most commonly isolated by ultracentrifugation. The four main lipoproteins and their functions are shown in Table 2.

Table 1 **Properties of some human apolipoproteins**

Apolipoprotein	Molecular weight	Site of synthesis	Function
A-I	28 000	Intestine, liver	Activates LCAT
A-II	17 000	Intestine, liver	-
B_{100}	549 000	Liver	Triglyceride and cholesterol transport Binds to LDL receptor
B_{48}	264 000	Intestine	Triglyceride transport
C-I	6600	Liver	Activates LCAT
C-II	8850	Liver	Activates LPL
C-III	8800	Liver	? Inhibits LPL
E	34 000	Liver, intestine, macrophage	Binds to LDL receptor and probably also to another specific liver receptor

LCAT = Lecithin: cholesterol acyl transferase
LPL = Lipoprotein lipase

METABOLISM

Lipoprotein metabolism (Fig. 2) can be thought of as two cycles, one exogenous and one endogenous, both centred on the liver. These cycles are interconnected.

Two key enzyme systems are involved in lipoprotein metabolism, e.g.:

- Lipoprotein lipase (LPL) releases free fatty acids and glycerol from chylomicrons and VLDL into the tissues.
- Lecithin: cholesterol acyl transferase (LCAT) forms cholesteryl esters from free cholesterol and fatty acids.

Table 2 **The four main lipoproteins and their functions**

Lipoprotein	Main apolipoproteins	Function
Chylomicrons	B_{48}, A -I, C-II, E	Largest lipoprotein. Synthesized by gut after a meal.Not present in normal fasting plasma. Main carrier of dietary triglyceride
Very low density lipoprotein (VLDL)	B_{100}, C-II, E	Synthesized in the liver. Main carrier of endogenously produced triglyceride
Low density lipoprotein (LDL)	B_{100}	Generated from VLDL in the circulation. Main carrier of cholesterol
High density lipoprotein (HDL)	A-I, A-II	Smallest but most abundant.Protective function. Takes cholesterol from extrahepatic tissues to the liver for excretion

The exogenous lipid cycle

Dietary lipid is absorbed in the small intestine and incorporated into chylomicrons which are secreted into the lymphatics and reach the bloodstream via the thoracic duct. In the circulation, triglyceride is gradually removed from these lipoproteins by the action of lipoprotein lipase. This enzyme is present in the capillaries of a number of tissues, predominantly adipose tissue and skeletal muscle. As it loses triglyceride, the chylomicron becomes smaller and deflated, with folds of redundant surface material. These remnants are removed by the liver. The cholesterol may be utilized by the liver to form cell membrane components or bile acids, or may be excreted in the bile. The liver provides the only route by which cholesterol leaves the body in significant amounts.

The endogenous lipid cycle

The liver synthesizes VLDL particles which undergo the same form of delipidation as chylomicrons by the action of lipoprotein lipase. This results in the formation of an intermediate density lipoprotein (IDL) which becomes low density lipoprotein (LDL) when further delipidated. LDL may be removed from the circulation by the high affinity LDL receptor or by other scavenger routes which are thought to be important at high LDL levels and the main way in which cholesterol is incorporated into atheromatous plaques.

HDL particles are derived from both liver and gut. They act as cholesteryl ester shuttles, removing the sterol from the peripheral tissues and returning it to the liver. The HDL is taken up either directly by the liver, or indirectly by being transferred to other circulating lipoproteins, which then return it to the liver. This process is thought to be anti-atherogenic, and an elevated HDL-cholesterol level has been shown to confer a decreased risk of coronary heart disease on an individual.

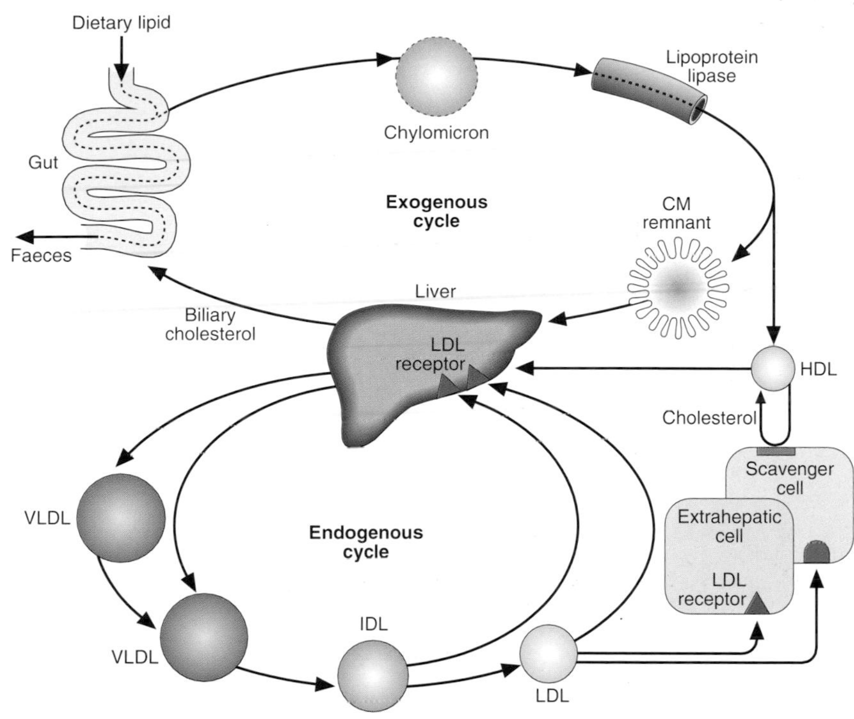

Fig. 2 **Lipoprotein metabolism.**

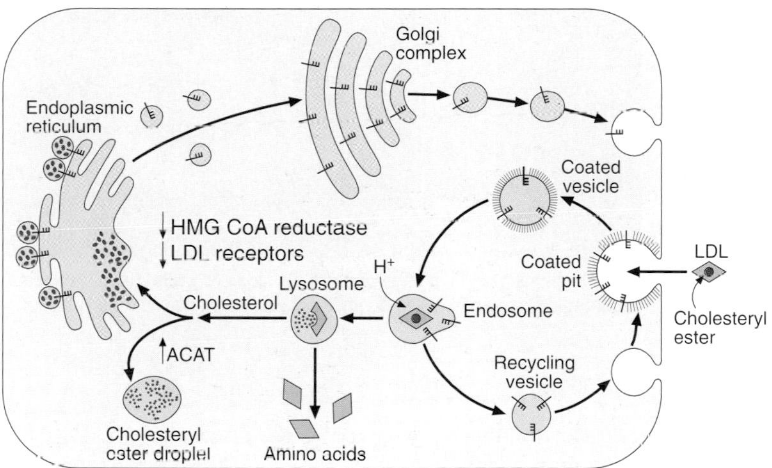

Fig. 3 **The LDL receptor pathway.**

APOLIPOPROTEINS

Apolipoproteins are the protein components of the lipoproteins (Table 1). They are important in:

- maintaining the structural integrity of the lipoproteins
- regulating certain enzymes which act on lipoproteins
- receptor recognition.

THE LDL RECEPTOR

The LDL receptor (Fig. 3), a glycoprotein present on the surface of all cells, spans the cell membrane and is concentrated in special membrane recesses, called 'coated' pits. It binds to lipoproteins containing apolipoprotein B and E, and internalizes them for breakdown within the cell. Receptors are then recycled to the cell surface. The number and function of receptors dictate the level of circulating LDL. When the cell has sufficient cholesterol, the synthesis of receptors is down-regulated; when the cell is cholesterol depleted, the receptors increase in number. Inherited malfunction or absence of these receptors leads to familial hypercholesterolaemia (FH).

A specific mutation of apolipoprotein B results in defective binding of LDL to its receptor and produces an identical clinical picture to FH called familial defective apo B (FDB).

Clinical note

About 25% of the UK population have plasma cholesterol levels above the desirable reference range. In most cases this is the result of diet and lifestyle.

Case history 52

A 3-year-old boy with a history of chronic abdominal pain was admitted as an emergency. His blood was noted to be pink in the syringe, and the serum was milky.

Na^+	K^+	Cl^-	HCO_3^-	Urea	Glucose
		mmol/l			
103	3.8	70	20	3.1	5.2

Serum osmolality was measured as 282 mmol/kg and amylase 1780 U/l. His triglyceride was reported to be >50 mmol/l.

- Why is there a discrepancy between the calculated and measured osmolality?
- What are the likely causes of the hypertriglyceridaemia?

Comment on page 157.

Lipoprotein metabolism

- Lipoproteins are complexes of lipid and proteins which facilitate lipid transport.
- Their metabolism can be thought of as two interconnected cycles centred on the liver.
- Lipoproteins are defined by their density and differ in composition, structure and function.
- Apolipoproteins have a functional as well as structural importance.
- Cholesterol can only be excreted from the body by way of the liver.

CLINICAL DISORDERS OF LIPID METABOLISM

Lipoprotein disorders are some of the commonest metabolic diseases seen in clinical practice. They may present with their various sequelae which include:

- coronary heart disease (CHD)
- acute pancreatitis
- failure to thrive and weakness
- cataracts.

Table 1 **Some genetic causes of dyslipidaemia**

Disease	Genetic defect	Fredrickson	Risk
Familial hypercholesterolaemia	Reduced numbers of functional LDL receptors	IIa or IIb	CHD
Familial hypertriglyceridaemia	Possibly single gene defect	IV or V	
Familial combined hyperlipidaemia	Possibly single gene defect	IIa, IIb, IV or V	CHD
Lipoprotein lipase deficiency	Reduced levels of functional LPL	I	Pancreatitis
Apo C-II deficiency	Inability to synthesize apo C-II (cofactor for lipoprotein lipase)	I	Pancreatitis
Abetalipoproteinaemia	Inability to synthesize apo B	Normal	Fat soluble vitamin deficiences, neurological deficit
Analphalipoproteinaemia (Tangier disease)	Inability to synthesize apo A	Normal	Neurological deficit Cholesteryl ester storage in abnormal sites

CLASSIFICATION

Currently there is no satisfactory comprehensive classification of lipoprotein disorders. Genetic classifications have been attempted but are becoming increasingly complex as different mutations are discovered (Table 1). *Familial hypercholesterolaemia* (FH) which presents with xanthelasma (Fig.1), tendon xanthomas, severe hypercholesterolaemia and premature coronary heart disease may be due to any of over 150 different mutations of the LDL receptor gene. Mutations of the apolipoprotein (apo) B gene can give an identical syndrome. *Familial hyperchylomicronaemia* which presents with recurrent abdominal pain and pancreatitis may result from genetic mutations of the lipoprotein lipase or apo C-II genes. Eruptive xanthomas (Fig. 2) are characteristic of hypertriglyceridaemia.

Until gene therapy and/or specific substitution therapy become more available, genetic classifications, while biologically very illuminating, are unlikely to prove very useful in practice. In practice, lipoprotein disorders are simplistically classified as being:

- *Primary*—when the disorder is not due to an identifiable underlying disease.
- *Secondary*—when the disorder is a manifestation of some other disease.

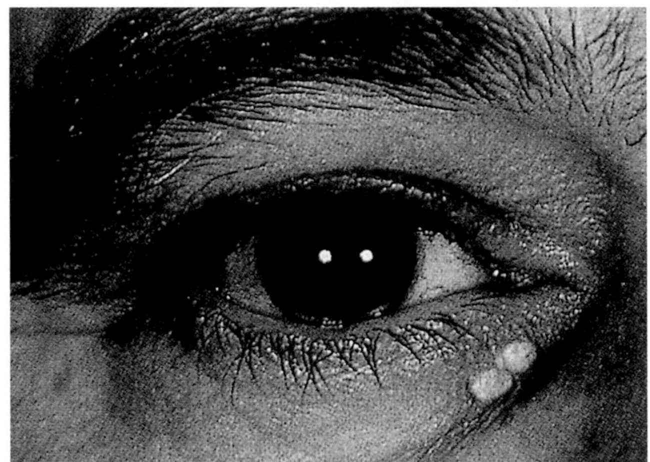

Fig. 1 **Xanthelasmas in younger individuals (age <40 years) usually indicate hypercholesterolaemia.** In the elderly they do not carry the same significance.

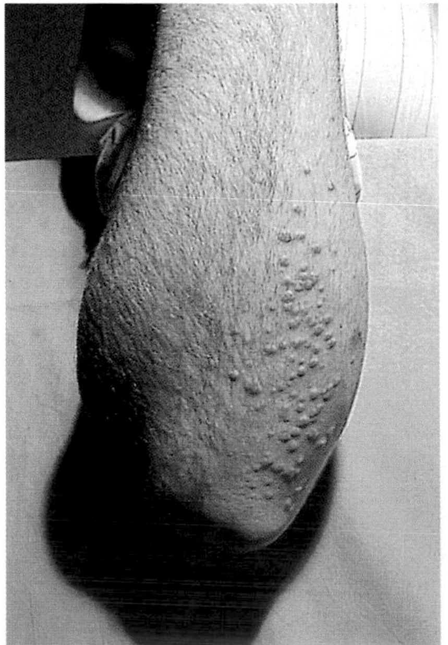

Fig. 2 **Eruptive xanthomas are characteristic of hypertriglyceridaemia.**

Primary

The Fredrickson or World Health Organization classification is the most widely accepted for the primary hyperlipidaemias (Fig. 3). It relies on the findings of plasma analysis, rather than genetics. As a result, patients with the same genetic defect may fall into different groups, or may change grouping as the disease progresses or is treated (Table 1). The major advantage of this classification is that it is widely accepted and gives some guidance for treatment.

The six types of hyperlipoproteinaemia defined in the Fredrickson Classification are not equally common. Types I and V are rare, while types IIa, IIb and IV are very common. Type III hyperlipoproteinaemia, also known as familial dysbetalipoproteinaemia, is intermediate in frequency, occuring in about 1/5000 of the population.

Table 2 **Common causes of secondary hyperlipidaemia**

Disease	Usual dominant lipid abnormality
Diabetes mellitus	Increased triglyceride
Alcohol excess	Increased triglyceride
Chronic renal failure	Increased triglyceride
Drugs, e.g. thiazide diuretics non-selective β-blockers	Increased triglyceride
Hypothyroidism	Increased cholesterol
Nephrotic syndrome	Increased cholesterol

Secondary

Secondary hyperlipoproteinaemia is a well-recognized feature of a number of diseases (Table 2) which divide broadly into two categories:

- Clinically obvious diseases such as renal failure, nephrotic syndrome and cirrhosis of the liver.
- Covert conditions which may present as hyperlipidaemia. These include hypothyroidism, diabetes mellitus and alcohol abuse.

ATHEROGENIC PROFILES

The casual association of certain forms of hyperlipidaemia and CHD is clearly the major stimulus for the measurement of plasma lipids and lipoproteins in clinical practice. The most common lipid disorder linked with atherogenesis and an increased risk of CHD is an elevated plasma LDL cholesterol level, but increasingly it is being recognized that individuals with low plasma HDL cholesterol and hypertriglyceridaemia are also at increased risk.

Type	Normal	Type I	Type IIa	Type IIb	Type III	Type IV	Type V
Sample							
Lipoprotein Chylomicrons	N	↑ Chylomicrons	↑ LDL ↑ VLDL	↑ LDL	↑ IDL	↑ VLDL ↑ VLDL	↑
Total Cholesterol	N	N or ↑	↑	↑	↑	N or ↑	N or ↑
Triglycerides	N	↑↑	N	↑	↑	↑	↑↑
LDL-CHOL	N	N or ↓	↑	↑	N or ↓	N	N
HDL-CHOL	N	N or ↓	N or ↓	N or ↓	N or ↓	N or ↓	N or ↓

Fig. 3 **Fredrickson (WHO) classification of dyslipidaemia.** This is based on the appearance of a fasting plasma sample after standing for 12 hours at 4°C and analysis of its cholesterol and triglyceride content.

Clinical note

The physical signs of the hyperlipidaemias are not specific for any particular disease and may sometimes be present in normolipidaemic patients, e.g. arcus senilis (Fig. 4). Their presence is, however, highly suggestive of raised lipids. Tendon xanthomas (Fig. 5) are particularly associated with familial hypercholesterolaemia.

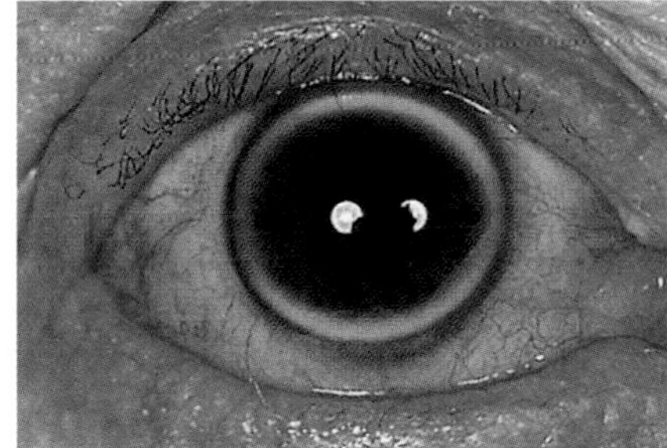

Fig. 4 **Arcus senilis.**

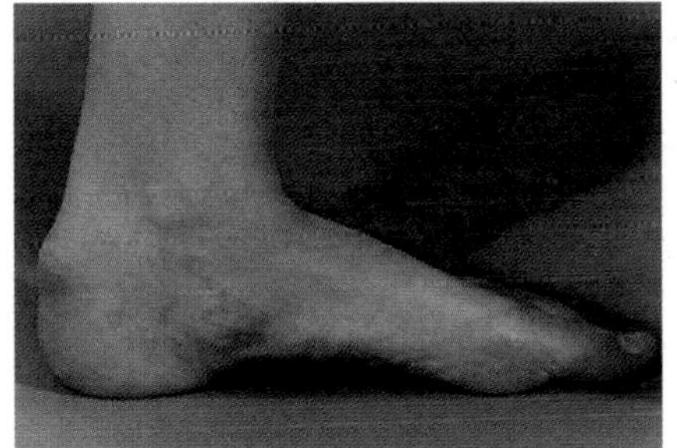

Fig. 5 **Tendon xanthomas.** These are pathognomic for familial hypercholesterolaemia and are often first seen on the achilles tendon as in this patient.

Case history 53

A 53-year-old male was found to have the following results on a fasting blood sample:

Total cholesterol	Triglyceride	Glucose	γGT
mmol/l			*U/l*
8.4	6.8	9.8	138

A non-smoker, his blood pressure was 145/95 mmHg and he was obese with central fat distribution.

- What other information and investigations would be helpful in this man's management?
- What treatment options would you consider in this case?

Comment on page 157.

Clinical disorders of lipid metabolism

- The Fredrickson classification is still commonly used to classify hyperlipoproteinaemias by phenotype.
- The genetic and environmental nature of many causes of primary hyperlipidaemia are, as yet, unknown.
- Secondary causes of hyperlipidaemia are common and include hypothyroidism, diabetes mellitus, liver disease and alcohol abuse.

MANAGEMENT OF HYPERLIPIDAEMIA

The management of hyperlipidaemia is an important aspect of coronary heart disease (CHD) risk factor correction. Modifying hyperlipidaemia together with the other non-lipid risk factors has been repeatedly shown to reduce the risk of developing CHD and to delay or even reverse the progression of established CHD. Risk factors for CHD (Table 1) fall into two groups: those which can be corrected (such as smoking, hypertension, hyperlipidaemia and obesity) and those which cannot be influenced (such as age, sex and family history).

Table 1 **Coronary heart desease risk factors**

Correctable	Non-correctable
Smoking	Age
Hyperlipidaemia	Sex
Hypertension	Family history of premature CHD
Obesity	Personal history of premature CHD
Lack of exercise	Diabetes mellitus
Excess alcohol	

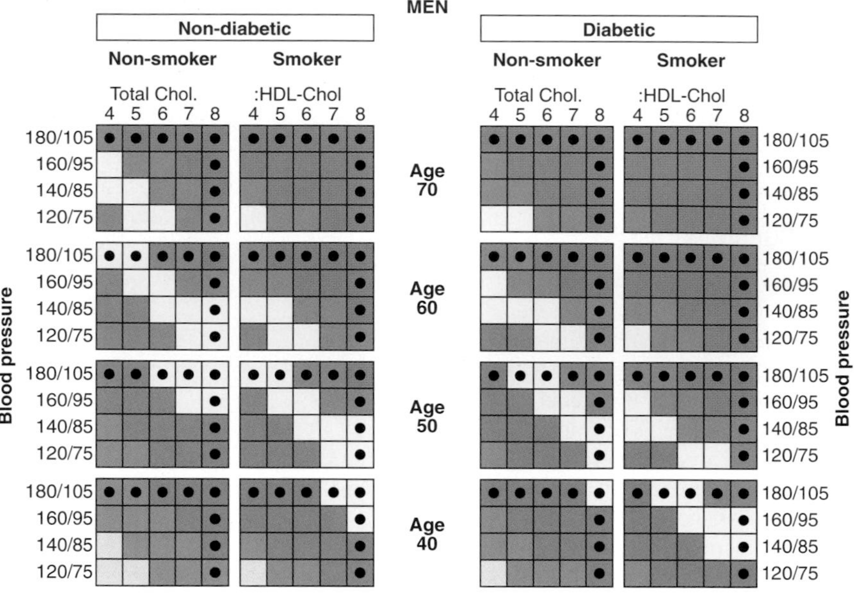

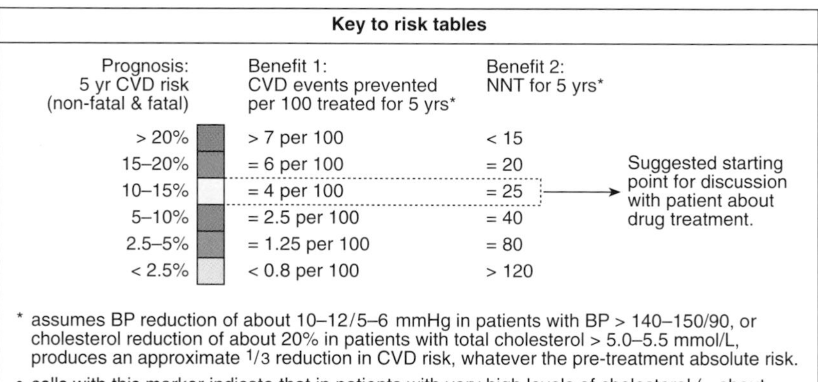

Fig.1 **Risk assessment table for men based on the National Health Committee New Zealand Guidelines 1997.**

CLASSIFICATION

Because the management of primary and secondary hyperlipidaemia is fundamentally different, the two groups of conditions must be distinguished. The main secondary hyperlipidaemias are due to:

- diabetes mellitus
- alcohol misuse
- hypothyroidism
- nephrotic syndrome.

MANAGEMENT GUIDELINES

There have been many published strategies for the management of a patient with primary hyperlipidaemia. Most modern guidelines advocate the overall CHD risk assessment of a patient when deciding to treat hyperlipidaemia. One tool for this risk assessment is shown in Figure 1. Here, knowledge of a patient's sex, age, smoking status, blood presure, diabetic status and total:HDL cholesterol ratio are integrated into a single score represented as the % risk of a major cardiovascular event over the next 5 years.

From this strategy it is clear that the decision to treat hyperlipidaemia relies heavily on biochemical results. The interpretation of these results and the action limits used for intervention are based on data from large studies where standardized methods were used to measure plasma cholesterol, triglyceride and HDL-cholesterol (HDL-C). It is, therefore, necessary that the laboratory analyzing the specimens follows strict quality control procedures, thus ensuring a high level of accuracy and precision. Because of gender differences in the incidence of CHD, most guidelines, including those in Figure 1, have different strategies for men and women.

DIETARY MANAGEMENT

The first-line management of any primary hyperlipidaemia should always be dietary modification. This may be time-consuming and difficult but its importance should not be underestimated. Dietary management as a sole therapy should be pursued for 3–6 months before its effect is evaluated. The principal dietary guidelines for reducing both plasma cholesterol and triglyceride are shown in Figure 2. This diagram illustrates the standard lipid-lowering dietary guidelines which are currently recommended, but these obviously require some translation for patient use.

In essence, it is recommended that red meat and dairy consumption be reduced while that of vegetables, fruit and pulses be increased together with more fish (especially oily fish such as mackerel, salmon and tuna). In addition to modifying the composition of the diet, weight reduction to achieve ideal body weight coupled with exercise are important as these will frequently improve glucose tolerance and lower blood pressure in addition to their effects on plasma lipids.

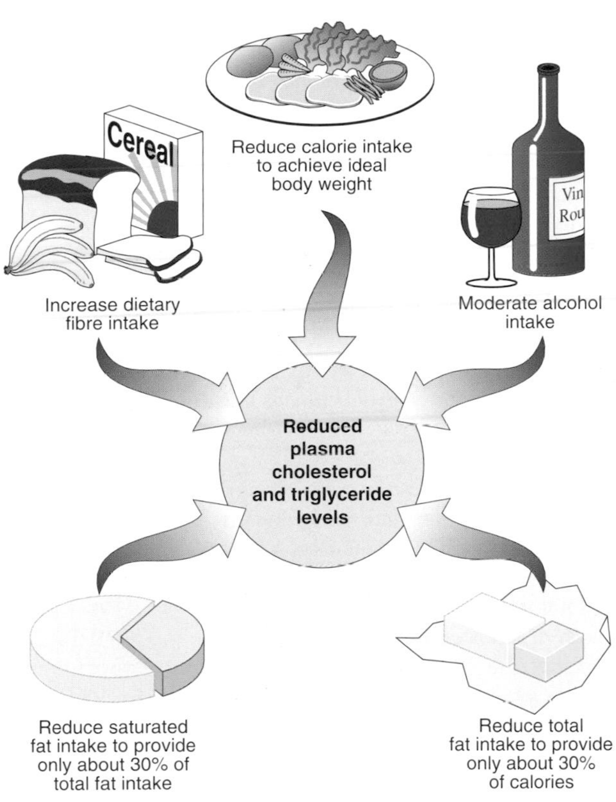

Fig. 2 **Lipid-lowering dietary guidelines.**

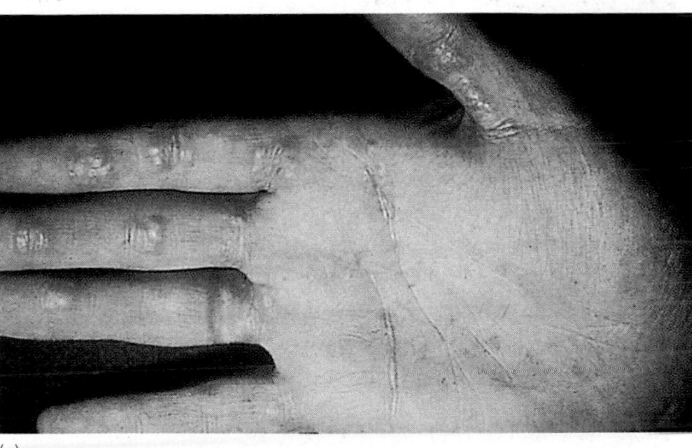

(a)

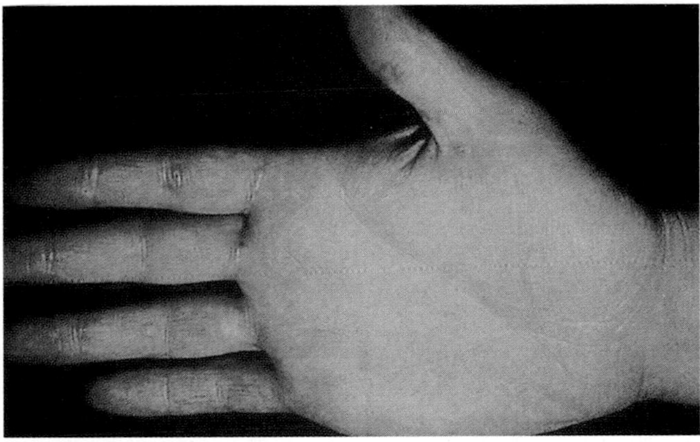

(b)

Fig. 3 **Palmar xanthomas before (a) and after (b) treatment.**

DRUG THERAPY

Drug therapy for hyperlipidaemia, if required, should be viewed as an adjunct to dietary management and other lifestyle changes. There is currently a range of lipid-lowering drugs available with a variety of actions (Table 2). The commonest drugs for the treatment of primary hypercholesterolaemia are the HMG CoA reductase inhibitors (the 'statins'). Two statins, pravastatin and simvastatin, have been conclusively shown to reduce coronary morbidity and mortality as well as all-cause mortality in large randomized controlled trials. The commonest drugs for the treatment of primary hypertriglyceridaemia or combined hyperlipidaemia are the fibrates. Figure 3 illustrates clinical improvement in a patient with combined hyperlipidaemia treated with lipid-lowering therapy.

Table 2 **Lipid-lowering drugs**

Drug group	Principal actions
Bile acid sequestrant resins	Block bile acid reabsorption and lower total and LDL cholesterol
HMG CoA reductase inhibitors	Inhibit cholesterol biosynthesis and lower total and LDL cholesterol
Fibrates	Activate lipoprotein lipase and lower triglyceride, total and LDL cholesterol. May increase HDL cholesterol

Case history 54

An asymptomatic 38-year-old woman was screened at a well-woman clinic and found to have a non-fasting plasma cholesterol level of 8.7 mmol/l.

- What other information and investigations would you require to help in the management of this woman?
- What would that management entail?

Comment on page 157.

Clinical note

It should not be considered too late for intervention, even if a patient has advanced coronary heart disease or has suffered a myocardial infarction. The benefits of secondary prevention are well established, particularly with statin therapy which has been shown to reduce all-cause mortality even in patients with apparently 'normal' total cholesterol levels.

Management of hyperlipidaemia

- At least two fasting lipid profiles should be performed before starting any form of lipid-lowering therapy.
- First-line therapy always consists of dietary modification.
- Drug therapy, if required, should be viewed as an adjunct to dietary therapy.
- Other risk factors for coronary heart disease must be managed along with hyperlipidaemia.

HYPERTENSION

Hypertension is defined as a chronically increased systemic arterial blood pressure. The World Health Organization criteria of hypertension is a systolic blood pressure of 160 mmHg or a diastolic blood pressure of 95 mmHg or more. Around one-quarter of the adult population of Europe and North America will have a blood pressure reading over this limit, although most will have a lower pressure on rechecking. It is important not to base clinical decisions on a single raised blood pressure reading. A diagnosis of hypertension should only be reached following repeated measurements of blood pressure over a number of weeks.

Serious complications of hypertension include:

- stroke
- heart disease (both cardiomegaly and coronary heart disease)
- renal failure.

Malignant hypertension describes severe hypertension which results in arterial damage characterized by retinopathy, papilloedema and progressive renal failure. Despite the confusing name, malignant hypertension is not due to cancer.

CAUSES OF HYPERTENSION

Hypertension can result from an increased cardiac output or an increase in peripheral resistance, or both. In practice, the main abnormality in most cases of hypertension is increased total peripheral resistance. In the majority of patients the cause of the hypertension is not known, with 95% of all hypertensive patients classified as having 'essential' or 'primary' hypertension. There is no doubt that hypertension is related to genetic and environmental factors. Obesity has a contributory role. Alcohol consumption is also commonly associated with hypertension.

By definition, the causes of secondary hypertension are known. The biochemistry laboratory has a role to play in the diagnosis of a variety of disorders which lead to secondary hypertension. These are discussed below.

Renal disease

Hypertension is a common feature of chronic renal disease and also of renal vascular problems. Unilateral or bilateral renal artery stenosis will lead to hypertension. The association of hypertension and the kidneys is outlined in Figure 1.

Drugs

The oestrogen and progestogen components of the oral contraceptive pill contribute to the hypertension which may develop in previously normotensive women.

Excess aldosterone secretion

Secretion of aldosterone from an adenoma in the glomerular zone of the adrenal cortex (primary hyperaldosteronism or Conn's syndrome) can cause hypertension (Fig. 2). The characteristic biochemical picture is that of a hypokalaemic alkalosis. Hypertension is also found in patients with Cushing's syndrome, where there is increased secretion of cortisol precursors which have mineralocorticoid activity. Congenital deficiency of the enzyme 11β-hydroxysteroid dehydrogenase which interconverts cortisol and cortisone results in the 'apparent mineralocorticoid excess' syndrome. This enzyme normally protects the mineralocorticoid receptor from binding and being activated by cortisol. Glycyrrhetinic acid, a component of liquorice, inhibits the 11β-hydroxysteroid dehydrogenase, and liquorice abuse produces a clinical picture which mimics primary aldosteronism.

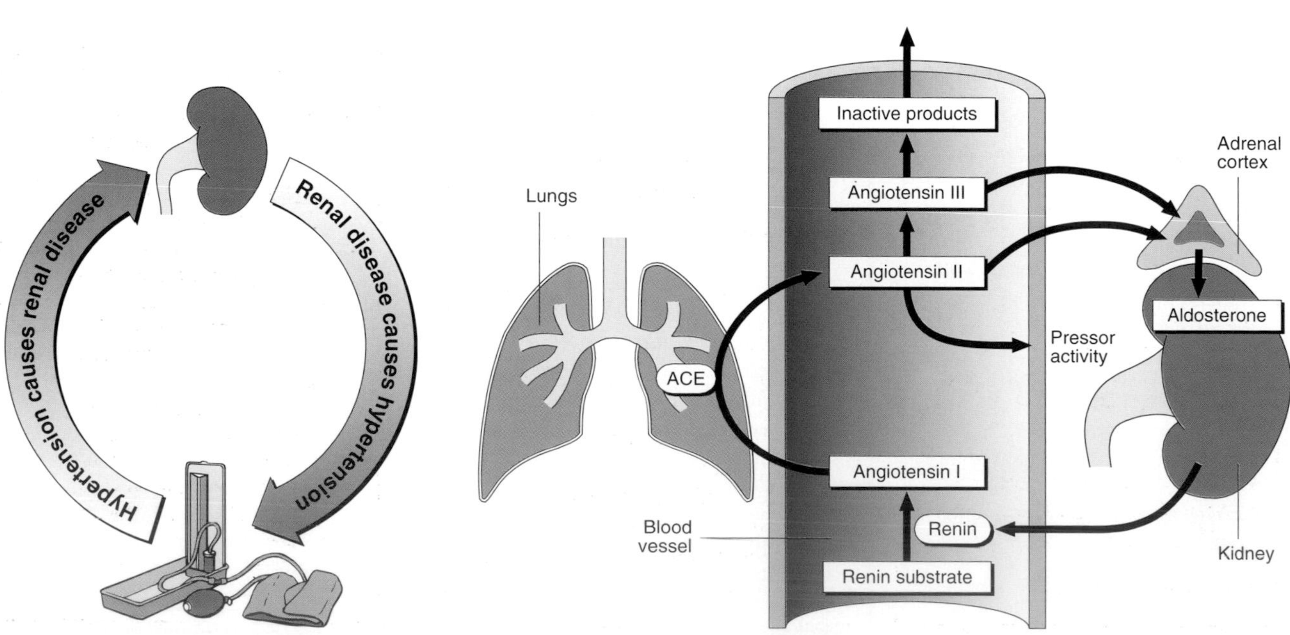

Fig. 1 **Hypertension and the kidney.**

Fig. 2 **Mechanism of primary hyperaldosteronism.**

Phaeochromocytoma

An increased production of catecholamines from a benign or malignant tumour causes vasoconstriction. The increased catecholamine production may not be easy to confirm, as phaeochromocytomas frequently secrete catecholamines episodically. Urinary catecholamine metabolites (Fig. 3) may not be elevated unless the patient has been symptomatic during the period of urine collection. Plasma adrenaline and noradrenaline concentrations are usually increased but these measurements are only available in a small number of centres.

Other endocrine diseases

Acromegaly and Cushing's syndrome are also associated with hypertension.

Pregnancy

The main feature of pre-eclampsia in pregnancy (pp. 142–143) is hypertension. A rising serum urate concentration is encountered early in the development of pre-eclampsia and is important for monitoring the condition, as is the urinary protein excretion and creatinine clearance.

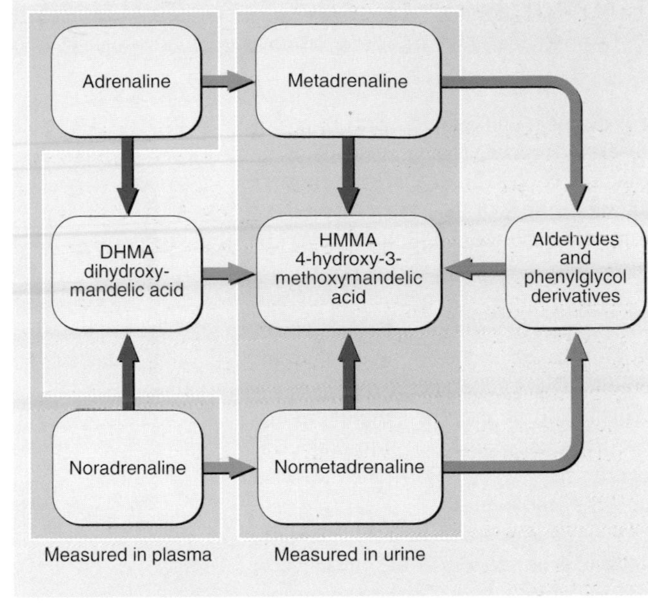

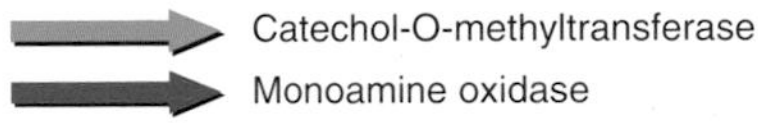

Fig. 3 **Pathway for production of catecholamine metabolites.**

INVESTIGATION OF THE HYPERTENSIVE PATIENT

Biochemical investigations in hypertension have three main roles:

- confirming that the condition is secondary to another disorder
- detecting and monitoring renal damage
- monitoring the biochemical effects of therapy, e.g. diuretic-induced hypokalaemia.

Table 1 **Anti-hypertensive drugs and their actions**

Drug	Action
Thiazide diuretics	Initial natriuresis and prolonged fall in peripheral vascular resistance
Loop diuretics	Natriuresis
Potassium sparing diuretics	Aldosterone inhibitors or inhibitors of tubular potassium secretion
Beta blockers	Block peripheral and central sympathetic activity, thereby reducing cardiac output, inhibiting renin release, decreasing noradrenaline release and decreasing central vasomotor activity
Calcium channel blockers	Reduce entry of calcium ions into vascular smooth muscle, thereby reducing vascular tone and peripheral resistance
ACE inhibitors	Competitively inhibits converting enzyme that turns angiotensin I into the potent vasoconstrictor angiotensin II

TREATMENT

Should one of the causes of secondary hypertension be diagnosed, treatment directed at the disease may often lead to the resolution of the hypertension. Treatment of essential hypertension may involve lifestyle modifications and the use of anti-hypertensive drugs (Table 1). A decision to proceed to anti-hypertensive drug therapy should always balance the risks of the treatment against the benefits which will ensue.

Case history 55

A 40-year-old lawyer is found by his GP to have a blood pressure of 165/110 mm Hg. The patient's main complaint was of excessive sweating. Glucose was detected on examination of his urine.

- Suggest two possible diagnoses.
- What biochemical investigations should now be requested?

Comment on page 158.

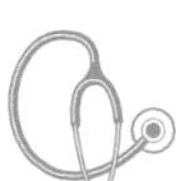

Clinical note

Measurement of blood pressure:

- Patient should be seated for at least 5 minutes.
- Rest arm on support at level of heart.
- Use appropriately sized cuff.
- Ensure mercury column is vertical.
- Inflate cuff above systolic level by palpating disappearance of radial pulse.
- Deflate cuff slowly and use the disappearance of sound (Korotkov phase V) as diastolic pressure.

Hypertension

- The overwhelming majority of patients with hypertension are found to have 'essential' or 'primary' hypertension, where no specific cause can be found.
- Hormone measurements may be necessary to exclude rare causes of hypertension such as phaeochromocytoma, Conn's syndrome, Cushing's syndrome and acromegaly.
- Biochemical tests are useful in detecting and monitoring renal damage which can be a cause of hypertension or a manifestation of it.
- Biochemical tests are useful in monitoring the biochemical effects of anti-hypertensive drugs, e.g. hypokalaemia.

CANCER AND ITS CONSEQUENCES

In Western societies one death in five is caused by cancer. The effects of tumour growth may be local or systemic (Fig. 1). If tumour growth is not countered by treatment, the consequences may be obstruction of blood vessels, lymphatics or ducts, damage to nerves, effusions, bleeding, infection, necrosis of surrounding tissue and eventual death of the patient. The cancer cells may secrete toxins locally or into the general circulation. Both endocrine and non-endocrine tumours may secrete hormones or other regulatory molecules.

A tumour marker is any substance which can be related to the presence or progress of a tumour. The use of tumour markers is covered on pages 130 – 131.

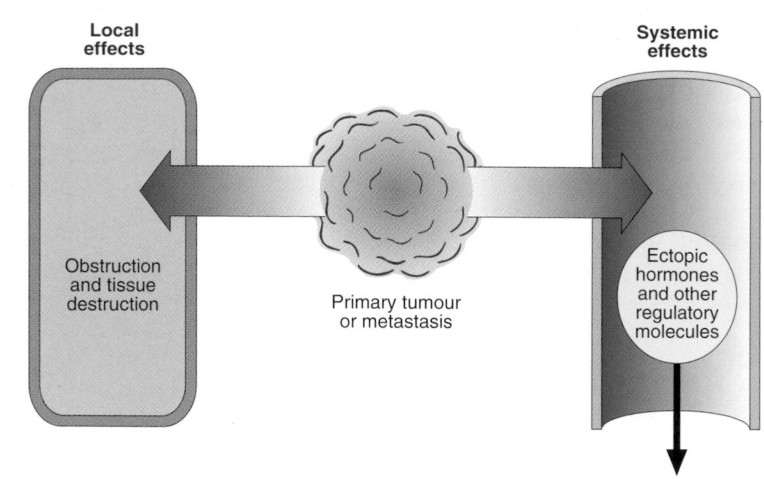

Fig. 1 **Biochemical effects of tumour growth.**

LOCAL EFFECTS OF TUMOURS

The local growth of a tumour can cause a wide range of abnormalities in commonly requested biochemical tests. This may be a consequence of obstruction of blood vessels or ducts, e.g. the blockage of bile ducts by carcinoma of head of pancreas causes elevated serum alkaline phosphatase activity, and sometimes jaundice. The symptoms which result from such local effects may be the first sign to the patient that something is wrong, but there may be no initial suspicion that there is an underlying malignancy.

The liver is often the site of metastatic spread of a tumour. An isolated increase in the serum alkaline phosphatase or γGT is a common finding when this occurs. Even with significant liver involvement, there may be no biochemical abnormalities. Modest increases in the activities of the aminotransferases, ALT and AST, are observed if the rate of cell destruction is high.

Metastatic spread of a tumour to an important site may precipitate complete system failure. For example, destruction of the adrenal cortex by tumour causes impaired aldosterone and cortisol secretion, with potentially fatal consequences.

Rapid tumour growth gives rise to abnormal biochemistry. Leukaemia and lymphoma are often associated with elevated serum urate concentrations due to the rapid cell turnover. Serum lactate dehydrogenase is often elevated in these patients reflecting the high concentration of the enzyme in the tumour and the cellular turnover. Large tumours may not have an extensive blood supply and the tumour cells meet their energy needs via anaerobic glycolysis. This may result in the generation of a lactic acidosis.

Renal failure may occur in patients with malignancy for the following reasons:

- obstruction of the urinary tract
- hypercalcaemia
- Bence-Jones proteinuria
- hyperuricaemia
- nephrotoxicity of cytotoxic drugs.

CANCER CACHEXIA

Cancer cachexia describes the characteristic wasting often seen in cancer patients. The features include anorexia, lethargy, weight loss, muscle weakness, anaemia and pyrexia. The development of cancer cachexia is due to many factors and is incompletely understood. Certainly, there is an imbalance between dietary calorie intake and body energy requirements. This results from a combination of factors:

- *Inadequate food intake.*
- *Impaired digestion and absorption.*
- *Competition between the host and tumour for nutrients.* The growing tumour has a high metabolic rate and may deprive the body of nutrients, especially if it is large. One consequence of this is a fall in the plasma cholesterol level in cancer patients.
- *Increased energy requirement of the cancer patient.* The host reaction to the tumour is similar to the metabolic response to injury, with increased metabolic rate and altered tissue metabolism.

Tumour spread may cause infection, dysphagia, persistent vomiting and diarrhoea, all of which may contribute to the overall picture seen in cancer cachexia. The observation that small tumours can have a profound effect on host metabolism suggests that cancer cells secrete, or cause the release of, humoral agents which mediate the metabolic changes of cancer cachexia. Some of these, such as tumour necrosis factor, have been identified. This cytokine is secreted by activated macrophages and acts on a variety of tissues including muscle, adipose tissue and liver.

ECTOPIC HORMONE PRODUCTION

It is a characteristic feature of some cancers that they secrete hormones, even though the tumour has not arisen from an endocrine organ. Referred to as ectopic hormone production, hormone secretion by tumours has frequently been invoked but rarely proven (Fig. 2). Small cell carcinomas are the most aggressive of the lung cancers and are the most likely to be associated with ectopic hormone production. Ectopic ACTH secretion causing Cushing's syndrome, an overproduction of cortisol, is the most common. However, the classic clinical features of Cushing's syndrome are not usually apparent in the rapidly progressing ectopic ACTH disorder. Biochemical features include hypokalaemia and metabolic alkalosis and these may be the sole indicators of the problem.

Not infrequently, patients with malignancy develop the syndrome of inappropriate antidiuresis (SIAD). Water is retained and patients present with hyponatraemia. This is probably the commonest biochemical abnormality seen in patients with cancer and is almost invariably due to pituitary AVP secretion in response to non-osmotic stimuli. SIAD is often, incorrectly, attributed to ectopic AVP secretion, which is in fact very rare.

Some cancers may cause hypercalcaemia. In many cases this is due to the secretion of parathyroid hormone related protein, PTHrP, so-called because of its relationship with PTH both in its structure and function.

CONSEQUENCES OF CANCER TREATMENT

Anti-tumour therapy can have serious effects. Gonadal failure arising from radiotherapy or chemotherapy is frequently encountered. Hypomagnesaemia and hypokalaemia may be a consequence of the use of the cytotoxic drug, cisplatin. Patients treated with methotrexate may become folate deficient.

Hyperuricaemia is the consequence of the massive cell death which occurs in the treatment of some tumours with cytotoxic drugs, particularly lymphomas and some leukaemias, and is known as tumour lysis syndrome.

(a)

Condition resolves after surgical removal of tumour or irradiation. Good evidence, but may be due to tumour secretion of a releasing factor, e.g. secretion of growth hormone may be due to the production of growth hormone releasing hormone.

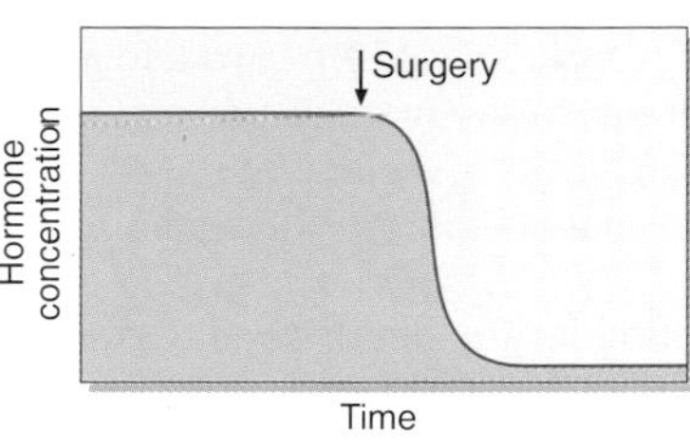

(b)

Demonstration that hormone level in arterial supply to tumour is less than in venous drainage. Good evidence, especially if combined with (a).

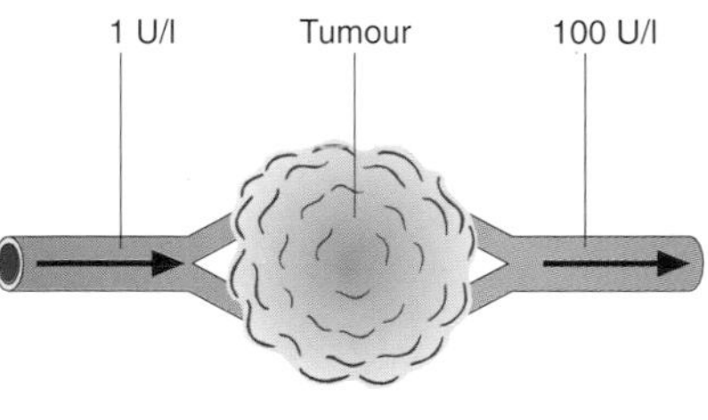

(c)

Hormone may be extracted from tumour. Good evidence, but may be due to absorption of hormone by tumour.

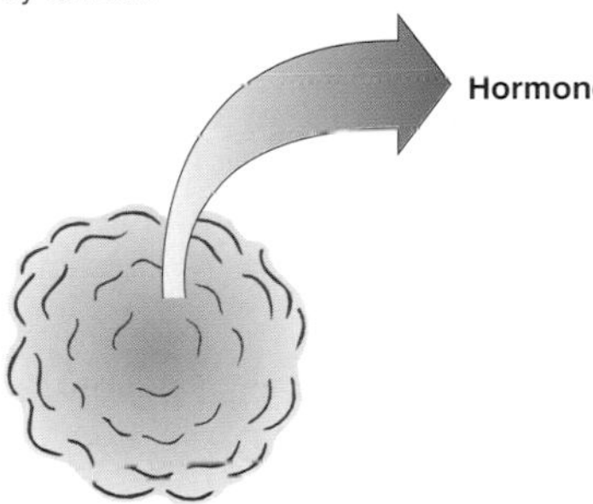

(d)

Histochemical demonstration of hormone in tumour cell secretory granules and mRNA for hormone in tumour. Definitive evidence.

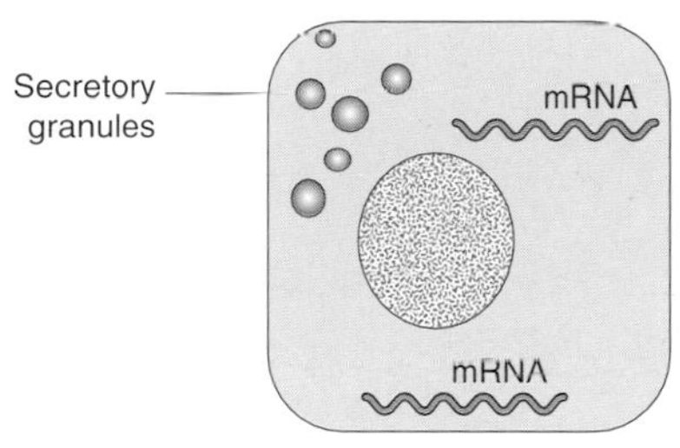

Fig. 2 **Evidence for ectopic hormone production.**

Clinical note

The measurement of oestrogen and progesterone receptors in biopsy material has been used to determine which breast cancer patients will respond to endocrine therapy, e.g. with the anti-oestrogen tamoxifen. As the synthesis of progesterone receptors is dependent on oestradiol, the presence of both receptors indicates the integrity of the oestrogen receptor mechanism in the tumour cells (Fig.3). The prognostic value of such receptor measurements is still controversial.

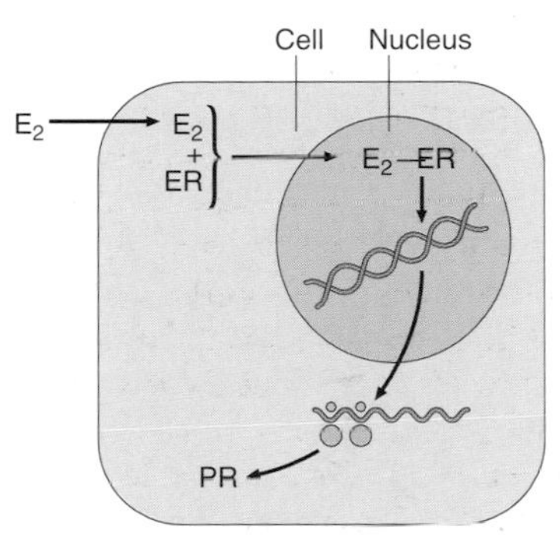

E_2 — Oestradiol
ER — Oestrogen receptor
PR — Progesterone receptor

Fig. 3 **Progesterone receptor synthesis is dependent on the integrity of the oestrogen receptor pathway**.

Case history 56

SI, a 37-year-old male, presented to his GP complaining of nocturia, frequency of micturition and polydipsia. On examination, he had mild truncal obesity, plethora, and ankle oedema. He had purpura of his arms but no striae. His blood pressure was 185/115 mm Hg. Biochemistry results in a serum specimen showed:

Na^+	K^+	Cl^-	HCO_3^-	Urea	Creatinine	Glucose
mmol/l					*μmol/l*	*mmol/l*
146	2.1	96	34	7.0	135	8.5

- What is the most likely diagnosis?
- What further biochemistry tests should be requested?

Comment on page 158.

Cancer and its consequences

- Cancer may cause clinical signs and symptoms in patients by causing obstruction, exerting pressure or destroying normal tissue.
- Cancer cachexia is characterized by anorexia, lethargy, muscle wasting, weight loss and anaemia.
- Some non-endocrine tumours secrete hormones, e.g. lung cancers may secrete ACTH.
- Hyponatraemia, due to water retention, is the commonest biochemical abnormality seen in patients with cancer.

TUMOUR MARKERS

A tumour marker is any substance which can be related to the presence or progress of a tumour. In practice, the clinical biochemistry laboratory measures markers which are present in blood, although the term 'tumour markers' can also be applied to substances found on the surface of or within cells fixed in frozen or paraffin sections. A tumour marker in plasma has been secreted or released by the tumour cells. Such markers are not necessarily unique products of the malignant cells, but may simply be expressed by the tumour in greater amount than by normal cells.

Tumour markers fall into one of several groups: they may be hormones, e.g. human chorionic gonadotrophin (HCG) secreted by choriocarcinoma; or enzymes, e.g. prostatic acid phosphatase in prostate carcinoma; or tumour antigens, e.g. carcinoembryonic antigen (CEA) in colorectal carcinoma.

THE USE OF TUMOUR MARKERS

Tumour markers can be used in different ways. They are of most value in monitoring treatment and assessing follow-up (Fig. 1), but are also used in diagnosis, prognosis and screening for the presence of disease.

Monitoring treatment

Treatment monitoring is the area in which most tumour markers have found a useful role. The decline in concentration of the tumour marker is an indication of the success of the treatment, whether that be surgery, chemotherapy, radiotherapy, or a combination of these. However, the rate of decline of marker concentration should match that predicted from knowledge of the marker's half-life. A slower than expected fall may well indicate that not all the tumour has been eliminated.

Assessing follow-up

Even when a patient has had successful treatment, it is often valuable to continue to monitor the marker long after the levels have appeared to stabilize. An increase indicates recurrence of the malignancy. Detection of increasing marker concentration allows second-line therapy to be instituted promptly. The frequency of sampling, with the attendant cost implications, is much discussed.

Diagnosis

Markers alone are rarely used to establish a diagnosis. Their detection in blood when there is clinical evidence of the tumour as well as radiological and, perhaps, biopsy evidence, will often confirm the diagnosis.

Prognosis

To be of value in prognosis, the concentration of the tumour marker should correlate with tumour mass. For example, HCG correlates well with the tumour mass in choriocarcinoma, HCG and alphafetoprotein (AFP) correlate with the tumour mass in testicular teratoma, and paraproteins correlate with the tumour mass in multiple myeloma.

Screening for the presence of disease

Tumour markers should not, in routine clinical practice, be used to screen for malignancy, however appealing this might be in theory.

The exception to this rule is the screening of specific high risk populations. For example, the hormone calcitonin, which is increased in patients with medullary carcinoma of thyroid, may be used to screen close relatives. Prophylactic thyroidectomy may then be advised if any are found to have elevated calcitonin concentrations.

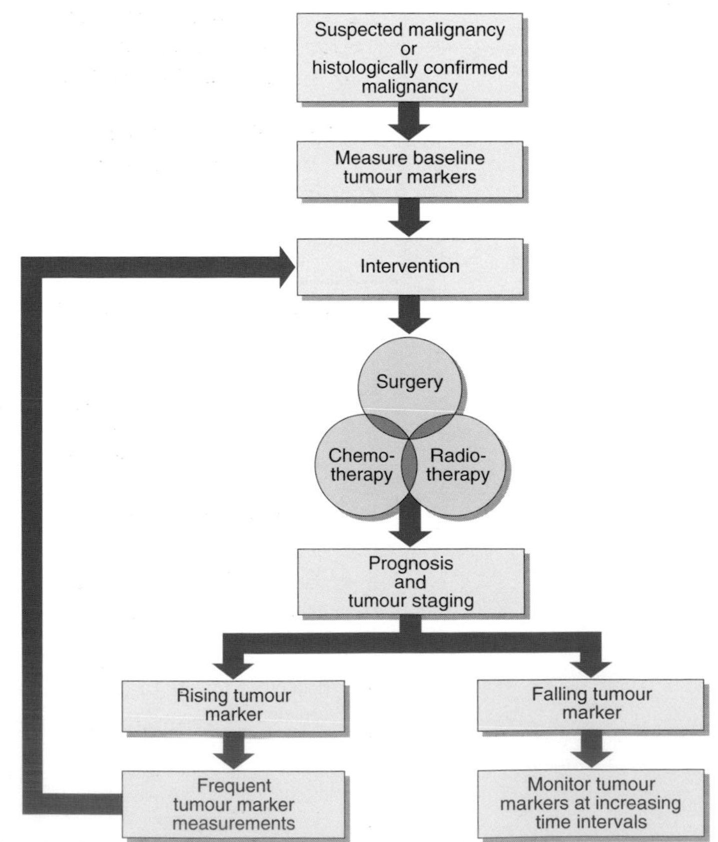

Fig. 1 **The use of tumour markers.**

A PRACTICAL APPLICATION OF TUMOUR MARKERS

Some of the uses of tumour markers discussed above can be illustrated with reference to Figure 2. This shows how the tumour marker AFP was helpful in the management of a young man with a malignant teratoma. The presence of AFP together with the hormone HCG confirmed the diagnosis. Between 75–95% of all patients presenting with testicular teratoma have abnormalities in one or both of these markers. The very high concentration of AFP (>10 000 kU/l) indicated that the prognosis was not good, and that it was likely there would be tumour recurrence after treatment. In fact, AFP concentrations fell in response to chemotherapy, but when the levels reached a plateau, surgery was carried out. Thereafter, chemotherapy was continued, and AFP fell to very low levels. Continued monitoring of AFP levels in such a patient would provide early warning of tumour recurrence.

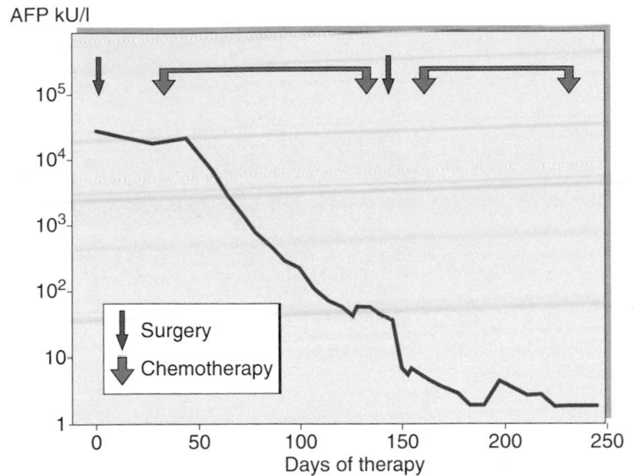

Fig. 2 **The use of AFP measurements in the management of a patient with a testicular teratoma.**

TUMOUR MARKERS WITH ESTABLISHED CLINICAL VALUE

Markers play a major role in the management of germ cell tumours and choriocarcinoma. Unfortunately, there are many cases in which markers are available but the tumours are resistant to chemotherapy, so their use is not mandatory. Table 1 shows which markers have gained an established place in the repertoire of tests commonly offered by the clinical biochemistry laboratory.

THE FUTURE

Monoclonal antibodies raised against tumour cells and their membranes have led to the development of many new tumour marker assays, although few have as yet gained an established place in the management of patients with cancer. There is no doubt that tumour markers are an efficient and cheap way to monitor treatment. The search goes on for the 'perfect' marker which could be used in population screening, diagnosis, prognosis, monitoring treatment and for follow-up of tumour recurrence. However, the capacity for tumours to alter the expression of their surface antigens may make this goal unattainable.

Table 1 **Clinical situations where tumour markers have been found to be useful**

Marker	Tumour	Screening	Diagnosis	Prognosis	Monitoring	Follow-up
AFP	Germ cell		✓	✓	✓	✓
AFP	Hepatoma	✓	✓		✓	✓
HCG	Germ cell		✓	✓	✓	✓
HCG	Choriocarcinoma	✓	✓	✓	✓	✓
CA 125	Ovarian		✓		✓	✓
Acid phosphatase	Prostate		✓		✓	✓
Prostate specific antigen (PSA)	Prostate		✓		✓	✓
CEA	Colorectal				✓	✓
Calcitonin	Medullary carcinoma of thyroid	✓	✓		✓	✓
Hormones	Endocrine		✓		✓	✓
Paraprotein	Myeloma		✓		✓	✓

Clinical note

Sometimes a man may act as a negative control when his partner uses a pregnancy test kit at home. Teratoma of the testis has a peak incidence in men in their twenties, and this tumour frequently secretes large amounts of HCG. This will give rise to a positive pregnancy test in the man! Such a finding should be taken very seriously and followed up immediately.

Case history 57

KS, a 72-year-old male, had complained of pains in his lower chest and abdomen for two months. His general practitioner detected dullness at both lung bases and referred him to a chest physician. On 23 June he was admitted to hospital. Examination revealed an enlarged liver. He had been a heavy drinker. Biochemistry results were:

Date	Bilirubin	ALP	AST	ALT	LDH	γGT
	μmol/l			*U/l*		
23/6	24	1540	83	98		719
1/7	25	2170	80	107	430	1020

- What is your differential diagnosis in the light of the liver function test results?
- How might AFP be of help in this case?

Comment on page 158.

Tumour markers

- The main use of tumour markers is in monitoring treatment, although they may also be of use in screening, diagnosis, prognosis, and in long-term follow-up.
- Calcitonin is used to screen the relatives and family of a patient with medullary carcinoma of thyroid.
- AFP, paraproteins, prostate specific antigen and a variety of hormones are helpful in establishing the diagnosis of certain tumours.
- AFP and HCG are of value in predicting the outcome of non-seminomatous germ cell tumours.

GUT HORMONES AND MULTIPLE ENDOCRINE NEOPLASIA

GUT HORMONES

More than 30 different molecules have been identified as having regulatory roles in the function of the gastrointestinal tract (Table. 1). Some are classical hormones, although the endocrine cells of the gut are not grouped together in discrete organs but are widely dispersed through the gastrointestinal tract. Others are local paracrine regulators or neurotransmitters. Some of these biochemical regulators act in all three ways. For example, somatostatin has an endocrine function, and is present in neurones, but it also has paracrine activity in the antrum of the stomach. The functions of many of these regulatory molecules remain unclear, but oversecretion is sometimes the cause of a specific clinical disorder.

Table 1 **Selected molecules which regulate gastrointestinal function**

Substance	Type of regulator	Major action
Gastrin	Hormone	Gastric acid and pepsin secretion
Cholecystokinin (CCK)	Hormone	Pancreatic enzyme secretion
Secretin	Hormone	Pancreatic bicarbonate secretion
Gastric inhibitory polypeptide (GIP)	Hormone	Enhances glucose mediated insulin release. Inhibits gastric acid secretion
Vasoactive intestinal polypeptide (VIP)	Neurotransmitter	Smooth muscle relaxation. Stimulates pancreatic bicarbonate secretion
Motilin	Hormone	Initiates interdigestive intestinal motility
Somatostatin	Hormone Neurotransmitter Paracrine	Numerous inhibitory effects
Pancreatic polypeptide (PP)	Hormone Paracrine	Inhibits pancreatic bicarbonate and protein secretion.
Enkephalins	Neurotransmitter	Opiate-like actions
Substance P	Neurotransmitter Paracrine	Contraction of smooth muscle

GASTROINTESTINAL DISORDERS

GASTRIN AND THE ZOLLINGER –ELLISON SYNDROME

Gastrinomas secrete large amounts of gastrin which stimulate excessive acid secretion in the stomach and cause ulceration. These peptic ulcers are refractory to therapy. The severity of the ulceration is a much greater threat to the patient in the short term than the malignant growth and spread of the tumour. Hypergastrinaemia together with acid hypersecretion is diagnostic of the Zollinger–Ellison syndrome. Although the pancreas does not contain many gastrin-secreting cells, most gastrinomas are, surprisingly, found as islet cell carcinomas. Gastrinomas often occur in association with other tumours.

VIPOMAS AND THE WATERY DIARRHOEA SYNDROME

Endocrine causes of chronic diarrhoea are rare. The syndrome which includes watery diarrhoea and extreme weakness due to potassium depletion is most often related to an overproduction of vasoactive intestinal polypeptide (VIP). Provided that other causes of diarrhoea such as infection, malabsorption or laxative abuse have been excluded, the presence of severe watery diarrhoea and hypokalaemia with normal or low gastric acid secretion is suggestive of a VIPoma. The diagnosis can be confirmed by the finding of an elevated VIP concentration in plasma. The tumours are usually found in the pancreas. Surgical resection is the treatment of choice.

GLUCAGONOMAS

Glucagonomas are rare. They are usually malignant tumours which arise in the pancreatic islets. The clinical features include a characteristic dermatitis, mild diabetes mellitus and low amino acid concentrations in plasma. Diagnosis may be confirmed by the demonstration of an elevated plasma glucagon concentration. Surgery is indicated, although many tumours are inoperable.

SOMATOSTATINOMAS

Somatostatinomas are rare pancreatic islet cell tumours which are usually malignant. The clinical features include mild diabetes mellitus, diarrhoea, malabsorption and gallstones. Diagnosis may be made by finding increased plasma concentrations of somatostatin. Surgery is an option if the tumour is localized, otherwise chemotherapy is the likely treatment.

TUMOURS SECRETING PANCREATIC POLYPEPTIDE (PPOMAS)

Tumours secreting pancreatic polypeptide are rare. The clinical effects are usually due to the local effects of the tumour rather than to the secretion of the hormone.

CARCINOID TUMOURS AND THE CARCINOID SYNDROME

Carcinoid tumours are found in the gastrointestinal tract, most frequently in the appendix and ileocaecal regions. They may also occur in the lungs or ovaries, and occasionally occur at multiple sites. Tumour behaviour varies with location. Most of those which arise in the appendix are benign, whereas those in the ileum or jejunum are often malignant. Many but not all patients with carcinoid tumours develop the carcinoid syndrome, which is characterized by flushing and diarrhoea. These symptoms are related to the secretion of serotonin, although other tumour products such as histamine may be involved. Serotonin is a vasoconstrictor which is present in high concentration in platelets and released during blood clotting. The diagnostic test is measurement of 5-hydroxyindoleacetic acid, a metabolite of serotonin, in urine (Fig. 1). Measurement of serotonin concentration in plasma is also possible. Drugs are often necessary to control the diarrhoea and flushing, and surgery is the treatment of choice.

Ectopic ACTH production from carcinoid tumours is a well-recognized cause of Cushing's syndrome.

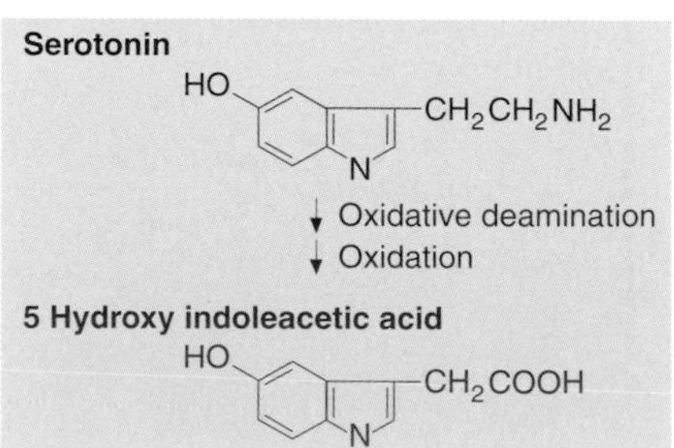

Fig. 1 **Serotonin and its urinary metabolite 5-hydroxyindoleacetic acid.** Certain foodstuffs such as bananas and tomatoes contain 5-hydroxyindoleacetic acid and may interfere with the urinary determination.

MULTIPLE ENDOCRINE NEOPLASIA (MEN)

Multiple endocrine neoplasias are inherited disorders. The syndromes are usually transmitted in an autosomal dominant pattern. The endocrine glands most often affected are the parathyroid, pituitary, pancreas, thyroid and adrenal. It is postulated that the cell types involved in these tumours have a common embryological precursor. There are three well-defined multiple endocrine neoplasia syndromes (Fig. 2).

MEN type I is characterized by hyperparathyroidism, together with pituitary and pancreatic tumours. Hypercalcaemia caused by excess PTH secretion is the dominant feature in this syndrome. The most common pituitary tumour is a non-functioning chromophobe adenoma which, although it does not secrete a hormone itself, may have effects on the secretion of other anterior pituitary hormones. The most common pancreatic tumour in MEN type I is an islet cell tumour secreting gastrin. The secretion of gastrin may lead to gastric ulceration.

In *MEN type IIa*, medullary carcinoma of thyroid is present with hyperparathyroidism and bilateral adrenal phaeochromocytomas. Medullary carcinoma of thyroid is diagnosed on the basis of elevated calcitonin concentrations in serum, although provocation tests, such as a calcium infusion and/or administration of pentagastrin, may be necessary to demonstrate the abnormal calcitonin regulation (Fig. 3). Diagnosis of phaeochromocytoma is not easy (p. 126).

Medullary carcinoma of thyroid, phaeochromocytoma, and multiple mucosal neuromas are present in *MEN type IIb*. The presence of these neuromas on the tongue, lips or buccal mucosa is the most consistent feature. Neuromas are also often found in the gastrointestinal tract and may be responsible for difficulties in swallowing, diarrhoea or constipation.

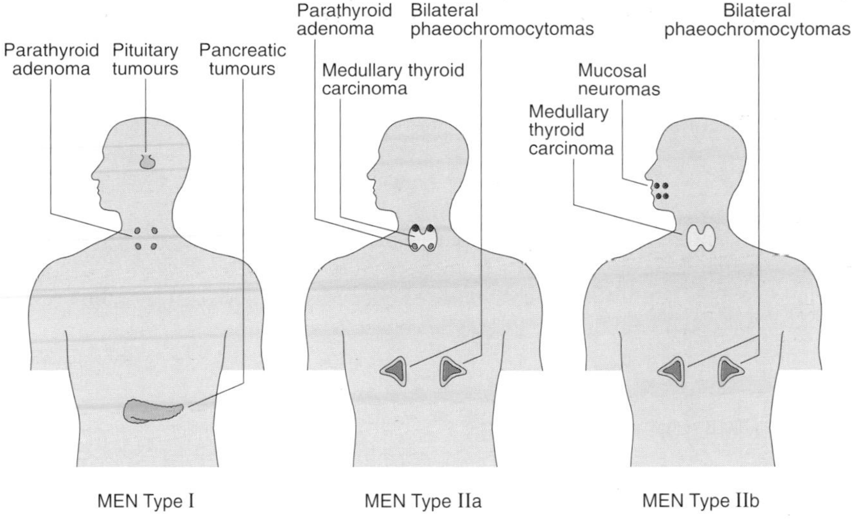

Fig. 2 **Classification of MEN syndromes.**

Treatment

Excessive hormone production seen in MEN syndromes gives rise to the expected clinical effects. Where possible, surgery is the treatment of choice. The three lesions of MEN type IIa are all individually potentially lethal, and early diagnosis and operation is vital if treatment is to be curative. An essential part of clinical management of any patient who is found to have a MEN syndrome will be the investigation of other family members. Provocation tests, such as that shown in Figure 3, can determine the presence of medullary carcinoma of thyroid even when baseline calcitonin concentrations are within the reference range. This will allow early surgical treatment.

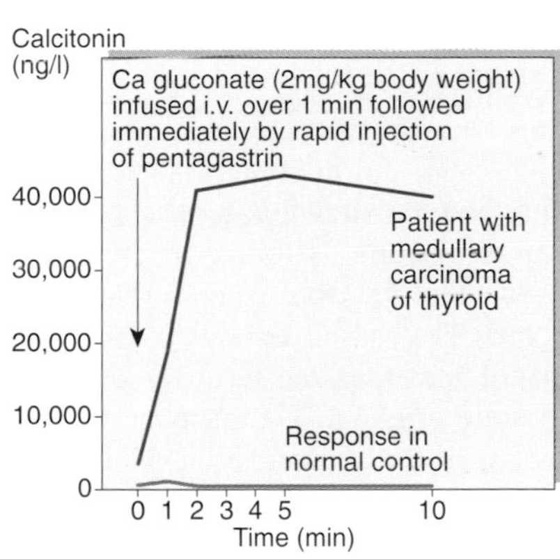

Fig 3 **Calcium and pentagastrin provocation test of calcitonin secretion.** There is an exaggerated response to combined calcium and pentagastrin provocation in a patient with medullary carcinoma of the thyroid.

Case history 58

DC, a 50-year-old man, was referred to a neurologist after complaining of a six-month history of severe headache. He was found to be slightly hypertensive. U and Es and LFTs were unremarkable. The only abnormality initially noted was a serum adjusted calcium concentration of 2.80 mmol/l.

- What further investigations are required in this patient?

Comment on page 158.

Clinical note

The H_2 receptor antagonists such as cimetidine are widely used to treat peptic ulcers. They may cause an increase in plasma gastrin concentrations to values which might suggest the presence of a gastrinoma. These drugs should be stopped before samples are taken for gastrin measurements.

Gut hormones and multiple endocrine neoplasia

- Clinical disorders involving regulatory peptides of the gastrointestinal tract are uncommon.
- Gastrinomas secrete gastrin which causes gastric acid hypersecretion and ulceration.
- VIPomas are a rare cause of chronic diarrhoea and potassium depletion.
- Some patients with carcinoid tumours develop flushing and diarrhoea, most probably due to an overproduction of serotonin.
- Multiple endocrine neoplasia syndromes are inherited disorders characterized by abnormal function of a number of endocrine glands.
- Management of MEN syndromes is by surgical treatment of the specific neoplasms wherever possible.
- Investigation of the patient's family is indicated in multiple endocrine neoplasia.

HYPERURICAEMIA

Nucleic acids contain bases of two different types, pyrimidines and purines. The catabolism of the purines, adenine and guanine, produces uric acid. At physiological hydrogen ion concentration, uric acid is mostly ionized and present in plasma as sodium urate (Fig. 1). An elevated serum urate concentration is known as hyperuricaemia. Uric acid and urate are relatively insoluble molecules which readily precipitate out of aqueous solutions such as urine or synovial fluid (Fig. 2). The consequence of this is the medical condition, gout.

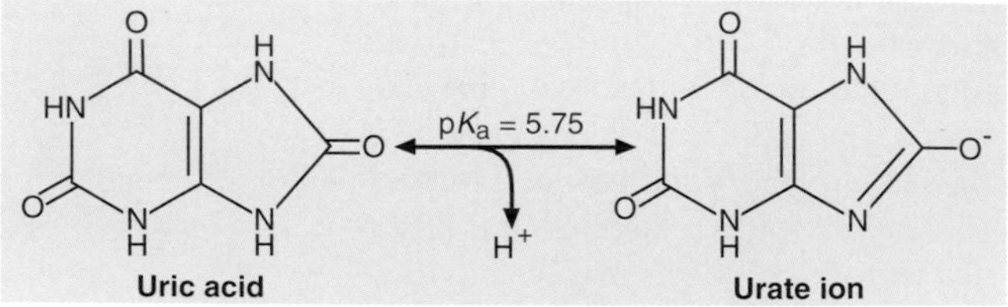

Uric acid $\xrightleftharpoons{pK_a = 5.75}$ Urate ion + H^+

Fig. 1 **Uric acid and urate.**

URATE FORMATION AND EXCRETION

Urate is formed in three ways. These are:

- by de novo synthesis
- by the metabolism of endogenous DNA, RNA and other purine containing molecules such as ATP
- by the breakdown of dietary nucleic acids.

Urate is excreted in two ways:

- *Via the kidney*. The majority of urate is excreted via the kidney. Renal handling of urate is complex. It is freely filtered at the glomerulus, but 99% is reabsorbed in the proximal tubule. The distal tubules also secrete urate, but again much is reabsorbed. The amount of urate excreted in the urine is around 10% of that filtered at the glomerulus.
- *Via the gut*. Smaller amounts of urate are excreted into the gut where it is broken down by bacteria. This process is called uricolysis.

Urate concentrations in serum are higher in men than women. Even within the reference range, serum urate is near its aqueous solubility limit. The presence of protein helps to keep the molecule in solution. A high serum urate may arise from increased urate formation, or from decreased excretion. The common causes of hyperuricaemia are summarized in Figure 3. Genetic causes of hyperuricaemia are known as primary disorders, and there are also secondary causes. Most primary causes are due to decreased excretion of urate (90% of cases) rather than increased production (10%).

Lesch–Nyhan syndrome

One genetic disorder which should be singled out is Lesch–Nyhan syndrome, an X-linked disorder caused by a deficiency of hypoxanthine-guanine phosphoribosyltransferase, an enzyme which is involved in salvaging purine bases for resynthesis to purine nucleotides. The syndrome is characterized clinically by excessive uric acid production, hyperuricaemia and neurological problems which include self mutilation and mental retardation.

GOUT

Gout is a clinical syndrome which is characterized by hyperuricaemia and recurrent acute arthritis. Whereas all patients who develop gout will have had hyperuricaemia at some point in the development of the disease, only a minority of patients with hyperuricaemia develop gout. The reason for this is not known.

Acute gout is triggered by the tissue deposition of sodium urate crystals which cause an inflammatory response. In the chronic situation, tophaceous deposits of sodium urate may form in the tissues (Fig. 4). Gout is exacerbated by alcohol. The reason for this is twofold. Ethanol increases the turnover of ATP and urate production. Ethanol in excess may cause the accumulation of organic acids which compete with the tubular secretion of uric acid. Disorders such as ethanol intoxication, diabetic ketoacidosis and starvation lead to elevations of lactic acid, β-hydroxybutyric acid and acetoacetic acid, and will cause hyperuricaemia.

Treatment

The symptoms of acute gout respond to anti-inflammatory drugs such as indomethacin, but it should be noted that these drugs have no direct effect on the serum urate level. Low-dose aspirin should be avoided as it inhibits renal urate excretion. Treatment must also be directed at the hyperuricaemia. Drugs such as probenecid which promote urate excretion can be used prophylactically. A diet which is low in purines and alcohol may be prescribed in an effort to reduce the plasma urate concentration. Allopurinol, a specific inhibitor of the enzyme xanthine oxidase which catalyzes the oxidation of hypoxanthine to xanthine and uric acid, may also be effective in reducing urate concentrations.

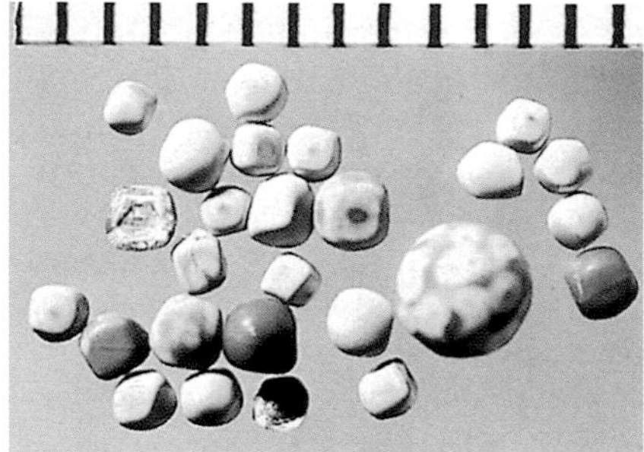

Fig. 2 **Urate stones from the urinary tract.**

A number of other crystalline arthropathies may present as gout but are not associated with hyperuricaemia. Most notably, pseudogout is due to the deposition of calcium pyrophosphate crystals.

RENAL DISEASE AND HYPERURICAEMIA

Renal disease is a common complication of hyperuricaemia. Several types of renal disease have been identified. The most common is urate nephropathy which is caused by the deposition of urate crystals in renal tissue or the urinary tract to form urate stones. This may be associated with chronic hyperuricaemia. Acute renal failure can be caused by the rapid precipitation of uric acid crystals which commonly occurs during treatment of patients with leukaemias and lymphomas. In the 'acute tumour lysis syndrome' (p. 129), nucleic acids are released as a result of tumour cell breakdown and are rapidly metabolized to uric acid.

URATE IN PREGNANCY

Serum urate is of value in the monitoring of maternal well-being in pregnancy associated hypertension (pre-eclampsia), alongside other markers such as blood pressure, urine protein excretion and creatinine clearance (p. 143).

NORMAL

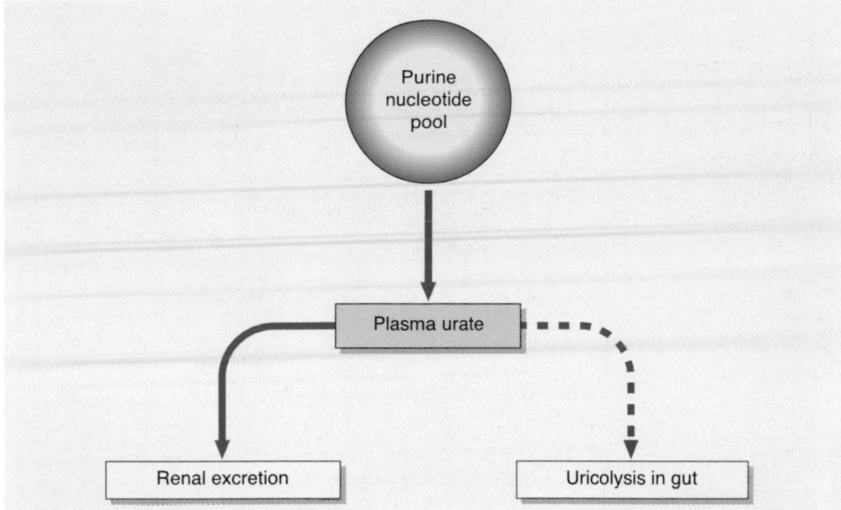

INCREASED PRODUCTION

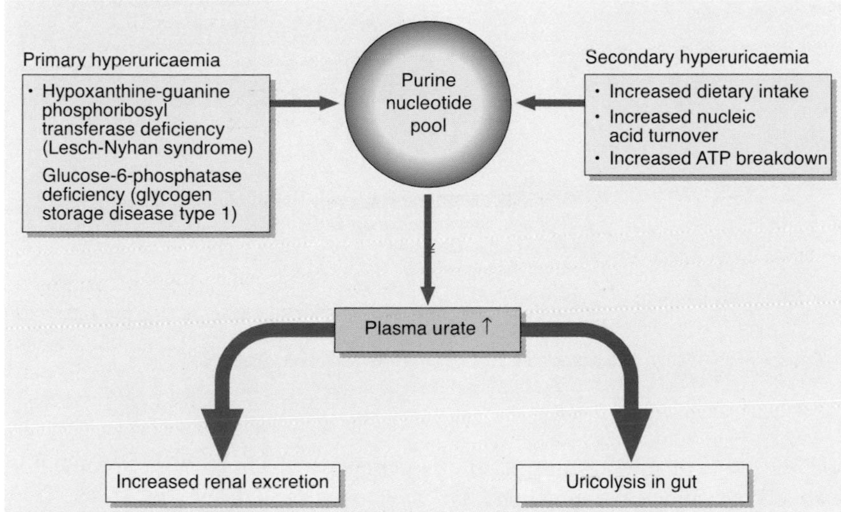

DECREASED EXCRETION

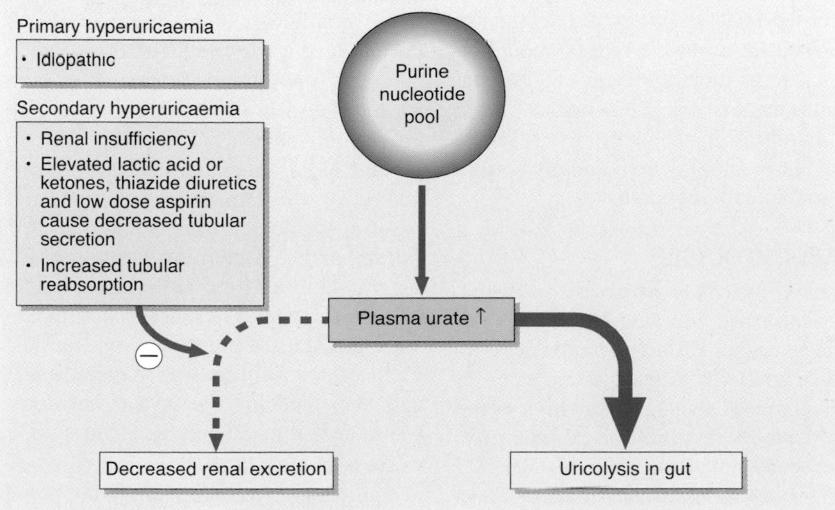

Fig. 3 **The causes of hyperuricaemia.**

Case history 59

A 50-year-old man was awakened by a severe pain in his left toe. He was shivering and feverish, and the pain became so intense that he could not bear the weight of the bedclothes.

- What biochemical tests would help make the diagnosis?

Comment on page 158.

Clinical note

Acute gouty arthritis may be diagnosed by examination of synovial fluid from an acutely inflamed joint. Sodium urate crystals will be observed within polymorphonuclear leukocytes viewed under polarizing light.

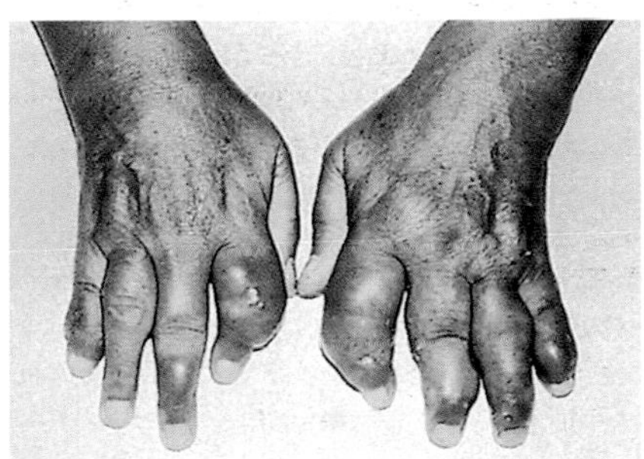

Fig. 4 **Tophaceous deposits of sodium urate in tissues.**

Hyperuricaemia

- Uric acid is formed from the breakdown of endogenous or exogenous purines.
- Hyperuricaemia may be caused by:
  - an increased rate of purine synthesis
  - an increased rate of turnover of nucleic acids, as in malignancies, tissue damage or starvation
  - a reduced renal excretion.
- Hyperuricaemia is a risk factor for gout which occurs when urate crystals are deposited in tissues.
- Hyperuricaemia is aggravated by a diet high in purines and alcohol.

SKELETAL MUSCLE DISORDERS

Myopathies are conditions affecting the muscles which lead to weakness and/or atrophy. They may be caused by congenital factors (as in the muscular dystrophies), by viral infection or by acute damage due to anoxia, infections, toxins or drugs. Muscle denervation is a major cause of myopathy. Muscle weakness can occur due to a lack of energy producing molecules or a failure in the balance of electrolytes within and surrounding the muscle cell necessary for neuromuscular function.

Normal muscle which is overused will end up weak or in spasm until rested. In severe cases of overuse, especially where movements are strong and erratic as might occur during convulsions, damage to muscle cells may result. Severely damaged muscle cells release myoglobin, a condition known as rhabdomyolysis.

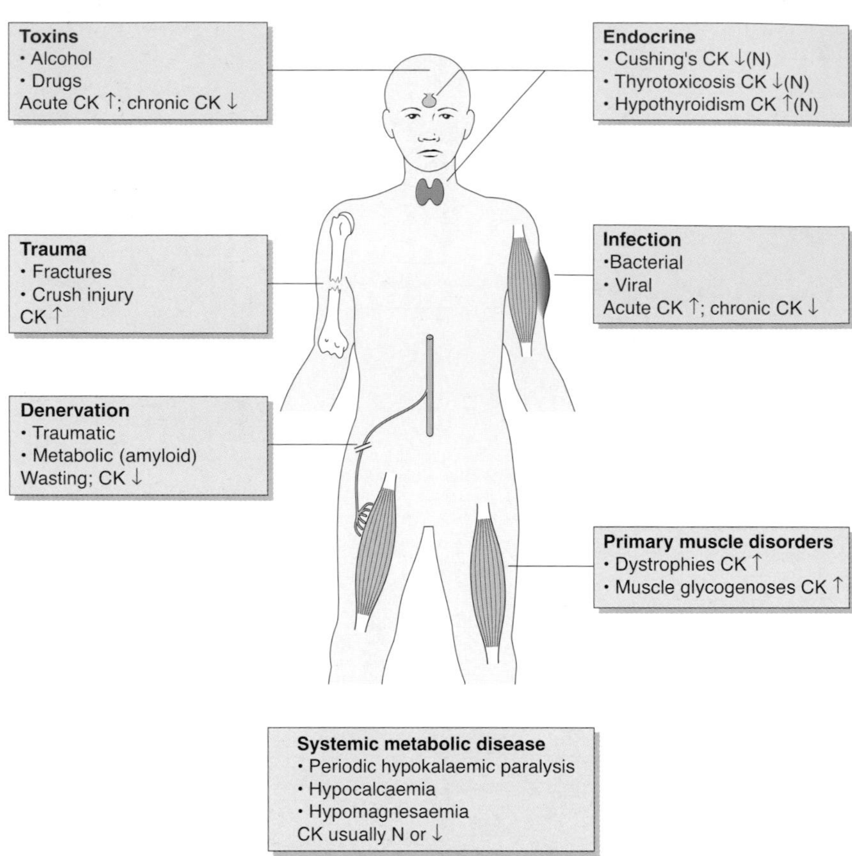

Fig. 1 **Causes of myopathy, with associated changes in serum creatine kinase (CK).**

MUSCLE WEAKNESS

Muscle weakness, which may or may not progress to rhabdomyolysis, has many causes (Fig. 1). Diagnosis of the condition will depend on the clinical picture and will include investigation of genetic disorders by enzymic or chromosomal analysis, endocrine investigations and the search for drug effects. Infective causes may be diagnosed by isolation of the relevant organism or its related antibody, but often no organism is detected. These cases, known as myalgic encephalitis (ME), post-viral syndrome or chronic fatigue syndrome, are relatively common and are now regarded as true diseases, whereas formally they were thought to be psychosomatic.

Investigation

In all cases of muscle weakness, serum electrolytes should be checked along with creatine kinase (CK). A full drug history should be taken to exclude pharmacological and toxicological causes, and a history of alcohol abuse should be excluded. Neuromuscular electrophysiological studies should be performed to detect neuropathies. Where a genetic cause is suspected, a muscle biopsy should be taken for histopathological studies and measurement of muscle enzymes (Table 1). In contrast to rhabdomyolysis, serum CK and myoglobin are frequently normal in patients with myopathy.

Table 1 **Cellular enzymes which may be measured in the investigation of muscle weakness**

Type of myopathy	Enzyme
Glycogen storage disease	Myophosphorylase Glycerol kinase Lactate dehydrogenase Phosphofructokinase Phosphoglycerate kinase Myoadenylate deaminase
Lipid diseases	Carnitine palmityl transferase

RHABDOMYOLYSIS

Muscle cells which are damaged will leak creatine kinase into the plasma. This enzyme exists in different isoforms. CK-MM or total CK is used as an index of skeletal muscle damage. Very high serum levels may be expected in patients who have been convulsing or have muscular damage due to electrical shock or crush injury. Creatine kinase concentrations may also be high in acute spells in muscular dystrophy. For these reasons, when CK is used as an indicator of myocardial infarction, it is better to measure the MB isoenzyme which is more specific for cardiac muscle damage (pp. 48–49).

The damaged muscle cells will also leak myoglobin. This compound stores oxygen in the muscle cells for release under conditions of hypoxia, as occurs during severe exercise. The dissociation curve of myoglobin is compared with haemoglobin in Figure 2. It delivers up its oxygen only when the PO_2 falls to around 3 kPa. When muscle cells become anoxic or are damaged by trauma, myoglobin is released into the plasma. It is filtered at the glomerulus. Urine containing myoglobin will be an orange or brown colour. The damaged muscle cells release large amounts of potassium ions into the extracellular fluid causing hyperkalaemia and also tend to take up calcium ions, reducing serum calcium concentration.

Severe muscle damage is frequently accompanied by a reduction in the blood volume. This may occur directly as a result of haemorrhage in severe trauma, or indirectly because of fluid sequestration in the damaged tissue. The resultant shock frequently causes acute renal failure.

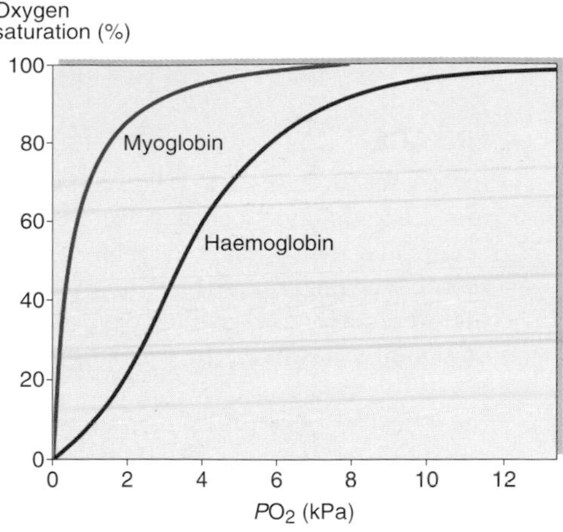

Fig. 2 **Comparison of oxygen saturation curves for haemoglobin and myoglobin.**

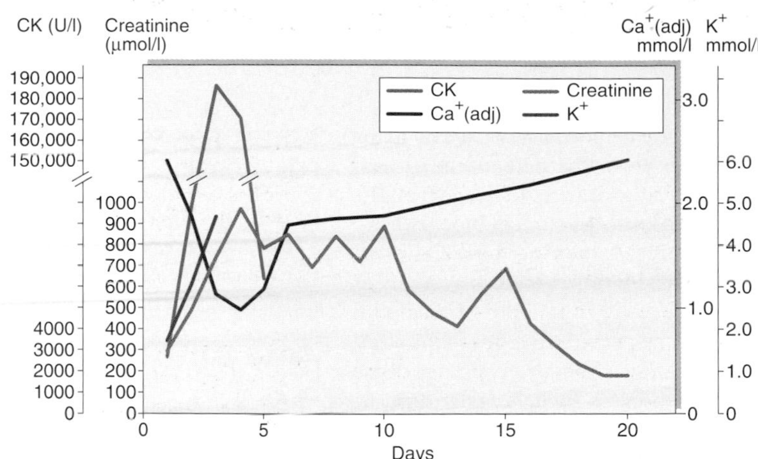

Fig. 3 **Biochemical results following rhabdomyolysis in a patient who had taken a drug overdose.**

Myoglobin itself is not nephrotoxic. Children with muscular dystrophy do not develop renal failure despite having increased levels of myoglobin in urine for many years.

Investigation and treatment

The biochemical tests which are of use in suspected rhabdomyolysis (Fig. 3) are:

- total creatine kinase in serum
- urine myoglobin
- serum potassium
- serum calcium
- serum creatinine.

Treatment is directed towards maintaining tissue perfusion and the control of electrolyte imbalances. It includes

- cardiac monitoring
- control of hyperkalaemia and hypocalcaemia.

Haemodialysis may be necessary where renal function is severely compromised.

OTHER CAUSES OF MYOGLOBINAEMIA AND MYOGLOBINURIA

Myoglobin is not specific for skeletal muscle and is also released following myocardial infarction, where it may be used as an early marker of myocardial damage (see pp. 48–49).

DUCHENNE MUSCULAR DYSTROPHY

This X-linked recessive disorder results from abnormalities in the dystrophin gene. Clinically, it is characterised by progressive muscle weakness, usually in boys, from the age of 5. Very high serum CK may precede the onset of symptoms but later in the disease the CK levels fall. Approximately 75% of female carriers also have raised CK levels.

Clinical note

Investigation of muscle weakness in an elderly patient should always include serum potassium, magnesium and calcium measurements. Hypokalaemia, hypocalcaemia and hypomagnesaemia may all develop insidiously. Correction can result in a dramatic improvement.

Case history 60

A 41-year-old labourer was admitted to hospital. He had collapsed and gave a four-day history of flu-like illness, with shivering, myalgia, headaches, dyspnoea, vomiting and diarrhoea.

Serum enzymes (on admission)

AST	ALT	LDH	CK
	U/l		
149	88	1330	6000

- What tissues could have contributed to the high serum enzymes activities?
- What tests may help identify the source(s) of enzyme elevation?

Comment on page 158.

Skeletal muscle disorders

- Muscle weakness is a common complaint with a wide variety of causes.
- Biochemical investigation of muscle weakness can provide rapid diagnosis and effective treatment where ionic changes are the cause.
- Intracellular enzyme analysis from muscle biopsies can provide a diagnosis in some inherited disorders.
- Severely damaged muscle cells release potassium, creatine kinase and myoglobin.
- Serum creatine kinase and myoglobin are frequently normal in patients with myopathy.
- Severe rhabdomyolysis, e.g. following injury, is an important cause of acute renal failure.

DNA DIAGNOSIS

Molecular genetics is a tool used by many disciplines and is the study of the expression and inheritance of genes at the molecular level. In clinical biochemistry this involves studying base pair sequence differences in the DNA. Analysis of a patient's DNA and the genes that it contains can provide diagnostic information. Mutations in single genes may cause inherited diseases such as cystic fibrosis, sickle cell anaemia, familial hypercholesterolaemia and Duchenne muscular dystrophy. Compound disorders involving several genes are thought to be important in common diseases such as coronary heart disease, diabetes mellitus and cancer.

THE HUMAN GENOME

Most of the human genome does not code for functional proteins; there are long untranslated regions between and even within genes. The genome is not identical from one person to the next, as on average every two hundredth base pair will be different. When a change occurs in the coding region, it may lead to the synthesis of an altered protein, defective in its function. Changes in the non-coding region are often neutral, but may be useful markers for the molecular geneticist. Recently, changes in non-coding DNA have been identified as the cause of such diseases as fragile X syndrome and myotonic dystrophy.

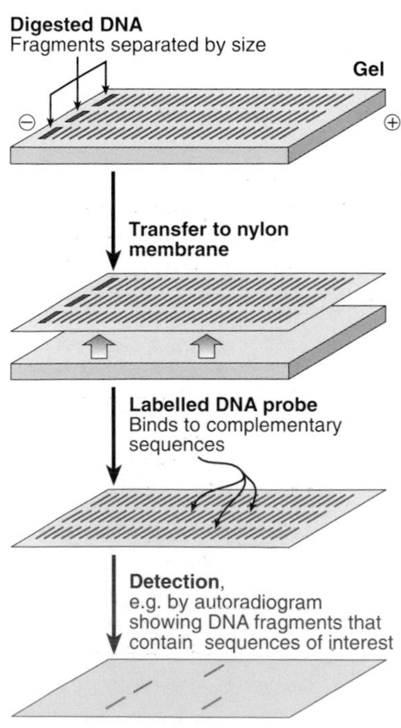

Fig. 1 **Southern blot analysis of human DNA.**

RESTRICTION FRAGMENT LENGTH POLYMORPHISMS

In the laboratory, DNA can be cut into small pieces by enzymes called restriction endonucleases. These enzymes are restricted to cutting the DNA at specific base pair sequences. The presence of polymorphic sites, where there are differences in the base pair sequence of the DNA, may create or abolish a cutting site for a particular restriction endonuclease. In these instances, the polymorphisms are known as *restriction fragment length polymorphisms* (RFLPs) as they lead to the production of DNA fragments of different lengths after enzyme action. DNA fragments may be separated by electrophoresis, transfered to a nylon membrane and hybridized with a DNA probe labelled with a radioactive or optically active marker. This is called Southern blot analysis (Fig. 1).

LINKAGE

In very few diseases, e.g. sickle cell anaemia, the mutation causing the disease occurs at a site which is recognized by a restriction enzyme. RFLP analysis is therefore immediately diagnostic. More commonly, however, the restriction site is not the mutation site. One then looks for a polymorphism in a restriction site which is close to the clinically important mutation site so that the two sites will remain linked during meiotic recombination. If the polymorphic restriction site and the mutation sought are closely linked then RFLP analysis will be highly informative, but as the distance between them increases the reliability of diagnosis decreases (Fig. 2).

VNTR POLYMORPHISM

RFLPs have the limitation that every individual has two copies of the relevant

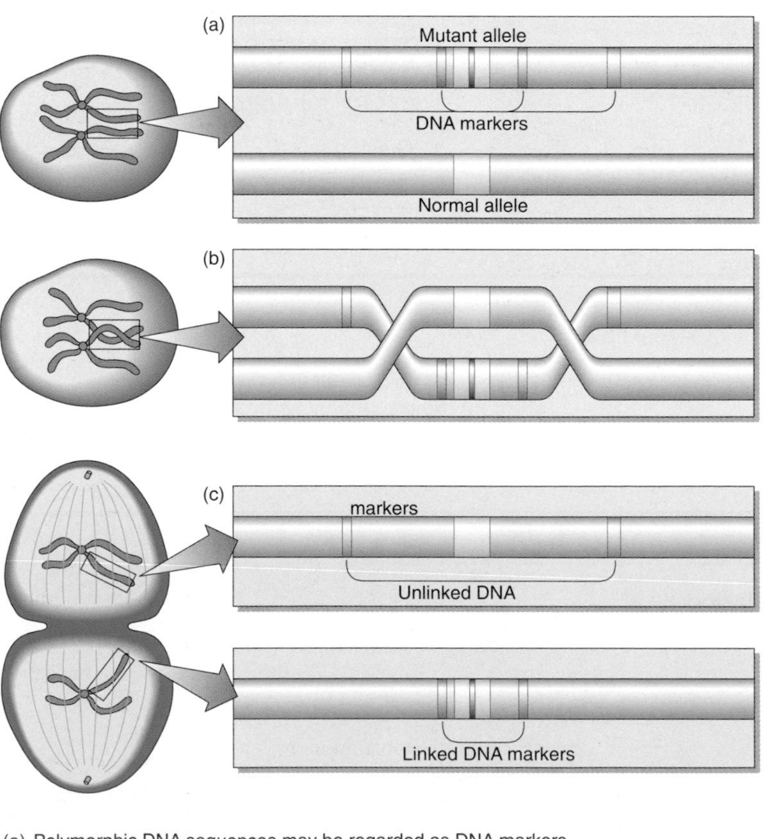

(a) Polymorphic DNA sequences may be regarded as DNA markers.

(b) During meiosis, chromatid crossover occurs and the DNA sequences are shuffled.

(c) Those markers that are physically close to the gene of interest remain linked, while those that are distant or on separate chromosomes are unlinked.

Fig. 2 **Linked and unlinked markers during meiotic recombination.**

section of the DNA (one inherited from each parent) and is either +/+ or +/- or -/- for the polymorphic site.

Another type of polymorphism is called a variable number tandem repeat (VNTR). Here the restriction sites flank a region of the genome whose length varies between individuals due to different numbers of copies of a specific sequence (a 'tandem repeat'). The restriction fragment pattern obtained using probes which identify different sequences is almost completely unique to an individual and can be used as a 'genetic fingerprint'.

POLYMERASE CHAIN REACTION

The polymerase chain reaction (PCR) (Fig. 3) has revolutionized the study of genes. PCR allows a small section of human genomic DNA to be amplified many times in the test tube. The technique is simple, fast, and requires as little as a single cell. DNA for analysis may be obtained from any nucleated cell; most commonly used are white blood cells, but hair roots, mouth scrapings or sperm can also be used. Such small samples have obvious advantages for prenatal and forensic diagnoses, but great care must be taken to avoid contamination with cells or DNA from the laboratory.

The primers chosen to amplify the DNA are identical to short lengths of the sequence of the genomic DNA which flank the area of interest. The double stranded DNA is first denatured by heating. Primers anneal to their complementary sequences and, by the action of DNA polymerase, extension occurs completing the first cycle. This newly synthesized DNA is also used as a template for the 2nd cycle and so on. By the 30th cycle, the region flanked by the two primers will have been amplified more than a million fold.

APPLICATIONS OF DNA DIAGNOSIS: CYSTIC FIBROSIS

Cystic fibrosis is relatively common, being encountered in 1/1600 Caucasian births. It is an autosomal recessive condition. Around one in twenty-two of the population are carriers, making the disease one of the most common serious genetic abnormalities. The disease affects exocrine secretions, and the onset of the disease may be at birth or later in childhood. Newborn screening has been largely unsuccessful, and traditional confirmation of the disease depended on the demonstration of an increased chloride concentration in a sample of sweat.

It is now possible to identify children who will be affected and also those who will be carriers so that genetic diagnoses and counselling can be given. The gene is on chromosome 7, and codes for a protein called cystic fibrosis transmembrane conductance regulator (CFTR). This regulates the function of a bicarbonate/chloride exchanger. DNA diagnosis of cystic fibrosis can be used in prenatal diagnosis. Furthermore, cystic fibrosis is now regarded as a target for gene therapy. This procedure in which missing or defective parts of the human genome are replaced or repaired heralds the beginning of a new era in medicine.

Other diseases in which DNA diagnosis could be of value include familial hypercholesterolaemia, alpha-1 antitrypsin deficiency, congenital adrenal hyperplasia and Wilson's disease.

Case history 61

A male infant has cystic fibrosis. He has two sisters and a brother. His mother and father are unrelated and appear well although his maternal uncle died as a child with the disease.

- Draw his family tree.
- How would this child have been diagnosed and how would you investigate his siblings?

Comment on page 158.

DNA diagnosis

- Analysis of a patient's DNA can provide the clinician with diagnostic information.
- The technology for studying DNA involves looking for the differences in the fragments formed when the DNA is digested by specific enzymes known as restriction endonucleases, or amplification of selected regions of the DNA by a technique called the polymerase chain reaction.
- Genetic analysis can now help diagnose children with cystic fibrosis and identify carriers of the disease.

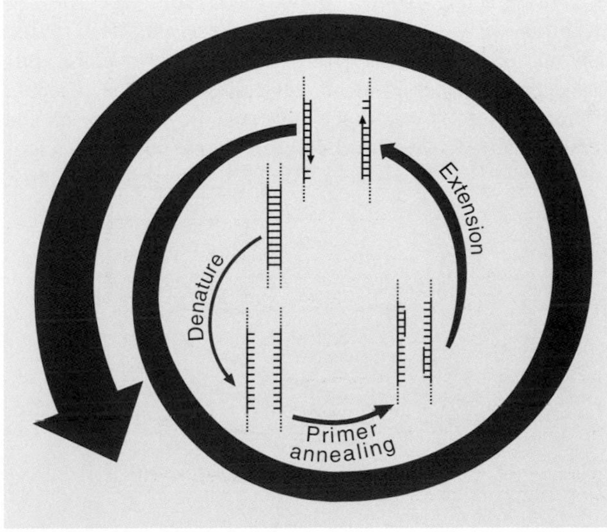

Fig. 3 **The polymerase chain reaction.**

Clinical note

In the investigation of inherited diseases, it is often useful to sketch a patient's family tree to illustrate at a glance his or her family history. The simple rules and conventions for constructing these diagrams are shown in Figure 4.

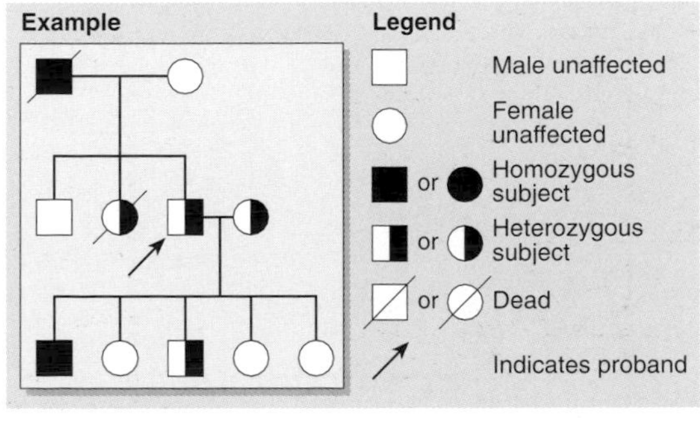

Fig. 4 **Family tree.**

FETAL MONITORING AND PRENATAL DIAGNOSIS

Biochemical tests have limited value in monitoring fetal development, but some components of maternal blood and urine and amniotic fluid may be measured to give evidence of pathology.

HUMAN CHORIONIC GONADOTROPHIN (HCG)

HCG is a glycoprotein produced by the chorionic cells of the developing embryo which is detectable by sensitive assays within days of conception. Measurement of HCG is used to confirm pregnancy, and forms the basis of pregnancy tests (p. 9). The protein's rapid rate of synthesis in early pregnancy provides systemic evidence of the blastocyst 24 h after implantation. HCG continues to be secreted by the developing placenta, and serum and urine concentrations increase during the first 9 weeks of pregnancy, then decline gradually until the third trimester (Fig. 1). The function of HCG is to maintain the activity of the corpus luteum, sustaining progesterone synthesis. Measurement of HCG is also of value in:

- Assessing fetal viability in threatened abortion.
- Detecting ectopic pregnancy. HCG fails to rise at the expected rate.
- Detecting and monitoring hydatidiform mole and choriocarcinoma. HCG may be used as a tumour marker for diagnosis and monitoring of these trophoblastic malignancies (pp. 130–131).

BIOCHEMICAL MONITORING OF FETOPLACENTAL FUNCTION

Human placental lactogen (HPL) is synthesized by the placenta. HPL concentration in maternal blood increases during pregnancy until term. It can be used to monitor placental function.

Oestriol is a steroid synthesized by the combined action of enzymes in the fetus and placenta. Concentration in maternal blood increases throughout pregnancy, and it can be assayed in maternal urine or blood. Oestriol was at one time commonly used to monitor fetoplacental function.

These two biochemical tests have been superseded by physical investigations such as ultrasound and cardiotocography.

PRENATAL DIAGNOSIS

Prenatal diagnostic techniques fall into two groups: invasive and non-invasive (Table 1). Prenatal diagnosis may be required because of increased risk of inherited disease. Neural tube defects cannot usually be predicted by family history, and pregnant women may be offered a screening test to detect these disorders.

Table 1 **Techniques for prenatal diagnosis**

Invasive	Amniocentesis Chorionic villus sampling Cordocentesis Fetoscopy Fetal skin biopsy Fetal liver biopsy
Non-invasive	Ultrasound Radiography

Alpha fetoprotein (AFP)

AFP is a small glycoprotein synthesized by the yolk sac and fetal liver and is a major fetal plasma protein. Because of its size it appears in fetal urine, and hence it is present in amniotic fluid and maternal blood. AFP concentrations increase in maternal blood until 32 weeks of gestation in a normal pregnancy (Fig. 2).

Detection of higher than normal AFP concentrations can suggest CNS defects such as anencephaly or spina bifida early in pregnancy, because such malformations of the neural tube are associated with leakage of plasma or CSF proteins into amniotic fluid and consequently maternal serum AFP concentrations increase. In some countries all pregnant women in antenatal care are given the opportunity to have their serum AFP measured between 16 and 18 weeks of gestation, with appropriate counselling. When a high result is obtained, the test must be repeated on a fresh sample. Once other possibilities for an elevated AFP, such as wrong dates or multiple pregnancies, have been excluded, an amniocentesis is performed and the AFP determined in amniotic fluid. High levels suggest the presence of a neural tube defect.

Amniotic fluid acetylcholinesterase (an enzyme found in high concentrations in neural tissue) is also used in some centres to detect fetal malformations.

Serum AFP and HCG concentrations and maternal age may be considered together to assess the risk that chromosomal disorders such as Down's syndrome are likely to be present. If the risk is high then amniocentesis may be performed to obtain cells for karyotyping.

Cells for study of inborn errors may be obtained either by biopsy of the chorionic villus, which is genetically identical to the fetus, or by culture of cells from amniotic fluid. The latter process takes 3–4 weeks. Both enzyme studies and, increasingly, DNA analysis may be carried out on these tissue samples.

Bilirubin

Bilirubin is measured in amniotic fluid to aid in the assessment of fetal risk in rhesus incompatibility. Incompatible red cell antigens can enter the maternal circulation either from the fetus at the time of delivery or, rarely, because of incompatible blood transfusion; specific red cell antibodies are stimulated in the mother. If, as in rhesus disease, the antibodies are IgG, they cross the placenta and react with specific antigens on the fetal red cell membrane causing haemolysis (Fig. 3). This is unusual in a first

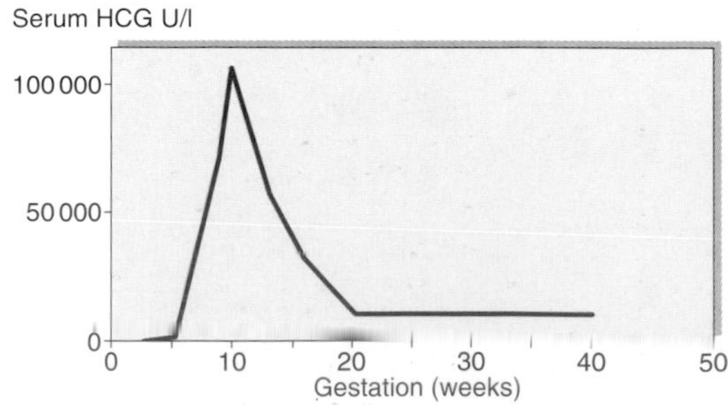

Fig. 1 **HCG concentration in maternal blood in early pregnancy.**

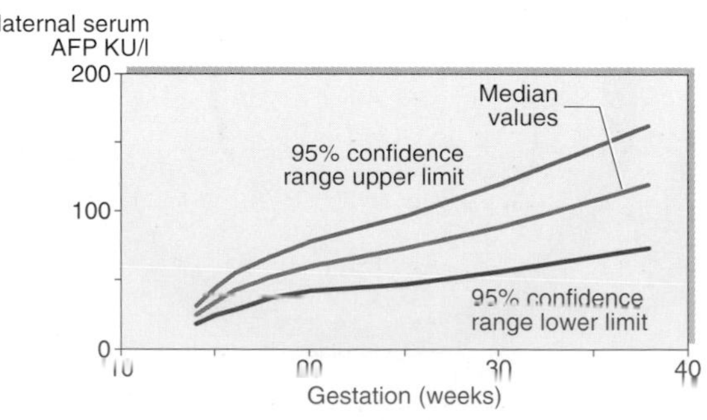

Fig. 2 **AFP in maternal blood during pregnancy.**

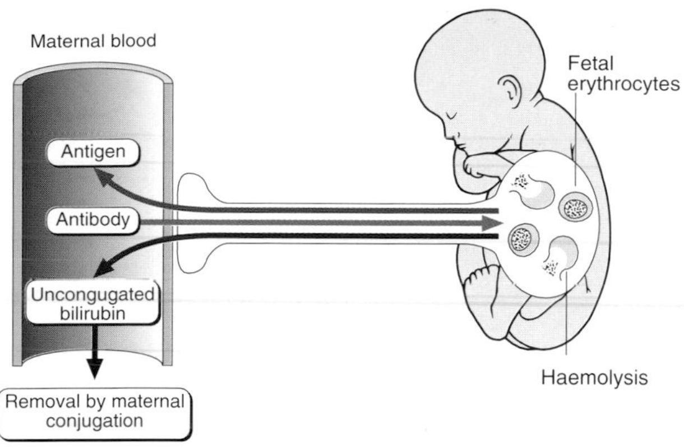

Fig. 3 **Hyperbilirubinaemia in rhesus incompatibility.**

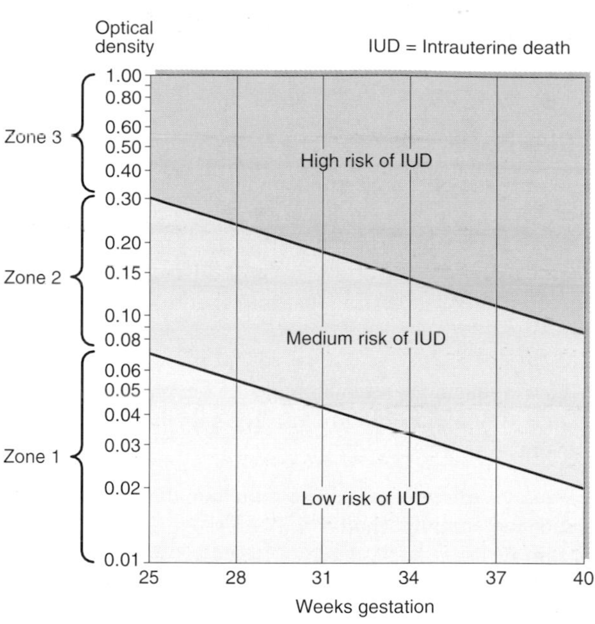

Fig. 4 **Liley graph.** Bilirubin absorbs light of 450 nm. The absorbance is directly related to its concentration and this enables the risk of intrauterine death to be estimated.

pregnancy but may be a feature of subsequent pregnancies. Excess breakdown of red cells leads to anaemia, overproduction of bilirubin and, eventually, oedema.

During fetal life, unconjugated bilirubin crosses the placenta and is removed by the mother, so the baby may not be born with obvious jaundice. However, the baby will rapidly become jaundiced in the days immediately after birth. In utero, the level of bilirubin in the amniotic fluid can be used to predict the severity of the fetal condition. Amniocentesis is performed on women who have previously had an affected fetus and on women who show a high and rising Rh titre. The severity of the problem can be assessed by reference to a nomogram which relates bilirubin levels to gestational age, such as that in Figure 4. Fetal exchange blood transfusion or early delivery may be considered.

Rhesus incompatibility is much less common nowadays since susceptible women are given an intravenous injection of anti-rhesus antibody at the time of delivery to eliminate fetal red blood cells which may have entered the maternal circulation. As a consequence they do not survive long enough to be recognized as foreign antigens in the mother. However, haemolytic disease of the newborn cannot be completely eliminated, because it may be caused by other blood group incompatibilities.

Phospholipids

In the immature lung, failure of surfactant production leads to the respiratory distress syndrome (see p. 148). This was the major cause of death in premature babies and is still the major indication for assisted ventilation. In certain circumstances, it is necessary to know if the fetal lungs are mature, and to assess the feasibility of an early delivery. The ratio of lecithin to sphingomyelin in amniotic fluid is measured and a ratio < 2 indicates immaturity. The absence of phosphatidyl glycerol also indicates that the lungs are not mature. These tests are rarely used now that surfactant is available as a treatment for at risk babies and gestational age can be accurately assessed by ultrasound.

Fetal blood gases

Hydrogen ion concentration, blood gases and serum lactate concentration can be measured in fetal blood. Such measurements are only requested when non-invasive investigations have indicated that the fetus is at risk. Fetal blood can be obtained by the technique of cordocentesis, where the blood is sampled from the umbilical cord through a fine needle inserted through the abdomen under ultrasound guidance.

Hydrogen ion concentration can also be measured in fetal blood to assess fetal distress during labour. Capillary blood samples can be obtained directly from the baby's scalp once the cervix is sufficiently dilated. Fetal hypoxia causes a lactic acidosis and elevated hydrogen ion concentration. Measurement of fetal PO_2 can be obtained directly using a transcutaneous oxygen electrode.

Case history 62

A 30-year-old woman who had previously delivered one live child and had one miscarriage attended for antenatal care. She was known to be rhesus negative. At 30 weeks gestation she was found to have a high titre of anti-D antibodies.

- What investigations are needed now?

Comment on page 158.

Clinical note

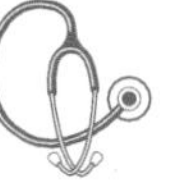

Fetal ultrasound scanning, related to time of conception and/or sequential measurements, has become the best way of monitoring fetal growth. This technique has superseded many biochemical tests of fetal well-being which were once commonly performed.

Fetal monitoring and prenatal diagnosis

- Confirmation of pregnancy is by detection of human chorionic gonadotrophin in maternal urine.
- Elevated concentrations of alpha fetoprotein in maternal blood and amniotic fluid may indicate the presence of a fetus with a neural tube defect.
- Amniotic fluid bilirubin measurements are of value in the detection of risk in rhesus incompatibility.

PREGNANCY

MATERNAL PHYSIOLOGY

Maternal physiology changes so dramatically during pregnancy that reference ranges for biochemical tests in non-pregnant women are often not applicable. The main differences in the commonly requested tests are shown in Table 1. These differences should not be misinterpreted as indicating that some pathology is present.

Weight gain

The mean weight gain in pregnancy is 12.5 kg, but there is a very large standard deviation (about 4 kg). The gain in weight is made up of several components:

- *The products of conception.* These include the fetus, placenta and amniotic fluid.
- *Maternal fat stores.* These may account for up to 25% of the weight increase.
- *Maternal water retention.* Total body water increases by about 5 litres, mostly in the extracellular fluid. The volume of the intravascular compartment increases by more than a litre.

Respiratory function

Mild hyperventilation occurs from early pregnancy, probably due to a centrally mediated effect of progesterone, and PCO_2 falls. However, blood hydrogen ion concentration is maintained within non-pregnant limits, since the plasma bicarbonate falls due to an increased renal excretion of bicarbonate. Oxygen consumption increases by about 20%, but PO_2 is relatively unchanged.

Renal function

Because of increases in plasma volume and cardiac output, renal blood flow increases. The GFR rises early in pregnancy, and creatinine clearance may be 150 ml/min or more by 30 weeks. Serum urea and creatinine concentrations fall. Tubular function alters and, in particular, there is a reduction in the renal threshold for glucose. Glycosuria may be present in up to 70% of pregnancies. Tubular reabsorption of uric acid and amino acids alters, and their excretion in urine increases.

Carbohydrate metabolism

The fasting blood glucose falls early in pregnancy, probably because of substrate utilization. The response to a standard carbohydrate challenge is altered in late pregnancy.

Protein metabolism

Serum albumin concentration falls gradually from early pregnancy and this is related to ECF expansion. The concentrations of many other proteins increase, particularly placental proteins such as alkaline phosphatase of placental origin, transport proteins such as transferrin, hormone-binding glycoproteins such as thyroxine-binding globulin, and fibrinogen.

Hormonal changes

Oestrogens and progesterone are secreted in greater amounts early in pregnancy, and protein hormones such as HCG and HPL are produced by the placenta.

PREGNANCY ASSOCIATED PATHOLOGY

Morbidity during pregnancy may be due to pre-existing medical conditions in the mother such as diabetes mellitus, hypertension, renal disease, thyrotoxicosis, or due to pregnancy-associated conditions.

Table 1 **Reference ranges in the third trimester of pregnancy, and how they compare with non-pregnant controls**

Serum / blood measurements	Pregnant	Non-pregnant
Sodium (mmol/l)	132–140	135–145
Potassium (mmol/l)	3.2–4.6	3.4–4.9
Chloride (mmol/l)	97–107	95–105
Bicarbonate (mmol/l)	18–28	21–28
Urea (mmol/l)	1.0–3.8	2.5–8.0
Glucose (fasting) (mmol/l)	3.0–5.0	4.0–5.5
Calcium (mmol/l)	2.2–2.8	2.2–2.6
Magnesium (mmol/l)	0.6–0.8	0.7–1.0
Albumin (g/l)	32–42	40–52
Bilirubin (μmol/l)	3–14	3–22
Alanine aminotransferase (U/l)	3–28	3–55
Aspartate aminotransferase (U/l)	3–31	12–48
Alkaline phosphatase (U/l)	175–400	80–280
Blood H^+ (nmol/l)	34–42	35–45
Blood PCO_2 (kPa)	3.0–5.0	4.4–5.6

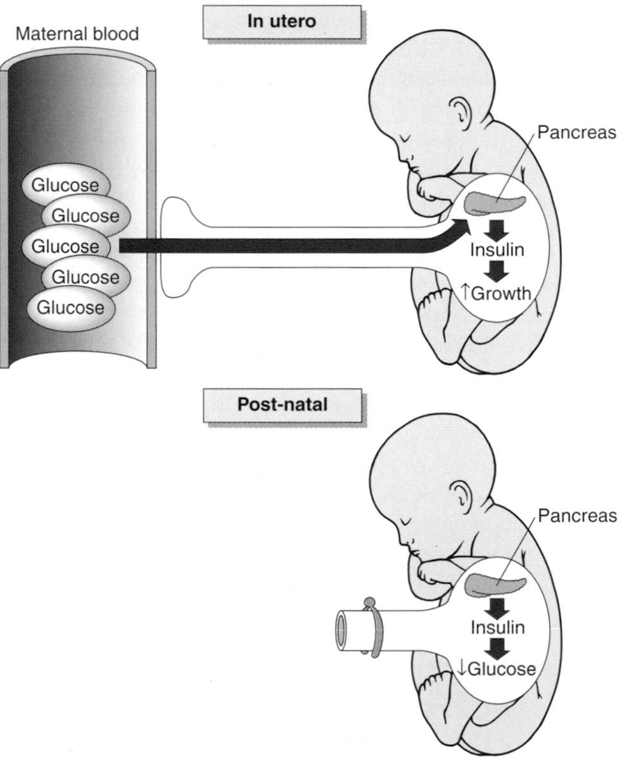

Fig. 1 **Diabetes mellitus in pregnancy is associated with fetal hyperinsulinaemia.** In utero this leads to increased growth, while post-natally the persisting hyperinsulinaemia causes neonatal hypoglycaemia.

Diabetic pregnancy

Pregnancy in a diabetic patient, whether she is known to be diabetic before pregnancy or when diabetes mellitus manifests itself during pregnancy, is associated with increased fetal mortality and morbidity. Maternal hyperglycaemia promotes hyperinsulinism in the fetus (Fig. 1). Insulin is a growth factor, and babies of poorly controlled diabetic patients are large and bloated. Adequate control of diabetes mellitus during pregnancy decreases complications. The baby of a diabetic mother has an increased probability of developing respiratory distress syndrome.

Increased frequency of micturition, and glycosuria, may cause concern that a pregnant woman has developed diabetes during pregnancy. These findings are common and do not necessarily indicate pathology.

Hypertension

The patient who develops hypertension in pregnancy—a condition described variously as pre-eclampsia or pregnancy-induced hypertension—is at increased risk of placental insufficiency and consequent fetal intrauterine growth retardation. The hypertension is thought to be the causative factor of eclampsia, a severe illness which usually occurs in the second half of pregnancy and is characterized by generalized convulsions, extreme hypertension and impaired renal function including proteinuria. This disease is a significant cause of maternal death, which occurs most commonly as a result of cerebral haemorrhage.

The features of pre-eclampsia are shown in Figure 2. Diagnosis depends on several of these features being present. The hypertension and a rising serum urate concentration are encountered early in the development of the condition. The aetiology of the vasoconstriction which is responsible for the hypertension is not known. Fluid retention which leads to oedema is often, but not always, a feature. As most women with normal pregnancies have oedema by term, this is not diagnostic of pre-eclampsia. There is a greater chance of pre-eclampsia in the patient who was known to be hypertensive before becoming pregnant.

It is important to monitor blood pressure, serum urate, 24 h protein excretion in urine, creatinine clearance and also to assess fetoplacental function. Pre-eclampsia may progress very rapidly and medical treatment is of limited value. The only action which will reverse pre-eclampsia is delivery of the baby. Frequently it is difficult to decide on the optimum time for delivery which is best for both mother and child.

Drugs in pregnancy

Many women have, of necessity, to continue to take drugs during pregnancy. No drugs are without risk to the developing fetus, and drug levels should be kept as low as possible during gestation and thereafter if the mother is breast feeding, since many drugs are secreted in breast milk. Of particular concern are anticonvulsant drugs. Careful monitoring of levels is necessary to steer between the dangers of maternal seizures and potential fetal damage from the drug.

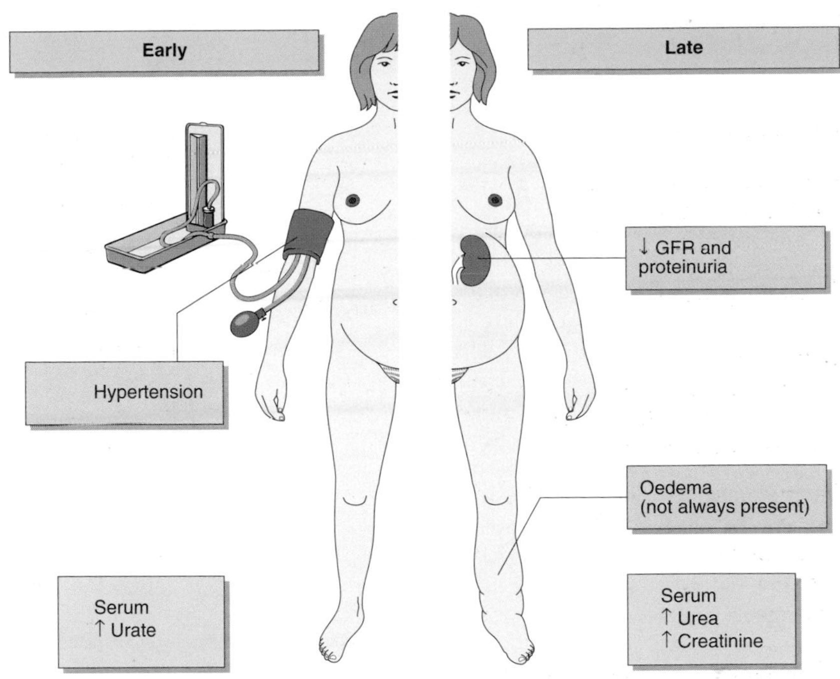

Fig. 2 **Clinical features of pre-eclampsia.**

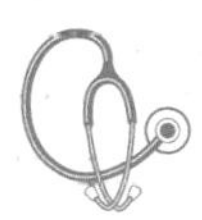

Clinical note

Pregnancy is the commonest cause of amenorrhoea in a woman of reproductive age. A pregnancy test should always be performed before other endocrine investigations of the cause of absent menstrual bleeding.

Case history 63

A 20-year-old woman in her first pregnancy was referred to hospital by her GP when she was 31 weeks pregnant. At 12 weeks pregnant she appeared well, had no oedema and her blood pressure was 110/70 mmHg. Now, she complained that she was unable to remove her wedding ring and that her vision was blurred. On examination ankle oedema was also observed and her blood pressure was found to be 180/110 mmHg.

- What is the most likely diagnosis?
- What sideroom test(s) should be performed?
- What biochemical investigations should be performed immediately?

Comment on page 159.

Pregnancy

- Physiological changes occur in pregnancy, altering many biochemical reference ranges. Do not be misled into believing that they indicate pathology.
- Diabetes in pregnancy is associated with increased fetal mortality and morbidity. Good diabetic control during pregnancy decreases complications. The baby of a diabetic mother has an increased probability of developing respiratory distress syndrome.
- Hypertension and a rising serum urate concentration are early features in the development of pre-eclampsia, a rapidly progressing condition which carries considerable risk to mother and fetus.

SCREENING THE NEWBORN FOR DISEASE

NEONATAL SCREENING PROGRAMMES

Many countries have programmes to screen for diseases at birth. A blood sample is collected from every baby around the seventh day of life. Capillary blood sampling in the neonate is best performed on the plantar aspect of the foot, especially on the medial aspect of the posterior third, as shown in Figure 1. A 'blood spot' is collected on to a thick filter paper card (Fig. 2). The specimen can be conveniently sent by mail to a central screening laboratory. The following questions are usually considered when discussing the cost-effectiveness of a screening programme.

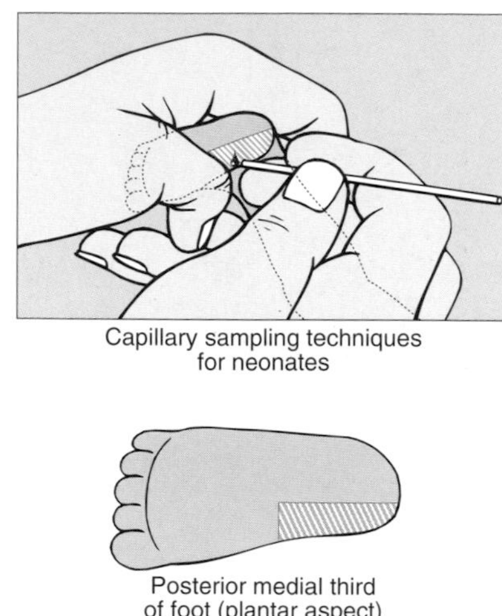

Fig. 1 **Capillary blood sampling in neonates.**

PKU BLOOD TEST
Print in Pencil or Ballpoint Pen
Baby's Name ______
Home Address ______
District Health Board ______
Place of Birth if not as above ______
G.P. Name ______
Address ______
Date of Birth ______ Sex ______
Date of Specimen ______
Date of first milk feeding ______
Type of feeding – Bottle ☐ Breast ☐
Tick if baby is premature ☐
FILL CIRCLES RIGHT THROUGH WITH BLOOD
○ ○ ○ ○

Fig. 2 **Filter paper card ('Guthrie card') for the collection of 'blood spots.'**

- Does the disease have a relatively high incidence?
- Can the disease be detected within days of birth?
- Can the disease be identified by a biochemical marker which can be easily measured?
- Will the disease be missed clinically, and would this cause irreversible damage to the baby?
- Is the disease treatable, and will the result of the screening test be available before any irreversible damage to the baby has occurred?

Neonatal screening programmes for hypothyroidism and phenylketonuria have been established in many countries. Both these disorders carry the risk of impaired mental development, which can be prevented by prompt recognition of the disease. Local factors, such as population mix, lead to the setting up of specific screening programmes. For example, the high incidence of congenital adrenal hyperplasia (1:500 live births) among the Yupik Eskimo is the stimulus for a screening programme for this disease in Alaska. In Finland, the incidence of phenylketonuria is low and neonatal screening is not carried out.

Disagreement on the benefits and risks of tests, the presence of public pressure and availability of funding are factors which continue to determine whether neonatal screening programmes are established.

Congenital hypothyroidism

Primary hypothyroidism is present in one in every three thousand five hundred births in the UK. There is often no clinical evidence at birth that the baby is abnormal, yet if congenital hypothyroidism is unrecognized and untreated, affected children develop irreversible mental retardation and the characteristic features of cretinism (Fig. 3). Most cases of congenital hypothyroidism are due to thyroid gland dysgenesis, the failure of the thyroid gland to develop properly during early embryonic growth. The presence of a high blood TSH concentration is the basis of the screening test (Fig. 4).

A positive result of a screening test should be confirmed by demonstration of an elevated TSH in a serum specimen obtained from the infant. When necessary, thyroxine treatment should be initiated as soon as possible after diagnosis. The initial dosage is 10 μg/kg and this can be gradually increased during childhood to the adult dosage of 100–200 μg per day by 12 years of age. The absence of clinical signs of hypothyroidism or hyperthyroidism, together with normal serum T_4 and TSH concentrations, provides evidence of the adequacy of treatment.

If a positive screening test is obtained, the mother's thyroid function is usually also assessed. Maternal autoantibodies can cross the placenta and block receptor sites on the fetal thyroid. In this rare situation, after an initial transient hypothyroidism just after birth, the baby's own thyroid function will usually develop normally.

TSH screening does not detect secondary hypothyroidism due to pituitary disease. This is a much rarer disorder than primary hypothyroidism, occurring in one in every one hundred thousand births.

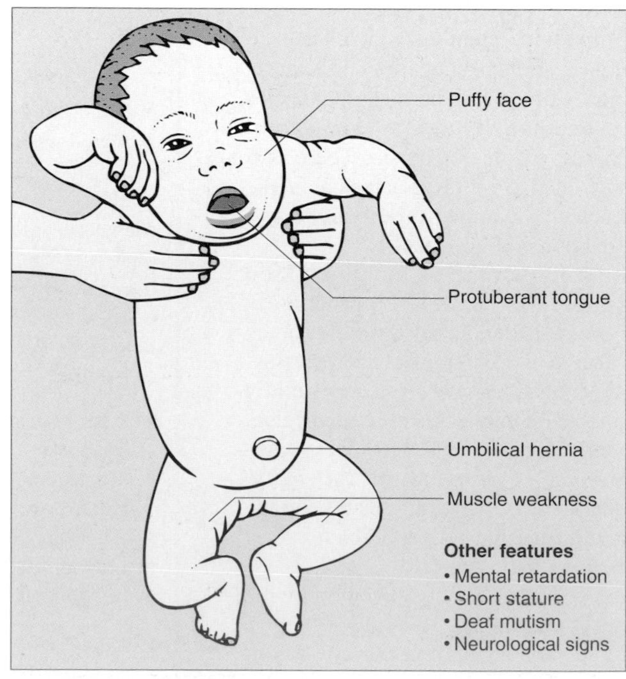

Fig. 3 **Features of cretinism.**

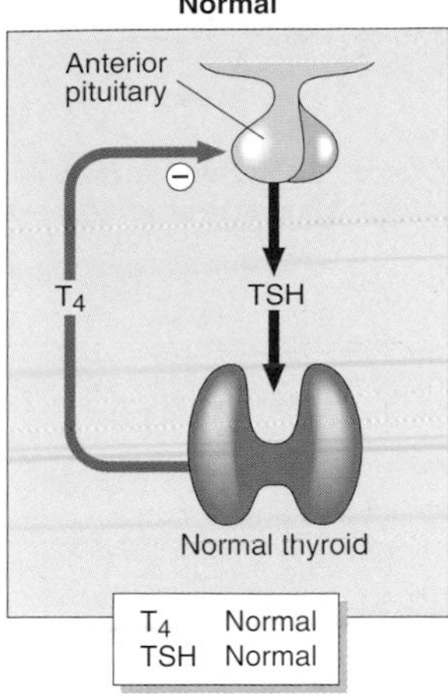

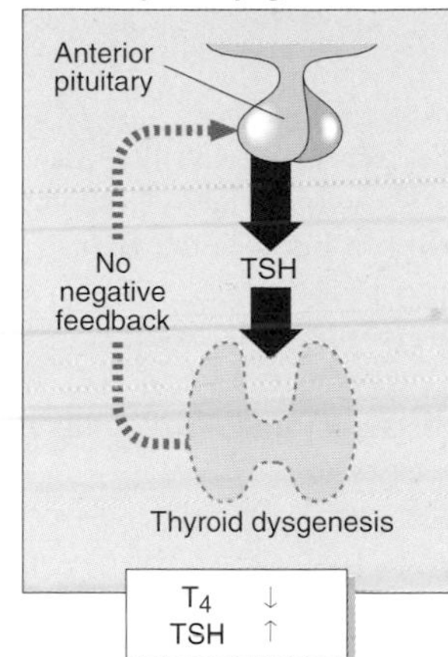

Fig. 4 **Control of TSH secretion.**

term which better describes the group of disorders.

The detection of phenylketonuria was the first screening programme to be established. The screening test is based on the detection of increased phenylalanine concentration in the blood spot.

The mainstay of the management of phenylketonuria is to reduce the plasma phenylalanine concentration by dietary control. Mental retardation is not present at birth, and can be prevented from occurring if plasma phenylalanine concentrations are kept low in the early years of life. It was thought that dietary control need only be followed for ten years or so but current views are that lifelong therapy is necessary.

Phenylketonuria

The incidence of phenylketonuria is around one in every ten thousand births in the UK. Phenylketonuria arises from impaired conversion of phenylalanine to tyrosine, usually because of a deficiency of phenylalanine hydroxylase. Figure 5 shows how phenylalanine, an essential amino acid, is metabolized. In phenylketonuria, phenylalanine cannot be converted to tyrosine, accumulates in blood and is excreted in the urine. The main urinary metabolite is phenylpyruvic acid (a 'phenylketone') which gives the disease its name. The clinical features include:

- irritability, poor feeding, vomiting and fitting in the first weeks of life
- mental retardation
- eczema
- reduced melanin formation in the skin, resulting in the classical fair haired, blue eyed appearance.

Phenylalanine hydroxylase uses tetrahydrobiopterin (BH4) as a cofactor. Defective BH4 supply or regeneration, due to deficiency of dihydropteridine reductase, have been identified as rare causes of 'hyperphenylalaninaemia', a

FOLLOW-UP OF SCREENING TESTS

A positive or equivocal result in a screening test should be followed up rapidly and efficiently. A clearly positive result will require immediate referral to a paediatrician. Requests for a repeat specimen because the result was borderline, or there was insufficient sample, or the analysis was unsatisfactory, must be handled tactfully. Parents frequently find it distressing if their child is suspected of a serious disorder even if subsequently the baby is found to be normal.

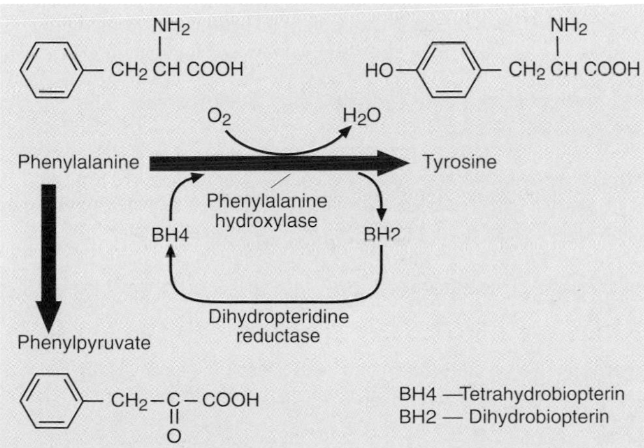

Fig. 5 **Metabolism of phenylalanine.**

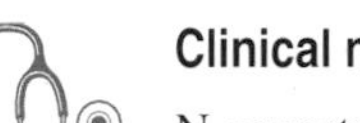

Clinical note

N-aspartylphenylalanine methyl ester (aspartame) is a commonly used artificial sweetener. It is broken down in the gut to phenylalanine. Patients with phenylketonuria must avoid any food containing this additive. It is particularly important that foodstuffs, including soft drinks, should be clearly labelled with a warning that they contain this artificial sweetener.

Case history 64

The 'blood spot' analysis on a 6-day-old baby girl indicated a high TSH, 28 mU/l. A second blood sample was quickly obtained for a repeat TSH estimation. The laboratory reported a TSH concentration of 6 mU/l.

- What further investigations should be carried out?

Comment on page 159.

Screening the newborn for disease

- In some countries screening programmes have been established to detect specific diseases in babies.
- Analyses are performed on blood spots obtained around one week after birth.
- Common diseases tested for in this way are congenital hypothyroidism and phenylketonuria.
- For it to be worthwhile to screen for a disorder the disease should have a relatively high incidence, be detectable within days of birth, result in serious consequences if missed clinically, and be treatable.

INHERITED DISORDERS

The feature of all inherited disorders is a genetic defect, often the result of a single base substitution or deletion in the DNA, which results in the reduced synthesis of a particular protein or in the synthesis of a protein with an altered amino acid composition. A classical inborn error of metabolism involves a missing or defective enzyme which causes a block on a metabolic pathway and the production of toxic metabolites. More than four thousand disorders involving single genes have been identified.

Inherited disorders may be detected at different stages during life:

- Heterozygote carriers of a disease may be found during screening, such as on family members of a patient with muscular dystrophy.
- Some inherited disorders can be detected before birth. The prenatal diagnosis of cystic fibrosis is described on pages 138–139.
- Neonatal screening can identify some disorders, such as phenylketonuria, in the newborn baby in the first days of life (pp. 144–145).
- Many disorders involving a single gene defect become apparent in the neonate, symptoms developing in the first week of life.
- Disorders such as familial hypercholesterolaemia (pp. 122–123) may not be recognized until adult life.

THE CHILD WHO FAILS TO THRIVE

The inherited disorders which are diagnosed in the first weeks of life usually involve central metabolic pathways such as amino acid metabolism, carbohydrate metabolism and storage, organic acid metabolism, steroid hormone biosynthesis or the urea cycle. Symptoms are often non-specific, e.g. vomiting, lethargy, poor feeding, fitting and hypotonia. Features which suggest the presence of an inherited disorder are shown in Table 1.

Table 1 **Clinical and biochemical features which strongly suggest presence of an inherited disorder**

Feature	Disorder
Unusual odour	Amino acid and organic acid defects
Cataracts	Galactosaemia
Metabolic acidosis and hyperventilation	Organic acid defects
Hyponatraemia	Congenital adrenal hyperplasia
Neurological dysfunction	Urea cycle defects

There may be information in the family history, perhaps even the death of a previous child.

Malformation in a newborn baby usually indicates either a genetic abnormality, or infection or drug exposure in utero. However, dysmorphism may also

Table 2 **Selected inherited disorders**

Disorder	Main feature
Acute intermittent porphyria	The porphyrias are disorders of haem biosynthesis. The acute porphyrias which present with abdominal pain and neurological features all have increased urinary porphobilinogen during an attack, and this is diagnostic
Adrenoleucodystrophy	This rare neurodegenerative disease is characterized by the impaired metabolism and subsequent accumulation of long chain fatty acids in plasma and tissues
Agammaglobulinaemia	There is a complete absence of immunoglobulin production. Selective IgA deficiency is more common with affected children presenting with recurrent respiratory infections
Alpha 1-antitrypsin deficiency	Patients with deficiency of the protease inhibitor, alpha 1-antitrypsin, may present with liver disease in childhood or with pulmonary emphysema in adults. All patients with genotypes associated with low alpha 1-antitrypsin in the serum are likely to develop emphysema if they smoke or are exposed to environmental pollutants
Biotinidase deficiency	A failure of biotin recycling results in an organic aciduria, developmental delay, seizures, alopecia, hypotonia and hearing loss
Congenital adrenal hyperplasia	This name is given to disorders of the enzymes involved in steroid hormone biosynthesis. The most common is lack of the 21 hydroxylase on the pathways which lead to cortisol and aldosterone (pp. 86–87)
Cystic fibrosis	See pages 138–139
Cystinuria	An increased excretion of the amino acids cystine, lysine, arginine and ornithine leads to an increased incidence of renal calculi. A defective carrier protein causes impaired renal tubular reabsorption of these amino acids from the glomerular filtrate
Cystinosis	This is a lysosomal storage disorder where there is a defect in the membrane transport of cystine. Cystine crystals are deposited in kidney, liver, spleen, bone marrow and cornea
Familial hypercholesterolaemia	See pages 122–123
Galactosaemia	This defect is present in approximately 1:100 000 babies in the UK. A deficiency of galactose 1-phosphate uridyl transferase means that the baby cannot utilize the galactose component of the lactose which is present in milk. Such infants may present with failure to thrive, vomiting and diarrhoea and if untreated may die in the neonatal period or go on to develop liver disease, mental retardation, cataracts and renal tubular damage

be related to the presence of an inherited metabolic disorder.

Basic biochemical tests may provide clues. Unexplained hypoglycaemia, hypocalcaemia, acid-base disturbances or liver dysfuncation indicate the need for further investigations. The diagnosis of an infection does not preclude the presence of an inherited metabolic disorder; sepsis commonly accompanies a metabolic defect.

In the severely ill infant, measurements of serum ammonia and lactate, urinary organic acids, urinary and serum amino acids and erythrocyle galactose 1-phosphate uridyl transferase will be required. If the baby has a problem which is apparent intermittently, then blood and urine should be collected for analysis during the acute phase.

Although, individually, inherited metabolic disorders are rare, collectively they present a major problem in management. The biochemical basis of disorders encompasses the breadth of metabolism and there is a multitude of specialized tests which are used to confirm the diagnosis. The specialist laboratory is the source of advice and assistance if an inherited defect is suspected.

Selected inherited disorders are outlined alphabetically in Table 2.

Clinical note

The diagnosis of many inherited disorders relies heavily on laboratory investigations. However, the presenting features of many inborn errors of metabolism are so non-specific that there is no substitute for the alert clinician in their detection. All newborn infants who are sick must be considered at risk of a genetic disorder.

Inherited disorders

- Inherited disorders are caused by gene defects which result in the synthesis of a reduced amount of a particular protein, or in the synthesis of a protein with an altered amino acid composition.
- An 'inborn error of metabolism' involves a missing or deficient enzyme which causes a block on a metabolic pathway.
- There are more than 4000 single gene defects, many of them rare, but collectively they present a challenge to both clinician and clinical biochemist.
- Some inherited disorders present in the first few weeks of life with non-specific symptoms.

Table 2 *Continued*

Disorder	Main feature
Glucose-6-phosphate dehydrogenase deficiency	This is an X-linked disorder associated with neonatal jaundice on the 2nd or 3rd day of life and drug-induced haemolytic crises (p. 149)
Glycogen storage disease (type I: von Gierke's)	Deficiency of glucose-6-phosphatase makes the glycogen stores of the body inaccessible. Children with this disorder have hepatomegaly and hypoglycaemia accompanied by hyperlipidaemia and lactic acidosis
Haemochromatosis	See pages 106–107
Homocystinuria	A deficiency of the enzyme cystathionine synthase leads to the accumulation of sulphur-containing amino acids. Affected children are normal at birth but develop eye problems, osteoporosis and mental retardation
Lesch-Nyhan syndrome	This is a severe form of hypoxanthine–guanine phosphoribosyltransferase deficiency, an enzyme involved in the metabolism of the purine bases (pp. 134–135)
Maple syrup urine disease	This defect in the decarboxylation of branched chain amino acids such as leucine, isoleucine and valine leads to severe brain damage and death during the first year of life
Mucopolysaccharidoses	This group of disorders is characterized by tissue accumulation of glycosaminoglycans such as heparin sulphate and dermatan sulphate. This results in skeletal deformities, mental retardation and premature death
Multiple endocrine neoplasias	See pages 132–133
Muscular dystrophy	See pages 136–137
Phenylketonuria	See pages 144–145
Propionic acidaemia	This is caused by deficiency of enzymes involved in the metabolism of propionyl coenzyme A
Urea cycle defects	Deficiency of enzymes of the urea cycle results in a build up of ammonia in the blood. Severe cases are often fatal in the first few days after birth
Vitamin D dependent rickets	See pages 70–71
Wilson's disease	This causes variable neurological and hepatic symptoms as a consequence of copper toxicity (pp. 108–109).

PAEDIATRIC BIOCHEMISTRY

The transition from intrauterine life to an independent existence requires changes in many biochemical systems. Mature function may not be attained for weeks, months or even years after birth.

RESPIRATORY FUNCTION

At birth the lungs must take over from the placenta as the organ where gas exchange takes place. 'Blood gases' are quite different in the fetus and in the newborn baby.

Fetal haemoglobin has a high oxygen affinity and the oxygen dissociation curve is moved to the left, which favours maternal–fetal transfer of oxygen (Fig.1). The fetal PO_2 is only about 4.6 kPa. However, there is a higher concentration of haemoglobin in fetal blood than in the adult, so that oxygen transport and tissue oxygenation are efficient. Maternal PCO_2 is lower than in the non-pregnant state, and fetal PCO_2 is higher, about 6.5 kPa. The fetal [H^+] is around 56 nmol/l.

During labour, the fetus can tolerate some degree of hypoxia and acidosis. The first respiratory movements inflate the lungs, and if they are mature and have adequate surfactant, there is a tenfold reduction in pulmonary vascular resistance. Gaseous exchange is quickly established so that PO_2 rises and PCO_2 falls.

Respiratory distress syndrome is caused by lack of surfactant (Fig. 2) and results from failure of alveolar expansion and subsequent alveolar collapse, decreased compliance and ventilation/perfusion abnormalities. Hypoventilation produces a respiratory acidosis, and hypoxaemia leads to a metabolic acidosis. The more immature the baby, the greater is the risk of respiratory distress syndrome.

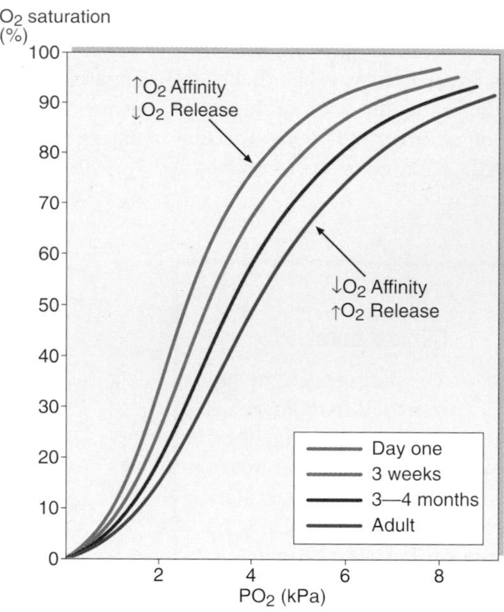

Fig. 1 **Oxygen dissociation curves for fetal and maternal haemoglobin.** At low PO_2 the fetal Hb delivers more oxygen to the tissues. For this reason the neonate can survive levels of hypoxia which would not be possible in an adult.

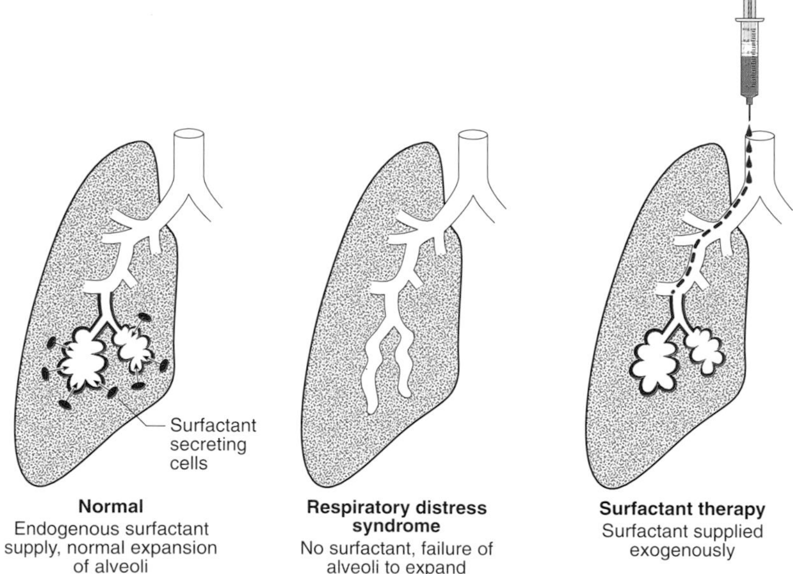

Fig. 2 **Surfactant and respiratory distress syndrome.**

RENAL FUNCTION

All glomeruli are formed by 36 weeks gestation, but because of reduced renal blood flow, the glomerular filtration rate is reduced at birth. Serum creatinine rises in the first few weeks of life and then falls at about 4 weeks and remains low for 5 years, when it gradually increases to adult levels.

Proximal tubular function is immature, and bicarbonate and glucose reabsorption is reduced. This leads to a low serum bicarbonate concentration. Glycosuria and aminoaciduria may be found in the normal neonate. A baby's ability to concentrate urine is poor. A urine osmolality of 600 mmol/kg is the maximum that can be produced. In the neonatal period, the kidney's ability to excrete water and electrolytes is limited. Thus, great care must be taken in the provision of intravenous fluids.

FLUID AND ELECTROLYTE BALANCE

The total body water of a newborn baby is around 75% of body weight, compared with 60% in the adult (Fig. 3). In the first week of life, the ECF contracts and this contributes to the weight loss which occurs normally at this time. By one year of age, the total body water is 60% and ECF 25% of body weight. It follows that fluids prescribed to sick children must be related to age and, particularly, to body weight.

Infants are very vulnerable to water loss because their renal tubular function is not fully mature. In addition, they are prone to fluid loss via the gastrointestinal tract due to diarrhoea. The dehydrated child is relatively more water depleted than sodium depleted because of the immature tubular function and larger body surface area relative to body weight.

Fluid depletion may be assessed by knowledge of clinical history and by clinical examination.

Mild dehydration, such as that caused by gastroenteritis, is often treated orally with solutions containing glucose and

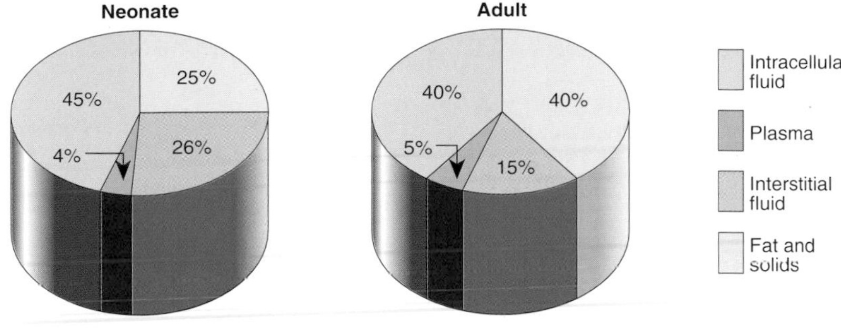

Fig. 3 **Body composition (% of bodyweight) in the neonate and adult.**

electrolytes. If the child is moderately or severely dehydrated, intravenous fluids may be required. The volume of fluid and the speed with which it is given will depend on the clinical condition. For example, dehydration due to severe diarrhoea may require urgent correction and plasma volume expansion.

The response to treatment must be carefully monitored by assessing fluid balance, urine output and state of hydration at frequent intervals. Body weight is a good simple index of hydration and should be regularly measured.

LIVER FUNCTION

The liver of a newborn baby may not be capable of conjugating all the bilirubin presented to it. The consequence is neonatal jaundice, and many babies become jaundiced during the first week of life. In full-term babies this usually resolves rapidly. In premature babies whose liver function is not fully mature the jaundice may be more severe and the bilirubin concentration takes longer to fall.

Jaundice during the first 24 hours of life is always pathological and most probably due to blood group incompatibility or infection. When there is increased destruction of red blood cells, as in rhesus or ABO incompatibility, there is an increase in unconjugated bilirubin. Unconjugated bilirubin binds to albumin, and when the albumin is saturated, the excess which is lipophilic is absorbed into cells. In particular it can cross the blood–brain barrier and bind to proteins in the brain where it is neurotoxic. The clinical syndrome of bilirubin-encephalopathy (kernicterus) may result in death or severe mental handicap.

Jaundice which lasts more than 10 days after birth should always be investigated. It may indicate galactosaemia, congenital hypothyroidism, cystic fibrosis or glucose-6-phosphate dehydrogenase deficiency.

Where the excess bilirubin is found to be conjugated, the pathology is different. The two most common causes are neonatal hepatitis, possibly contracted from the mother at birth, or biliary atresia where biliary drainage is disordered. This may require surgical intervention.

Case history 65

The baby of a diabetic mother weighed 1.64 kg (below 10th centile for weight) when born at gestational age of 32 weeks. The baby was well at birth, but her condition deteriorated within hours and she had respiratory problems.

- What biochemical determinations should be requested on this baby?
- Why is it important to consider each request carefully?

Comment on page 159.

ENERGY METABOLISM

Before birth, the chief source of energy for the fetus is glucose obtained from the mother via the placenta. Any excess glucose is stored as liver glycogen. Free fatty acids cross the placenta and are stored in fat. At birth, the baby must switch to gluconeogenesis and glycogenolysis to maintain blood glucose concentration, with lipolysis producing free fatty acids to provide the main energy source until feeding is established.

Neonatal hypoglycaemia is defined as a blood glucose below 2 mmol/l. This may be encountered particularly in:

- the light-for-dates baby, or preterm infant where the glycogen stores are depleted
- the infant of a diabetic mother, because of the fetal hyperinsulinaemia (see p. 142).

Clinical note

Newborn babies have low levels of vitamin K, which is involved in the synthesis of blood coagulation factors. To minimize the risk of intracerebral haemorrhage, it has been recommended that all newborn babies, particularly those who are breast fed, be given this vitamin.

GASTROINTESTINAL FUNCTION

Although the brush border disaccharidases (maltase, lactase, sucrase) are present at birth, for the first 7 days of life lactose may be absorbed unchanged and appear in the urine in the normal infant. The proteolytic enzymes, rennin and pepsin, are present in the neonatal stomach, but some protein may be absorbed without digestion.

CALCIUM

Particularly in the premature infant, there may be a transient, often asymptomatic, hypocalcaemia in the first few days of life when the infant's parathyroid glands appear not to respond adequately to the hypocalcaemia.

Neonatal hypocalcaemia is more likely to occur in preterm infants, infants with respiratory distress syndrome, asphyxiated infants and infants of diabetic mothers.

Paediatric biochemistry

- Respiratory distress syndrome is the consequence of lack of surfactant, which prevents expansion and aeration of pulmonary alveoli.
- Relative to adults, babies have increased total body water and extracellular water. Renal function changes with age. Guidelines for fluid and electrolyte replacement therapy in babies are quite different from those in adults.
- Jaundice is common in babies in the first week of life. In term babies, this usually resolves rapidly. Jaundice during the first 24 hours of life is always pathological.
- Neonatal hypoglycaemia may be encountered in the premature infant, the 'light-for-dates' baby or the infant of a diabetic mother.

BIOCHEMISTRY IN THE ELDERLY

By the year 2050 more than 20% of the world's population will be over 65 years of age. As the population ages, more clinical biochemical resources will need to be directed towards the problems of the elderly population.

There is considerable variation in the onset of functional changes in body systems because of age. Many organs show a gradual decline in function even in the absence of disease; but since there is often considerable functional reserve, there are no clinical consequences. The problem facing the clinical biochemist is how to differentiate between the biochemical and physiological changes which are the consequences of ageing, and those factors which indicate that disease is present. Just because the result of a biochemistry test in an elderly patient is different from that in a young person does not mean some pathology is present. Serum creatinine is an example. Renal function deteriorates with age (Fig. 1) but finding a creatinine of 140 µmol/l in an 80-year-old woman should not be cause for alarm. Indeed, this creatinine result may represent a remarkably good glomerular filtration rate considering the age of the patient.

The interpretation of biochemical measurements in the elderly requires that laboratories establish age-related reference ranges for many of the tests undertaken.

DISEASE IN OLD AGE

Some diseases are more commonly encountered in the elderly than in the young. In addition, common diseases may present in a different way to that in the young. Elderly patients may have more than one disease or may take several medications which mimic or mask the normal disease presentation.

The admission of a patient for geriatric assessment involves a degree of 'screening' biochemistry which may point towards the presence of disorders which may not be suspected (Table 1).

The metabolic diseases which occur most commonly in the elderly and may present in unusual ways include:

- thyroid disease
- diabetes mellitus
- renal disease
- pituitary disease
- impaired gonadal function
- bone disease.

Thyroid disease

Thyroid dysfunction is common in the elderly. Diagnosis may be overlooked since many of the clinical manifestations of thyroid disease may be misinterpreted as just the normal ageing process (Fig. 2). Unusual presentations are common e.g. elderly patients with hyperthyroidism are more likely than younger patients to present with the cardiac-related effects of increased thyroid hormone.

The interpretation of TSH, T_4 and T_3 results may not be straightforward in the elderly population as these patients usually have more than one active disease process. A patient with a severe non-thyroidal illness may show low T_4, T_3 and TSH (p. 83). A patient's thyroid function can only be satisfactorily investigated in the absence of non-thyroidal illness. Elderly patients may also be taking drugs which affect thyroid function (Table 2).

Hypothermia is often encountered in an elderly patient. It is important to establish if there is an underlying endocrine disorder such as thyroid disease, or even adrenal or pituitary hypofunction (Fig. 3).

Table 1 **Biochemical assessment in a geriatric patient**

Test	Associated conditions
Potassium	Hypokalaemia
Urea and creatinine	Renal disease
Calcium, phosphate and alkaline phosphatase	Bone disease
Total protein, albumin	Nutritional state
Glucose	Diabetes mellitus
Thyroid function tests	Hypothyroidism
Haematological investigation and faecal occult blood	Blood and bleeding disorders

Diabetes mellitus

Diabetes mellitus is common in old age (Fig. 4). Genetic factors and obesity contribute to the insulin resistance which underlies the development of NIDDM (pp. 56–57).

Glucose tolerance declines with age even in the absence of diabetes mellitus, and the renal threshold for glucose rises. These observations can make the diagnosis of diabetes mellitus difficult in an elderly patient.

Table 2 **Some common drugs known to affect thyroid action**

Effect	Drugs
Increase TBG	Oestrogens
Decrease TBG	Androgens, glucocorticoids
Inhibit TBG binding	Phenytoin, salicylates
Suppress TSH	L-DOPA, glucocorticoids
Inhibit T_4 secretion	Lithium
Inhibit T_4-T_3 conversion	Amiodarone, Propanolol
Reduce oral T_4 absorption	Cholestyramine, colestipol

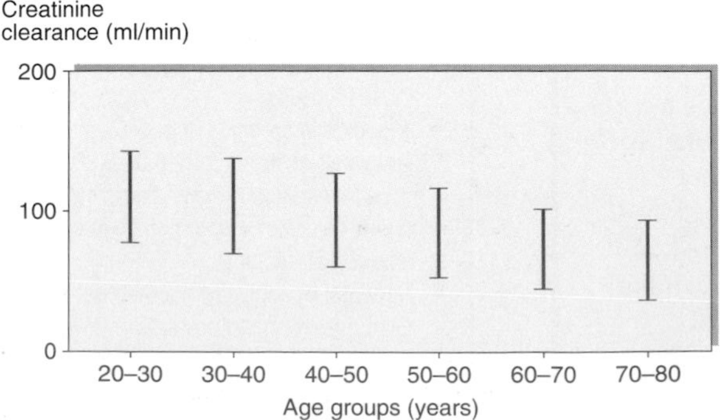

Fig. 1 **Age-related fall in the creatinine clearance reference range.**

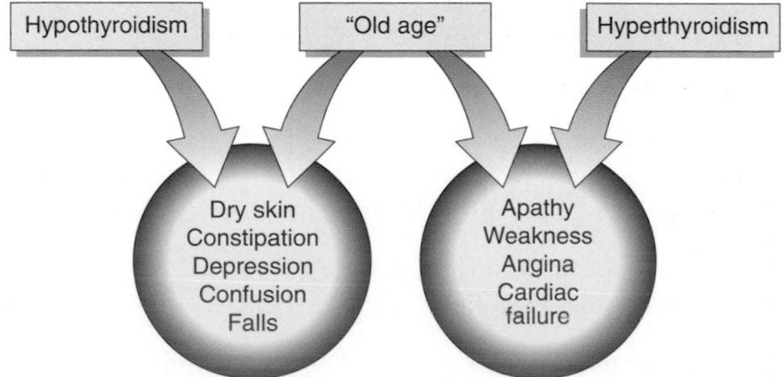

Fig. 2 **The clinical manifestations of thyroid disease may be misinterpreted as characteristics of "normal" ageing.**

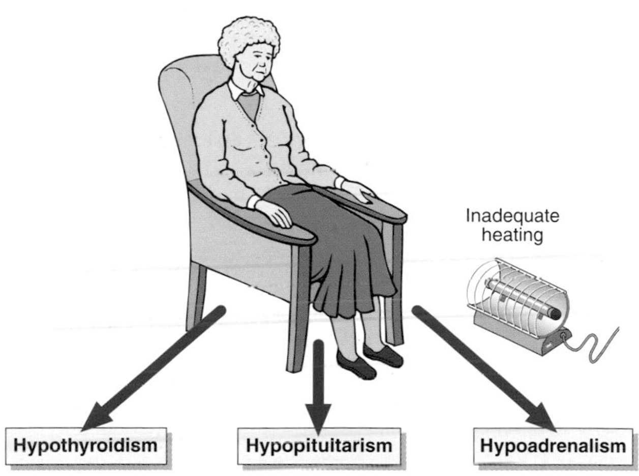

Fig. 3 **Possible endocrine reasons for hypothermia in the elderly patient.**

Renal disease

Renal function gradually deteriorates throughout life as shown by the increases in the upper limit of the age-related reference ranges for both urea and creatinine. Creatinine clearance falls even though the amount of creatinine produced decreases as a consequence of reduced muscle mass. A degree of cardiac insufficiency may enforce this fall. The ability of the kidneys to concentrate urine and to excrete a dilute urine both decline with age.

Pituitary disease

With increasing age the pituitary gland decreases in size, and the incidence of microadenomas and focal necrosis increases. Gonadotrophin and AVP secretion increase, and growth hormone secretion decreases. The significance of the latter is the subject of much current investigation.

Gonadal function

Both ovarian and testicular hormone secretion decline with age. The menopause in women may cause distressing symptoms in the short term, and serious bone disease in the long term. The benefits of post-menopausal hormone replacement therapy (HRT) are well established in relation to menopausal symptoms, and maintenance of bone structure, and may significantly reduce the risk of coronary heart disease.

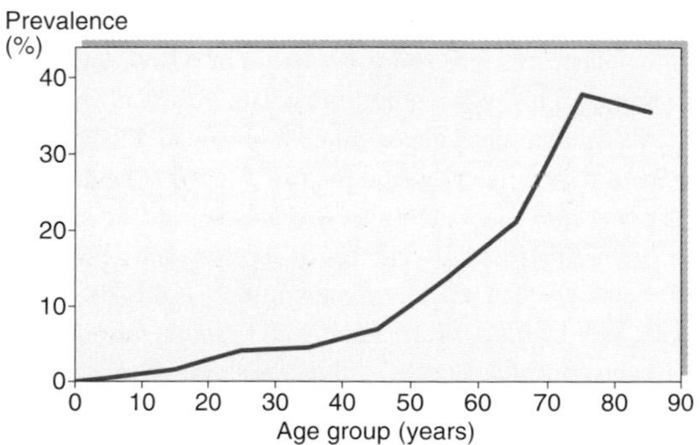

Fig 4 **Age specific prevalence of known diabetes mellitus.**

Bone disease

Bone disease in general is more common in elderly patients than in the young. Osteoporosis is the most common bone disease which occurs in the elderly (p.72). The risk of hip fracture increases dramatically with increasing age because of a reduction in bone mass per unit volume. Bone loss accelerates when oestrogen production falls after the menopause in women, but both sexes show a gradual bone loss throughout life. The common biochemical indices of calcium metabolism are normal in patients even with severe primary osteoporosis, and currently are of little help in diagnosis and treatment, except to ensure that other complicating conditions are not present.

Vitamin D deficiency remains a cause of osteomalacia in the elderly, housebound or institutionalized patients. Vitamin D status can be assessed by measurement of the main circulating metabolite, 25-hydroxycholecalciferol. In severe osteomalacia due to vitamin D deficiency, serum calcium will fall, and there will be an appropriate increase in PTH secretion. Alkaline phosphatase will be elevated.

Paget's disease is characterized by increased osteoclastic activity which leads to increased bone resorption. Bone pain can be particularly severe. Serum alkaline phosphatase is very high, and urinary hydroxyproline excretion is elevated.

Myeloma is frequently encountered in older patients. However, a sizeable proportion of the elderly population will have a paraprotein band on electrophoresis, but only a minority will have overt myeloma.

NUTRITION IN ELDERLY PATIENTS

Nutritional deficiencies are more common in the elderly, especially those who are neglected or who fail to eat a balanced diet. Recent evidence suggests that this is a factor in the reduced immune response found in all malnourished patients, which renders them more susceptible to infection.

Clinical note

When faced with a biochemical problem in an elderly patient it is important to remember that it is highly likely (in contrast to a young person) that more than one pathology is present.

Case history 66

A 72-year-old man presented to his GP in a confused state. On examination he was emaciated and had motor and sensory polyneuropathy. Alcohol could be smelt on his breath.

- What further tests should be undertaken?

Comment on page 159.

Biochemistry in the elderly

- The clinical biochemist must be aware of whether a change in a biochemical parameter is a normal occurrence of old age or indicates the presence of disease.
- Common diseases in elderly patients may present in a different way to that in younger patients.
- Elderly patients may be prescribed a number of medications which will complicate the interpretation of results.

CASE HISTORY COMMENTS

Case history 1

The delay in transporting the specimen to the laboratory was not known and the pattern of results obtained (serum urea = 11.8 mmol/l, sodium = 130 mmol/l and potassium = 6.7 mmol/l) suggest that the patient may be sodium depleted with pre-renal uraemia and hyperkalaemia. This pattern, if correct, is typical of Addison's disease, an endocrine emergency. However, a delay in separating the serum from the clot makes the potassium and sodium concentrations unreliable as these ions move out of and into the erythrocytes along their concentration gradients. Thus another specimen is required to establish the patient's true electrolyte status.

Case history 2

A serum potassium of 45 mmol/l is not compatible with life. This spurious result may have arisen as a result of a transcription error from the phone to the notes (the real result should have been 4.5 mmol/l). In an otherwise healthy and fit young subject with a serum urea and/or creatinine in the reference range, the likelihood of a serious electrolyte disturbance is very remote.

Case history 3

As is common in these circumstances the boy had consumed a large amount of refined carbohydrate—two cans of soft drinks, a jam doughnut and in excess of 200 g of assorted sweets over the preceeding 2 hours. Thus, it is to be expected that the blood glucose would be high and a diagnosis of diabetes mellitus should *not* be made.

Case history 4

After 2 days or so the kidneys adapt to the decreased input and would conserve sodium, potassium and water. However, he will continue to lose water insensibly and as a result the ICF and ECF will contract in equal proportion. After 3–4 days the contraction will become critical when the ECF may be insufficient to maintain the circulation and, if not corrected, will lead to death.

Many individuals in this situation will also be severely injured with significant blood loss. This would obviously further compromise the ECF volume and would make survival unlikely.

Case history 5

The biochemical results strongly suggest pre-renal uraemia, as there is a marked increase in the serum urea with a very modest increase in the serum creatinine. He has severe hypernatraemia and these two observations would indicate that the patient is primarily suffering from water depletion. The serum potassium is normal as is his anion gap. These results would, therefore, indicate the presence of profound uncomplicated water depletion.

In a case such as this it is essential to exclude non-ketotic, diabetic, precoma. His blood glucose was 9.2 mmol/l which excludes this diagnosis. Ketones were not detected, nor did he have an acidosis. It was rapidly established from the clinical history that the man did not have access to water for more than three days. A diagnosis of pure water depletion was therefore established on the basis of the history, clinical findings and biochemical features.

Case history 6

These urea and electrolytes are typical of dilutional hyponatraemia. Her normal blood pressure and serum urea and creatinine concentrations exclude significant sodium depletion. The absence of oedema excludes a significant increase in her total body sodium. These results are characteristic of the so-called syndrome of inappropriate antidiuresis (SIAD) and are due to secretion of AVP in response to non-osmotic stimuli. The ectopic production of AVP is extremely rare even in patients with malignant disease.

The urine osmolality is in keeping with the diagnosis of SIAD. However, any urine osmolality, other than a maximally dilute, urine of 30 mmol/kg, would support the diagnosis. When the urine is maximally dilute, the urine flow-rate is in excess of 500 ml/hour which is invariably clinically obvious. Thus, the measurement of the urine osmolality adds little to making a diagnosis in this case.

Case history 7

This is a classic presentation of severe sodium and water depletion with clinical evidence (hypotension, tachycardia, weakness) and biochemical evidence (pre-renal uraemia with a significant increase in the serum urea and a modest increase in the serum creatinine) which indicate severe contraction of the ECF volume. It is worth noting that a serum sodium concentration is a very poor guide to the presence, or absence, of sodium depletion. This patient requires both sodium and water as a matter of urgency. In view of his gastrointestinal symptoms this will need to be given intravenously as a 0.9% sodium chloride solution.

Case history 8

As in all cases of acute trauma the priorities are A, B, C: ensure a patent **A**irway, ensure the patient is **B**reathing and ensure that the patient's **C**irculation is intact. These are the basic principles of resuscitation.

From a biochemical point of view the patient has a dangerously high serum potassium. This is due to release of potassium from damaged tissues. This will require immediate treatment with calcium (given i.v. as calcium chloride or calcium gluconate) to counteract the dangers of hyperkalaemia, and then steps need to be taken to lower the potassium. This will involve the use of insulin and glucose infusions in the first instance and it is likely that such a patient may require to be dialysed. The other feature of note is the low serum bicarbonate and the high serum anion gap. From the history and these results one can confidently make a diagnosis of lactic acidosis due to tissue hypoxia. The treatment of the lactic acidosis will depend upon establishing a satisfactory circulation and tissue oxygenation.

Case history 9

This woman displays the features of severe sodium depletion and she is also likely to have a less severe degree of water depletion. The evidence for sodium depletion is her progressive weakness, her pre-renal uraemia and her hyponatraemia. While her glomerular filtration rate has decreased her tubular function appears satisfactory as demonstrated by her ability to form a concentrated urine and to conserve her urine sodium. This woman received inadequate intravenous fluid therapy post-operatively. Her treatment regimen was especially deficient in sodium which led to a contraction of her ECF and this caused her to develop pre-renal uraemia. The contraction in her ECF will also have stimulated AVP secretion and, thus, she conserved water and became hyponatraemic. The contraction in her ECF also stimulated aldosterone secretion which caused her renal tubules to conserve sodium.

In order to prescribe appropriate fluid therapy for this woman, one needs to estimate her sodium, potassium and water deficits from her fluid balance charts. Particular note must be taken of losses that are relatively rich in sodium, such as drainage fluid, losses from fistulae, stomas or by nasogastric aspiration. Insensible water loss and urinary losses must also be taken into account.

Case history 10

The creatinine clearance is calculated using the formula below where U is the urine creatinine concentration, V is the urine flow-rate and P is the plasma or serum creatinine concentration. As there are 1440 minutes in a day this man's urine flow-rate, $V = 2160 / 1440 =$ 1.5 ml/minute. His urinary creatinine must be in the same units as his serum creatinine. His urinary creatinine concentration: $U = 7.5$ mmol/l = 7500 µmol/l. His serum creatinine: $P = 150$ µmol/l. Thus,

$$\frac{UV}{P} = \frac{7500 \times 1.5}{150} = 75 \text{ ml/minute}$$

This is low for a young male.

When it was discovered that the urine collection was for 17 hours and not 24 hours his urine flow-rate was recalculated (2160 /1020): $V= 2.1$ ml/minute.

Recalculating his creatinine clearance:

$$\frac{UV}{P} = \frac{7500 \times 2.1}{150} = 105 \text{ ml/minute}$$

This is in the range one would expect in a young male. One can see, therefore, how errors in the timing and collection of urine significantly influence the calculation of the creatinine clearance. Errors in collection are by far the most common and serious errors encountered when estimating the creatinine clearance.

Case history 11

It would be unnecessary and even dangerous to attempt to perform a water deprivation test on this patient. It is worth noting that one can make a confident diagnosis of cranial diabetes insipidus from the history and the observation that she was producing large volumes of urine and complaining of thirst. Her blood glucose level excludes diabetes mellitus as a cause of her polyuria and her hypernatraemia accounts for her thirst. In normal circumstances a serum sodium concentration of 150 mmol/l will stimulate AVP production and cause the urine to be maximally concentrated. This patient's urine is, therefore, inappropriately dilute. Note that her serum urea is not increased. This reflects her high urine flow-rate despite her significant water depletion.

Case history 12

The marked increase in the serum urea with the modest increase in the serum creatinine would indicate the presence of pre-renal uraemia. Pyrexial patients are frequently hypercatabolic which will contribute to his high serum urea. His urine osmolality of 629 mmol/kg would support this, for if his pre-renal uraemia were purely due to dehydration his urine osmolality would be much higher. His low serum bicarbonate and high anion gap indicates that he has a metabolic acidosis. This acidosis will cause the potassium to move from the intracellular to the extracellular compartment. The reduction in his glomerular filtration rate results in his inability to maintain a normal serum potassium in the face of this efflux as both these factors contribute to his hyperkalaemia.

Case history 13

The serum urea in this case, though high, is relatively low in comparison to the serum creatinine. This would indicate a low protein intake. The serum bicarbonate is low indicating the presence of a metabolic acidosis. However, the anion gap is normal and, hence, it is unlikely that this patient's [H^+] will be grossly abnormal. The hyperkalaemia, therefore, is likely to be entirely due to the low glomerular filtration rate with the efflux of potassium from the intracellular to the extracellular compartment being of minor importance. The hyponatraemia in this case would reflect an increase in total body water. These results clearly indicate that the patient needs to continue with dialysis. This woman's serum calcium status should also be assessed. Hypocalcaemia should be excluded and a high serum alkaline phosphatase would indicate the presence of metabolic bone disease. Serum PTH concentrations are a very sensitive method of detecting hypocalcaemia and metabolic bone disease in patients with renal failure.

Case history 14

The low [H^+] and high bicarbonate concentration confirm that this patient has a metabolic alkalosis. This will have been caused by his severe vomiting which, in view of the history, is likely to be due to pyloric stenosis. Ingestion of bicarbonate would not lead to this degree of metabolic alkalosis though it will have aggravated the situation. The severe vomiting has led to dehydration and this is manifested by the presence of pre-renal uraemia. The hypokalaemia is due to a combination of potassium loss in the vomitus and the metabolic alkalosis causing the influx of potassium from the ECF to the ICF.

The urine results are typical of a patient with dehydration and metabolic alkalosis due to vomiting. Aldosterone is being secreted in an attempt to expand his ECF and the patient is conserving sodium despite his hypernatraemia. The hyperaldosteronism is promoting potassium loss despite his hypokalaemia and the patient has the classical paradoxical acid urine.

Case history 15

The high [H^+] and PCO_2 confirm the presence of a respiratory acidosis which, from the history, will have been expected. Note that the bicarbonate is not abnormally increased, which indicates that this is an acute development, and renal compensation for the respiratory acidosis has not had time to have a significant impact on the respiratory acidosis.

Case history 16

The [H^+] is at the upper end of the reference range. The PCO_2 is markedly elevated which would indicate the presence of a respiratory acidosis but the bicarbonate concentration is also markedly increased as the compensatory response for the respiratory acidosis. This man has type 2 respiratory failure.

Case history 17

The dominant feature in this patient's acid–base disorder is an alkalosis as the [H^+] is low. The bicarbonate concentration is in keeping with the presence of a metabolic alkalosis, which is the dominant disorder in this case. The PCO_2 is increased which may be partially due to a compensatory reaction to the alkalosis. However, the increase in PCO_2 is in excess of that associated with this degree of alkalosis. The patient had a long-standing history of respiratory disease.

The PO_2 indicates that the patient is satisfactorily oxygenating her blood.

This patient's hypokalaemia and metabolic alkalosis can be explained by profound potassium depletion due to the use of diuretics with an inadequate intake of potassium.The principles of therapy are potassium supplementation and alteration of her drug regimen to one that will ameliorate potassium loss, e.g. use of an ACE inhibitor.

Case history 18

By far the most likely diagnosis based on the information given is the nephrotic syndrome. In the nephrotic syndrome you would expect the serum albumin to be low and the urinary albumin to be high. The serum urea and electrolytes are frequently normal. Although the glomerular basement membrane may be damaged, the glomerular filtration rate is usually normal in the early stages of the nephrotic syndrome. Hypercholesterolaemia is a feature of the nephrotic syndrome. The history of recurrent infections suggests a degree of immune deficiency. This patient is likely to be losing immunoglobulin and some of the components of the complement system in her urine and this could lead to a relative immune deficiency.

Case history 19

This man is suffering from multiple myeloma. He is one of the approximately 20% of patients with myeloma that do not have a paraprotein in the serum but have Bence–Jones proteinuria. His renal function should be tested and hypercalcaemia should be excluded.

Case history 20

This man is likely to have suffered a myocardial infarction. However, with the history lasting an hour he may not, at this stage, have abnormal serum cardiac enzyme levels. One may wish to establish baseline values for his cardiac enzyme so that any subsequent change may be quantitated, but there is no definitive indication for doing biochemical investigations on this man.

Case history 21

Metastatic breast carcinoma is the most likely diagnosis in this case. The liver function tests indicate that there is little hepatocellular damage present and that bilirubin excretion is normal. These findings, however, do not exclude the possibility of hepatic metastasis, giving rise to localized areas of intrahepatic obstruction. If this were so, then the γGT would also be increased. A normal serum calcium does not exclude the possibility of bone metastasis, which is another source of the high alkaline phosphatase activity. This would be detected by doing alkaline phosphatase isoenzyme studies. A third possibility is that there may be a local recurrence with the tumour itself producing alkaline phosphatase, though this would be very unlikely. A bone scan would be very helpful in this case.

Case history 22

In this case, by far the most likely diagnosis is carcinoma of the head of the pancreas obstructing the common bile duct. This, classically, gives rise to severe, painless, deep jaundice which is in keeping with a bilirubin of 250 μmol/l. This is uncomplicated obstructive jaundice which is characterized by an alkaline phosphatase activity that is more than three times the upper limit of the reference range. The aspartate and alanine aminotransferase activities do not indicate severe hepatocellular damage. By far the most important further investigations to be performed on this patient would be to image the structures in the vicinity of the head of the pancreas and the common bile duct looking for the cause of the obstruction. This could be done by ultrasound or radiology.

Case history 23

The most striking features of these results are the marked increase in the aspartate and alanine aminotransferase activities. These indicate the presence of acute hepatocellular damage. The bilirubin is increased and there is a degree of cholestasis as indicated by the increase in the serum alkaline phosphatase activity. As the increase in alkaline phosphatase is less than twice the upper limit of the reference range, cholestasis is unlikely to be the dominant cause of the jaundice. The increase in the γGT is to be expected as this enzyme is increased in many forms of liver disease.

By far the most likely diagnosis in this case is that the woman has acute viral hepatitis.

Case history 24

(i) This man has diabetes mellitus confirmed by the presence of a fasting venous plasma glucose greater than 8.0 mmol/l and a two-hour glucose value in excess of 11 mmol/l.
(ii) Though this woman has a satisfactory fasting venous plasma glucose, she does have diabetes mellitus as her two-hour glucose is greater than 11.0 mmol/l.
(iii) This man does not have diabetes mellitus but he does have impaired glucose tolerance, as is demonstrated by his fasting and two-hour glucose levels.
(iv) This woman has impaired glucose tolerance.

Case history 25

By far the most likely diagnosis in this case is diabetic ketoacidosis. This may be precipitated by a number of conditions, such as infection. This may have caused anorexia and, thus, the patient may have omitted to take her insulin. Trauma can increase a patient's requirement for insulin but there is nothing to suggest that in this case. The blood glucose can be checked at the bedside as can a specimen of urine for the presence or absence of ketones. The laboratory tests which may be requested are urea and electrolytes to assess renal function, the presence or absence of hyperkalaemia and the serum sodium concentration. The patient's acid-base status should be assessed to quantitate the severity of the acidosis present, and the blood glucose should be accurately measured. These will influence the patient's treatment. It is essential in cases such as this that samples of blood and urine and, if appropriate, sputum are sent to the microbiological laboratory to look for the presence of infection.

Case history 26

Nocturnal hypoglycaemia is the most likely cause of this woman's symptoms. The diagnosis can be made by measuring her blood glucose while she is symptomatic. However, this can be distressing to patients and not always feasible. Indirect evidence of nocturnal hypoglycaemia may be obtained by measuring her urinary catecholamine excretion or urinary cortisol excretion overnight. A further clue may be obtained if the woman's glycated haemoglobin level indicates good diabetic control in the face of hyperglycaemia during the day. In many such cases a diagnosis of nocturnal hypoglycaemia is inferred if the symptoms are relieved by changing the insulin regimen or getting the patient to eat more food before she retires at night.

Case history 27

As renal failure is the most common cause of hypocalcaemia, her serum urea and electrolytes should be measured. Unsuspected renal failure is unlikely as her serum phosphate is normal. Her plasma PTH should be measured and if high (appropriate to the low calcium) then vitamin D deficiency is the most likely diagnosis, and the cause should be sought. An increased serum alkaline phosphatase would be compatible with vitamin D deficiency. The bone pain is due to the underlying osteomalacia.

A low PTH would indicate hypoparathyroidism. Other causes of hypocalcaemia would be unlikely in this case.

Case history 28

The two most likely diagnoses in this case are primary hyperparathyroidism and hypercalcaemia of malignancy. The most important biochemical investigation to be performed at this stage would be a plasma PTH measurement, which will be high in primary hyperparathyroidism and suppressed in hypercalcaemia of malignancy. In patients with hypercalcaemia of malignancy, the underlying disease is usually detectable by a careful clinical history and examination. There are however notable exceptions, multiple myeloma being one, and therefore a sample of serum and urine should be sent for protein electrophoresis to see if a paraprotein band can be identified. A blanket request for tumour markers such as CEA or AFP should not be requested unless there is a clear clinical indication for doing so. The patient's alkaline phosphatase activity should be measured and alkaline phosphatase isoenzyme studies may be indicated, especially if the plasma PTH concentration is suppressed.

The patient shows evidence of dehydration and has severe hypercalcaemia which should be treated by rehydration in the first instance.

Case history 29

Though this patient is hypocalcaemic, in view of the hypomagnasaemia one would expect the PTH to be suppressed.

This patient needs magnesium supplements. As magnesium salts cause diarrhoea they need to be given parenterally, especially in this case where there is established diarrhoea and malabsorption. It is likely that once the patient is magnesium replete, her original Vitamin D and calcium supplements will be sufficient to maintain her in a normocalcaemic state.

Case history 30

As Paget's disease can be considered a disorder of bone remodelling, the serum alkaline phosphatase, which is a good marker of osteoblastic activity, can be used to monitor the disease activity. It cannot, however, be used to demonstrate the involvement of a specific bone or deformity; this has to be done radiologically. If a patient is being given a bisphosphonate it is important to monitor the serum calcium, as hypocalcaemia is a well-recognized side-effect of these drugs.

Case history 31

The history and presentation indicate hypopituitarism. This causes an increase in insulin sensitivity due to the relative deficiency of glucocorticoids and growth hormone. It was correct, therefore, to use a lower dose of insulin.

In view of this man's marked increase in prolactin, which does not change significantly during the combined anterior pituitary function test, one can make a diagnosis of prolactinoma.

The hypoglycaemic stress induced in this patient did not cause the expected rise in serum cortisol. It is essential, therefore, that he is commenced on cortisol replacement before surgery. His low T_4 combined with the abnormal response in his TSH (i.e., the 60 min level being greater than the 30 min level) would support a diagnosis of secondary hypothyroidism. He should therefore also be commenced on thyroxine replacement. As prolactinomas frequently shrink dramatically in response to bromocriptine he may be treated with this drug pre-operatively to facilitate the surgical removal of the tumour.

Case history 32

There are many causes of short stature but in view of the documented fall off in the patient's growth rate over the past year and his delayed bone age, growth hormone deficiency is highly likely. The measure-ment of random blood growth hormone levels are unhelpful as one frequently gets false positive and false negative results with this test. Urinary growth hormone measurements appear to offer a useful screening test for physiological growth hormone assessment. However, the standard test for diagnosing growth hormone insufficiency remains the insulin stress test. This is a potentially dangerous test and should, therefore, only be performed in centres with specialist expertise in paediatric endocrinology.

Case history 33

This patient has a high serum T_4 because the oestrogen component of hormone replacement therapy stimulates the synthesis of thyroxine-binding globulin. Thus, to maintain a normal level of the physiologically active Free T_4 the total serum T_4 needs to be increased.

By far the most important investigation for this woman is a fine-needle aspiration biopsy of the thyroid nodule. Frequently, cystic lesions will be drained by this procedure and may not recur. It is important, however, that adequate thyroid epithelium be obtained to enable the diagnosis of thyroid cancer to be excluded or confirmed.

Case history 34

As the TSH is approximately 20 times the upper limit of the reference range and the serum T_4 is significantly decreased, this woman has severe hypothyroidism. Skeletal and cardiac muscles are involved in the hypothyroid process, causing the release of creatine kinase into the circulation. This, combined with a decrease in the catabolic rate of creatine kinase, will be sufficient to cause the creatine kinase to increase to the levels observed in this case. The aspartate aminotransferase is at the upper end of the reference range and this will fall along with the creatine kinase and cholesterol after a few weeks treatment with thyroxine. In view of the evidence of myocardial ischaemia it is prudent to proceed cautiously in this case with a low dose of thyroxine and gradually increase it in a step-wise manner.

Case history 35

It is likely that this patient has suffered a relapse of her thyrotoxicosis. This may not yet be clinically manifest, though one would expect a patient with a fully suppressed TSH and a T_4 in excess of 200 nmol/l to be symptomatic.

If the woman is pregnant or taking an oral contraceptive which contains a large amount of oestrogen this may cause an increase in her serum thyroxine-binding globulin sufficient to account for a serum T_4 of 210 nmol/l in a euthyroid woman. The TSH frequently remains fully suppressed in patients who are recovering from thyrotoxicosis when thyroid-stimulating immunoglobulins will contribute to the stimulation of the thyroid gland in addition to the patient's endogenous TSH production. If there is a doubt about the diagnosis of a relapse of her thyrotoxicosis, a serum T_3 or Free T_4 may be helpful in making the diagnosis. Both would be increased if she has suffered a relapse.

Case history 36

Whenever one encounters the combination of hyponatraemia with hyperkalaemia, adrenocortical failure must be suspected. There is a modest increase in the serum creatinine with a normal serum urea which is not typical of Addison's disease. In adrenal failure the patient usually has pre-renal ureamia which causes the serum urea to rise more than the creatinine. The low serum bicarbonate is a feature of adrenal failure.

It is essential that a Synacthen test is performed in this patient to exclude or confirm the diagnosis of adrenal failure. As the patient has severe skeletal muscle pain the creatine kinase should be measured as the hyperkalaemia may be due to potassium released from damaged muscle. If rhabdomyolysis were detected, it would be important to monitor renal function and calcium status carefully.

Case history 37

This presentation is classical of acute adrenal failure with characteristic symptoms, physical findings and electrolyte pattern. The diagnosis is confirmed by the Synacthen test.

On presentation, this woman was sodium depleted with pre-renal uraemia. As her ECF was expanded with 0.9% sodium chloride, this improved her glomerular filtration rate which is sufficient, even in the absence of aldosterone, to correct the hyperkalaemia by increasing her urinary potassium excretion. The reduction in this patient's blood volume will stimulate vasopressin secretion, giving rise to the hyponatraemia. The sodium chloride infusion by restoring her blood volume will inhibit AVP secretion, enabling her to correct the hyponatraemia.

Case history 38

Cushing's syndrome is the most likely diagnosis in this case. One can be confident of the diagnosis in view of the increased urinary cortisol:creatinine ratio, the absent diurnal rhythm, failure to suppress with low-dose dexamethasone and the failure of the insulin-induced hypoglycaemia to stimulate cortisol secretion.

Establishing a diagnosis of Cushing's syndrome is insufficient as it is essential to discover the underlying cause to enable the correct treatment to be given. This patient should have a high-dose dexamethasone suppression test with serum cortisol and ACTH being measured. Suppression of the cortisol would point to the pituitary-dependent Cushing's syndrome as would an abnormally increased ACTH concentration. An adenoma should be actively sought in her pituitary and adrenal glands by CT or MRI scanning. If her ACTH is abnormally increased she may undergo selective venous catheterisation to locate the source which may be due to a carcinoid tumour of the lung.

Case history 39

This clinical presentation combined with the biochemical findings of increased LH and testosterone are typical of the polycystic ovarian syndrome. Ultrasound examination of her ovaries would confirm the diagnosis.

Case history 40

An accurate measurement of height and serial measurements of weight are the most important means of monitoring the nutritional progress of such a patient. Patients are at risk of developing micronutrient deficiency if they experience difficulty in swallowing and, as a consequence, alter their diet to one which may be deficient in one or more components. For example, fresh fruit and vegetables may be sacrificed in favour of highly processed foods, thus causing vitamin C deficiency. Another alternative that has to be considered in these patients is that because of the relentless, incurable, nature of their disease they may ingest excessive amounts of vitamin and trace element supplements in the vain attempt to halt the progression of their disease. A careful dietary assessment should be made in this man and, if suspected, vitamin or trace element deficiencies or excesses tested for biochemically.

Case history 41

Measuring the serum vitamin B_{12} concentration is inappropriate in patients on parenteral treatment. A routine blood count is much more appropriate. In a patient with pernicious anaemia feeling 'run down', hypothyroidism should also be suspected and thyroid function assessed. The incidence of carcinoma of the stomach is increased among patients with pernicious anaemia and this diagnosis should also be borne in mind.

Case history 42

This patient has insufficient small bowel to enable him to be fed enterally. He will, therefore, require long-term parenteral nutrition. It is important that he is encouraged to take some oral fluids and nutrients to maintain the integrity of his remaining bowel.

The caloric and nitrogen requirements to restore and maintain his skeletal muscle and body mass should be assessed. It is important to assess his baseline micronutrient status so that any deficiencies can be corrected. As he will receive the bulk of his nutrition parenterally in the future, his micronutrient status will need to be monitored. Once he is stable this should be formally checked at six-monthly intervals along with his weight, skin-fold thickness and skeletal muscle mass.

Case history 43

In a patient such as this in ITU the biochemical measurements that are most frequently helpful are:

- *serum urea and electrolytes* to monitor renal function and *serum potassium* as he may become hyperkalaemic as a result of tissue damage
- *pulse oximetry* to assess tissue oxygenation
- *blood gas analysis* and *plasma lactate* to detect and quantify acid–base disorders that may arise
- *serum muscle enzymes* such as CK may help detect a compartment syndrome or monitor rhabdomyolysis.

Case history 44

Recurrence or metastatic spread of the breast cancer would need to be excluded in this woman by imaging her liver and skeleton. Alkaline phosphatase isoenzyme studies should be performed. However, if the increase is due to an increased bone activity, this does not necessarily represent metastatic spread of the tumour. In view of the history and symptoms, osteomalacia due to malnutrition or malabsorption may be the reason. If the patient has malabsorption or malnutrition she may have a macrocytic anaemia due to folate or B_{12} deficiency and may be deficient in other micronutrients such as zinc and other vitamins. Malabsorption is often difficult to detect clinically and she should undergo tests of malabsorption such as faecal fat measurement.

Case history 45

This patient has the classic symptoms and signs of iron deficiency anaemia. The finding of a low serum ferritin with a low serum iron and per cent transferrin saturation are typical of this condition. However, if iron deficiency anaemia is suspected, the most important and usually the only investigation required is to demonstrate the presence of a hypochromic microcytic anaemia by examining the blood film.

Case history 46

The finding of a high liver copper concentration would indicate that the patient died from Wilson's disease which is an autosomal recessive disorder. The patient's sister (and brothers if any) should be screened for Wilson's disease. Serum copper, caeruloplasmin and urinary copper excretion may indicate if she also has the disease. A liver biopsy may be indicated to confirm the diagnosis and allow treatment to be initiated. DNA analysis is becoming available to assist in the diagnosis.

Case history 47

This patient has symptoms of digoxin toxicity. This is in keeping with the plasma digoxin concentration which is high though such levels are not always a reliable means of detecting digoxin toxicity as its action is influenced by other factors such as the $[H^+]$ and serum potassium concentration. This patient had developed pre-renal uraemia which resulted in a decrease in her digoxin excretion and, as a result, she developed digoxin toxicity on a dose that had previously been appropriate in her case.

Case history 48

These results would indicate that the man has taken an overdose of salicylate. The plasma salicylate of 4.6 mmol/l will contribute to his relatively high anion gap of 18 mmol/l. Salicylate poisoning is associated with a metabolic acidosis and a respiratory alkalosis due to the direct effect of salicylate on the respiratory centre. The $[H^+]$ and PCO_2 indicate that the respiratory alkalosis is dominant at this stage in the patient.

In all cases of salicylate overdose the plasma paracetamol should also be measured as many proprietary analgesics contain aspirin and paracetamol. In the early stages of paracetamol poisoning, when treatment is effective, patients will not display any specific signs or symptoms.

Case history 49

Many imported cosmetic agents contain lead. Not infrequently children will ingest these agents accidentally and may develop lead poisoning. It is, therefore, appropriate to measure the whole blood lead and erythrocyte protoporphyrin levels.

Case history 50

A high serum γGT is not diagnostic of alcohol abuse. γGT is induced by a number of enzyme-inducing agents such as phenytoin and phenobarbitone which this boy was taking. Currently, there is no biochemical test to confirm alcohol abuse. However, the combination of an increased serum γGT and urate with a macrocytosis is strongly suggestive of alcohol abuse.

The alkaline phosphatase of 520 U/l is entirely appropriate for a teenager during his pubertal growth spurt. It should not be taken as indicative of liver disease.

Case history 51

Hypoglycaemia is by far the most common cause of acute coma in insulin-dependent diabetics. It is essential that this patient's blood glucose be measured and, if hypoglycaemic, he should be given glucose. It is possible that the combination of hypoglycaemia, with or without alcohol intoxication, may have caused him to have an accident which could result in a head injury causing his coma. Thus, in addition to monitoring his vital signs and grading his coma, it is essential to look for any superficial or neurological signs suggestive of head injury. It is essential that this be done even if he is demonstrated to be hypoglycaemic and rapidly recovers when given glucose, as the complications of a head injury such as a subdural haematoma may not be immediately apparent.

Case history 52

This boy's calculated osmolality is approximately 206 mmol/kg. Thus, the osmolal gap is approximately 76 mmol/lkg. This has arisen because of his severe hyperlipidaemia which has caused pseudohyponatraemia. In severe hyperlipidaemia the plasma water concentration is decreased due to the abnormally high contribution of the lipoproteins to the plasma volume. As a result, the concentration of sodium per litre of serum is decreased as the sodium is not present in the lipoproteins but will have a normal concentration in the serum water.

Severe hypertriglyceridaemia in a child may be caused by a decrease in lipoprotein lipase activity. This may result from genetic defects in the enzyme itself or in the enzyme's cofactor, apolipoprotein CII. Lipoprotein lipase is essential for the normal catabolism of chylomicrons and VLDL.

Case history 53

This man has diabetes mellitus which is the most likely cause of his hyperlipidaemia. His γGT is high which may be due to the presence of a fatty liver, a common finding in non-insulin dependent diabetics on presentation. The high γGT may also be due to a high alcohol intake which may contribute to his hypertension. However, the combination of diabetes mellitus with central obesity and hypertension would suggest insulin resistance or the so-called Syndrome X.

Details of his family history with respect to coronary heart disease should be obtained. Palmar or tuberous xanthomas should be looked for and, if present, would suggest Type III hyperlipidaemia. His Apo E genotype should then be established.

This patient should be treated by dietary measures. Particular attention should be paid to his alcohol intake. Liver disease should be excluded as its presence would preclude the use of metformin which would be an appropriate drug to treat his diabetes, or the use of fibric acid derivatives to treat his hyperlipidaemia.

Case history 54

Though the plasma cholesterol level is not significantly altered in non-fasting blood samples, this woman's hypercholesterolaemia should be confirmed on a fasting plasma sample in which her triglyceride and HDL cholesterol should also be measured. Secondary causes of hyperlipidaemia such as hypothyroidism and diabetes mellitus should be excluded. If her plasma triglyceride is normal and she has primary hypercholesterolaemia, a likely diagnosis is familial hypercholesterolaemia (FH).

If FH is diagnosed, her children and other members of her family should be screened for the condition. Treatment is based on diet which, in patients with FH, almost invariably needs to be combined with cholesterol-lowering drugs such as the HMG CoA reductase inhibitors and/or the bile acid sequestrant resins.

Case history 55

This man is most likely to have essential hypertension, but it is important to consider other secondary causes especially in a relatively young patient. Acromegaly and phaeochromocytoma may present with the combination of hypertension, excessive sweating and glycosuria. Once considered, the signs and symptoms of acromegaly are usually readily recognized. However, phaeochromocytoma may not have any symptoms or signs suggestive of the diagnosis apart from the episodic nature of the sweating. The patient's fundi should be checked for any evidence of malignant hypertension.

In suspected phaeochromocytoma, urinary catecholamines or their metabolites should be measured. If the patient does not experience symptoms during the period of collection these tests may be normal. Hyperglycaemia and hypercalcaemia are other recognized consequences of excessive catecholamine secretion in patients with phaeochromocytomas. If a phaeochromocytoma is diagnosed then the possibility of familial disease should be considered and family members screened.

Case history 56

In males at this age, the most likely diagnosis is Cushing's syndrome due to carcinoma of the lung with ectopic ACTH production. As this disease is usually very aggressive, patients tend to develop florid metabolic features of the disease compared with the physical signs which may be minimal. His serum urea and electrolytes indicate that he has developed profound hypokalaemic alkalosis and glucose intolerance. These can all be attributed to hypercortisolism. Cortisol will also cause muscle wasting which, combined with hypokalaemia, will lead to weakness. The nocturia and polyuria can cause profound potassium depletion.

Cushing's syndrome should be confirmed by measuring his urinary cortisol output or demonstrating an increased serum cortisol in the early morning and late evening with the absence of the normal circadian rhythm. His plasma ACTH concentration should be grossly elevated. In such cases, if carcinoma of the lung is demonstrated radiologically and/or by bronchoscopy, the diagnosis of ectopic ACTH production is made without necessarily confirming it biochemically. Conn's syndrome and other conditions which may give rise to hypokalaemia with hypernatraemia are much rarer.

Case history 57

Though he is not clinically jaundiced the high alkaline phosphatase and γGT with modest increases in the AST and ALT would suggest cholestasis. This may be due to liver cirrhosis or malignant disease affecting the liver, both of which would be likely diagnoses in this case.

An AFP level may be helpful as it is a good tumour marker for hepatocellular carcinoma which is also a likely diagnosis in this case. In Western society, alcohol-induced cirrhosis of the liver is the most common predisposing factor to the development of hepatocellular carcinoma.

Case history 58

The patient's plasma PTH should be measured and, if increased, a diagnosis of primary hyperparathyroidism can be made. However, hyperparathyroidism with a serum calcium of 2.8 mmol/l is usually asymptomatic and thus another cause for his hypertension, headaches and anxiety should be sought. If the symptoms were episodic this would suggest the possibility of a phaeochromocytoma which is associated with hyperparathyroidism in families with MEN. The patient should have his urinary catecholamines measured and, if the diagnosis is made, it is important that other members of his family be screened for hyperparathyroidism and phaeochromocytoma.

Case history 59

Acute severe pain in the metatarsophalangeal joint is the classic presentation of gout. The serum urate level is usually high in gout, but only a minority of patients with hyperuricaemia develop gout and frequently patients with acute gout may have a normal serum urate level. The presence of fever would be compatible with septic arthritis. The joint should be aspirated and, in addition to looking for urate crystals which would confirm a diagnosis of gout, some of the aspirate should be sent for microbiological studies to exclude the possibility of infection.

Case history 60

The large increase in the CK and LDH relative to the AST and ALT would indicate that muscle is the major tissue contributing to the increase in serum enzyme activities. However, muscle does not contain ALT which comes from the liver. AST and LDH are found in muscle, liver and erythrocytes. Thus, the tissues which could have contributed to the serum enzyme activities include muscle (either skeletal or cardiac), the liver or erythrocytes.

Muscle is the only source of CK and by measuring the isoenzyme CK-MB one can determine whether or not cardiac muscle is involved. If the liver is involved then the serum γGT should be increased as this is one of the most sensitive indicators of liver disease. LDH isoenzyme analysis will help identify erythrocyte damage as a possible source for some of the LDH and AST activity. In haemolytic disorders, one would expect a reticulocytosis and intravascular haemolysis will lead to a low serum haptoglobin level. These investigations will help identify whether or not erythrocytes have contributed to the serum enzymes.

Case history 61

Family tree

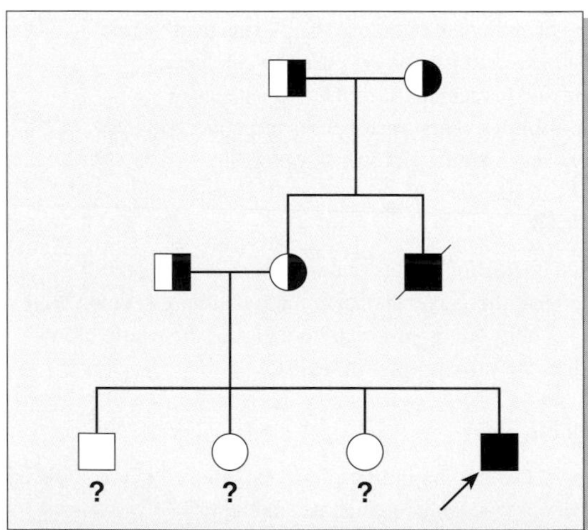

This child should have a sweat test as it remains the definitive test to confirm the diagnosis of cystic fibrosis (CF). The concentration of chloride in sweat is high in cases of CF. It would be appropriate to perform the same test on his siblings though the test cannot be used to detect heterozygote carriers. DNA diagnosis of both those with CF and heterozygous carriers is possible, and such tests may be used if the sweat test is equivocal in the proband. It can also be used to test the carrier status of his sibs or for prenatal diagnosis in future pregnancies. Although over 170 mutations of the CFTR gene have been described, a single deletion mutation, designated ΔF 508, accounts for up to 75% of CF in people of North European origin.

Case history 62

This woman should have an amniocentesis performed with bilirubin being measured in her amniotic fluid. In Rhesus incompatibility the amniotic fluid bilirubin concentration will rise because of the destruction of fetal red cells.

Case history 63

This woman's signs and symptoms are typical of pre-eclampsia, which is the most likely diagnosis. The most appropriate side room test to perform would be to test for albuminuria. Biochemical investigations that should be performed on this woman are:

- *Serum urate*, as this is a sensitive indicator for pre-eclampsia.
- *Serum urea and electrolytes* should be measured as she may be developing renal failure.
- *Serum albumin* and *liver function tests* should be measured to detect liver disease.
- *Glomerular filtration rate* should be measured as should urinary protein excretion to monitor her condition.

Case history 64

No other investigations should be performed but the parents should be reassured that their daughter does not have congenital hypothyroidism.

Over 99% of all six-day-old children will have a TSH of <10 mU/l while the majority of patients with congenital hypothyroidism will have a TSH >100 mU/l. Babies with a blood TSH between 15-40 mU/l on their first test are considered to have an equivocal result. If in a second sample a normal result is obtained, as is usually the case, no further investigation need be made.

Case history 65

This baby's blood gas status should be assessed as she is at risk of developing the respiratory distress syndrome. In view of her maternal history, weight and gestational age, she may be hypoglycaemic so her blood glucose should be measured. Hypocalcaemia is another possibility that should be considered, so her serum calcium should be measured.

The total blood volume in neonates is small and could be less than 100 ml in this baby. It is, therefore, very important not to collect too much blood from neonates as they can become anaemic if a large number of investigations are performed.

Case history 66

Elderly people living on their own frequently have an inadequate diet. This is particularly true of men if they are unused to cooking for themselves. This patient may have a number of micronutrient deficiencies but, acutely, the most important would be possible thiamine deficiency. This can be detected by demonstrating an increase in the percentage activation of erythrocyte transketolase *in vitro* by the addition of thiamine or the measurement of thiamine pyrophosphate in erythrocytes. These investigations are usually unavailable in the acute situation and patients are usually treated empirically with multivitamin preparations. When micronutrient deficiency is suspected, the diagnosis can only be confirmed if the appropriate samples are collected before the patient is given supplements.

INDEX

A

B

C

D

E

F

G

H

I

Q

R

S

T

U

V

W

X

Z